Trauma-informed Care for Nursing Education Fostering a Caring Pedagogy, Resilience & Psychological Safety

Authored By

Kathleen Stephany

Faculty of Health Sciences
Douglas College
New Westminster, BC
Canada

Trauma-informed Care for Nursing Education Fostering a Caring Pedagogy, Resilience & Psychological Safety

Author: Kathleen Stephany

ISBN (Online): 978-981-5223-76-7

ISBN (Print): 978-981-5223-77-4

ISBN (Paperback): 978-981-5223-78-1

© 2024, Bentham Books imprint.

Published by Bentham Science Publishers Pte. Ltd. Singapore. All Rights Reserved.

First published in 2024.

need for a court order if at any point you breach any terms of this License Agreement. In no event will any delay or failure by Bentham Science Publishers in enforcing your compliance with this License Agreement constitute a waiver of any of its rights.

3. You acknowledge that you have read this License Agreement, and agree to be bound by its terms and conditions. To the extent that any other terms and conditions presented on any website of Bentham Science Publishers conflict with, or are inconsistent with, the terms and conditions set out in this License Agreement, you acknowledge that the terms and conditions set out in this License Agreement shall prevail.

Bentham Science Publishers Pte. Ltd.
80 Robinson Road #02-00
Singapore 068898
Singapore
Email: subscriptions@benthamscience.net

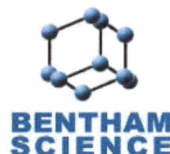

BENTHAM SCIENCE

CONTENTS

FOREWORD

"Real change is not the sole domain of leaders and so-called heroes; rather, change is driven forward by the choices and actions of each and everyone one of us."

-Jodie Wilson-Raybould (2022, p. 23)

We are at a pivotal time in our world, perched at the confluence of historically significant movements and events with an ever-increasing awareness of the impacts of our decisions on others and the environment. The Covid-19 pandemic has indelibly changed the landscape of healthcare and continues to affect individuals and teams who care for people, including those who have experienced intentional and unintentional trauma. Research on trauma, and our knowledge of this complex and highly subjective experience, continue to grow and evolve.

As nurses work in many areas beyond acute care settings, including in the community, long-term care, assisted living facilities, forensic systems, and postsecondary institutions, developing an awareness of the prevalence and impacts of trauma, while building on a strengths-based approach that prioritizes psychological safety, is crucial in helping all nursing professionals to work effectively and compassionately. Any client in any healthcare context, and any of our colleagues, may have experienced trauma. Since nursing practice is grounded in connection, it is vitally important we root our praxis in an understanding of how trauma can shape individual experiences and responses, while extending our gaze to consider how the systems in which we practice can more effectively support the physical, cultural, and emotional safety of people accessing care, as determined by clients themselves.

Within postsecondary education, estimates vary, but it is believed that as many as 89% of college students have potentially experienced at least one traumatic event, with the peak age of trauma exposure occurring between the ages of 16-20. Women, particularly racialized women, also report higher rates of trauma (Valdez, 2023). Students experiencing traumatic stress may have difficulties with learning and memory, attention and focus, problem-solving, and executive function, resulting in higher rates of absenteeism (Levi-Gigi, 2012). Therefore, it is vital that educators consider the experiences of learners to help mitigate the potential for retraumatization in the classroom, and help students learn within psychologically safe environments, all the while fostering resilience and building on a learner's strengths.

This new year will mark a two decade-long milestone since graduating with my nursing degree and starting my first clinical role at a busy trauma and neurosurgery unit at an inner-city hospital in Toronto, ON. I have been reflecting on how much my own understanding of nursing as a profession, and of myself as a nursing professional, has shifted over time. It was during my graduate studies that I started to become aware of the need for creating trauma-and-violence-informed and culturally safe environments for clients, families, and healthcare providers alike while working with Indigenous women who had experienced violence after listening to their experiences of seeking healthcare. As I pursued additional education in forensic sciences, completing my Forensic Nurse Death Investigator micro-credential [FNDI-MC] in 2023, I have developed a keen awareness of how the very systems meant to support and care for people can instead perpetuate violence and retraumatize them. As a society, and especially as nurses, we must move away from blaming survivors and victims of trauma, both in subtle and overt ways, and instead be cognizant of how our understanding of trauma shapes how we show up and engage with clients, colleagues, and society more broadly.

It has been suggested that a career in nursing requires openness, humility, and the ability to embrace the inherent complexity of healthcare systems and relationships. As human beings we integrate and assess vast amounts of information every day and our brains are primed for maximum efficiency. Yet, busy healthcare and teaching environments can create conditions that leave us all vulnerable to bias, stereotyping, and assumptions (Persaud, 2019). In turn, our implicit biases can create barriers to safe and equitable classrooms and healthcare environments even though that may not be our intent (Newlove, 2021) - this is why it is important to continually address and unpack our assumptions, and to operate from a place of moral courage, empathy, and respect.

Learning about trauma has been critical for me not only in my professional roles but in the volunteer work that I do as an investigator supporting families of missing persons. As the current Decolonizing Lead for a nursing program at a postsecondary institution in BC, I have been working closely with other faculty students, and staff in advancing Truth and Reconciliation within our program. Through this work, I have developed a renewed appreciation of the importance of self-compassion, mindfulness, self-awareness, and self-reflection in how I engage and help to lead this work under the guidance of indigenous elders, knowledge-keepers, scholars, and collaborators. The recent indigenous cultural safety, cultural humility, and anti-racism standard from the British Columbia College of Nurses and Midwives [BCCNM], for example, draws attention to the expectations of the regulatory body for registrants on providing culturally safe and anti-racist care for indigenous clients. The standard considers Canada's shameful history of colonialism and the legacy of intergenerational trauma that continues to reverberate through Indigenous communities negatively impacting healthcare experiences and outcomes for many Indigenous peoples (In Plain Sight, 2020). Developing awareness of the various forms of trauma, and how trauma impacts health, benefits not only everyone seeking care but is also deeply transformative for healthcare providers. It is crucial that all nurses be willing to learn and unlearn while leaning into the discomfort of how we are complicit in some of the healthcare policies and practices that continue to perpetuate trauma and violence, and in doing so, cause harm.

I very much appreciate how the opportunity for deep reflection and engagement is woven throughout the pages of this book, and how Dr. Stephany provides numerous opportunities for readers to consider specific examples to help bring the concepts and ideas she explores within its pages to life. There are questions for further consideration that educators can build on for rich classroom discussions, as well as recommended strategies that help provide readers with helpful scripts and actions they can incorporate into their communication with peers, instructors, and clients. In my experience as an educator, providing learners and faculty with opportunities to consider and work through examples can help consolidate learning, and over time, shift one's practice. Dr. Stephany also centers on self-care in this book, normalizing some of the more challenging aspects of nursing school and providing an affirmative, validating, and thoughtful approach by focusing on strengths, resilience, and on finding joy in one's work. While there can be a tendency to pathologize trauma in some of the literature, I have found a more useful reframe to look at trauma as a normal response to abnormal events (Haskell & Randall, 2009) as Dr. Stephany does in this book as well.

Being a nurse has been an honour and a privilege. My life has been forever changed in innumerable positive ways by the beautiful mosaic of connections and experiences I have had with colleagues, clients, and learners throughout my career. I am delighted to say that nearly twenty years on, I continue to learn and grow with every new role I take on and I am certainly never bored. Despite the many challenges within healthcare and postsecondary settings, it is an exciting time to be a nurse and a nurse educator. The opportunity and potential for nurses to follow their curiosities and their passions and to create the nursing roles of tomorrow are limited only by our imaginations.

I finished reading Dr. Stephany's book with a renewed sense of possibility and inspiration and I am grateful that someone with her training and expertise, and her heart, is doing this work. I found her approach to this book both compelling and timely. Engaging with the book's content will help readers start to build an awareness of the complexity of trauma and trauma experiences while appreciating the role of the nurse's unique and privileged position in providing compassionate, non-judgemental care that extends its focus beyond the individual to the broader systems at large. Much work remains to be done and I remain ever hopeful as to what we can achieve when we all work together.

REFERENCES

Haskell L., Randall M.. Impact of trauma on adult sexual assault victims: What the criminal `justice system needs to know (January 1, 2019). Available at SSRN: https://ssrn.com/abstract=3417763 [http://dx.doi.org/ssrn.3417763/10.2139]

In Plain Sight report (2020). Addressing Indigenous-specific racism and discrimination in BC health care. Retrieved from: https://engage.gov.bc.ca/app/uploads/sites/613/2020/11/In-Plain-Sight-F-ll-Report-2020.pdf

Levy-Gigi, E. Kéri S., Myers CE., (2012). Individuals with post traumatic stress disorder show a selective deficit in generalization of associative learning. *Neuropsychology, 26*(6), 758-767. [http://dx.doi.org/10.1037/a002936122846034]

Newlove, T. (March 2021). Partnering for pediatric pain: Why what we think matters. Pain BC – Symposium Presentation Notes. Vancouver, BC.

Persaud, S. (2019). Addressing unconscious bias: A nurse leader's role. *Nurs Admin Q, 43*(2), 130-137. [http://dx.doi.org/10.1097/NAQ.00000000000034830839450]

Valdez, C. in Stromberg, E. (ed). (2023). *Trauma-informed pedagogy in higher education: A faculty guide for teaching and learning.* New York: Routledge.

Wathen, C.N. & Varcoe, C. (eds). (2023). *Implementing trauma-and-violence informed care: A handbook.* Toronto: University of Toronto Press.

Wilson-Raybould, J. (2022). *True reconciliation: How to be a force for change.* McLelland & Stewart: Penguin Random House Canada.

Angela Heino
BA, BScN, MSN, RN, FNDI-MC
January 5, 2024
New Westminster, British Columbia

PREFACE

"Although the world is full of suffering, it is also full of the overcoming of it. My optimism, then, does not rest on the absence of evil, but on a glad belief in the preponderance of good and a willing effort always to cooperate with the good, that it may prevail." Helen Keller, American Author and Educator.

When I was completing a mandatory course in Trauma Counselling during Graduate School, I was exposed to the types of adversity that exist in the world, their prevalence, and the personal stories of endless human suffering. I felt overwhelmed with sadness and started to view the world as a cruel place of indifference. I confided in the professor teaching the course at the time about my feelings of despondency. He quoted the message relayed above by Helen Keller. Helen Keller was a blind and deaf woman who persevered despite obstacles, got a degree, became a writer, educator, and advocate, and believed in the capacity of good to overcome evil. Helen's words of wisdom helped me to understand that although the world is full of anguish, it also is full of opportunities to help alleviate suffering. I subsequently felt compelled to integrate theories associated with caring into my practice, especially the ethic of care, and the therapeutic merits of empathy and compassion because I believe that they are the hallmarks of nursing. I was thrilled when I was introduced to trauma-informed care because, for people who have experienced adversity, it offers hopeful and useful strategies that facilitate healing and assist them in living more fulfilling lives.

As a nurse educator, I was eager to teach trauma-informed care to students because as future practitioners they needed these skills when caring for people who have been traumatized. However, what became apparent was that nursing students were also a risk group for trauma because they may have a history of personal loss and are in danger of developing secondary trauma during training while caring for the injured, seriously ill, or dying. These revelations became the impetus for this book with the goal of equipping student nurses with the tools to care for people who have been traumatized, but also ensuring that we make their learning experiences more psychologically safe. In the planning and design of this work, I purposely incorporated caring strategies into each Chapter because taking care of others is the essence of what we do as nurses, and it is an integral component of trauma-informed care. I also encouraged self-awareness through ongoing reflection to assist nurses and student nurses in becoming more aware of inherent biases, so they can purposefully transform them into tolerance and acceptance. A caring pedagogy that integrates caring components into teaching, that are engaging, inclusive, genuine, and student-centered, is also an essential theme of this book. At the end of each chapter, strategies are recommended that promote self-care. However, these ideas are not intended as a substitute for medical or psychological advice. Furthermore, some of the material presented in this book may negatively impact the reader, and if that occurs you are strongly advised to reach out for professional support.

Kathleen Stephany
Faculty of Health Sciences
Douglas College
New Westminster, BC
Canada

ACKNOWLEDGEMENTS

I would like to acknowledge past, current, and future nursing students. I wrote this book with all of you in mind.

CONSENT FOR PUBLICATION

Not applicable.

CONFLICT OF INTEREST

The author declares no conflict of interest, financial or otherwise.

Kathleen Stephany
Faculty of Health Sciences
Douglas College
New Westminster, BC
Canada

DEDICATION

I dedicate this book to my beloved cousin and retired nurse Kathleen Palmer who recently left us. You were an amazing role model for all nurses due to your genuine capacity to care.

CHAPTER 1

The Prevalence and Impact of Trauma and Why Trauma-informed Care is Needed in Nursing Education

Abstract: Chapter one explores the reasons why student nurses need to be educated in trauma-informed care. Trauma-informed care endeavours to help people who have experienced trauma and targets change at the organizational and clinical level with the aim of improving client/patient outcomes. Various forms of adversity that exist are presented, and we are informed that trauma is not merely a childhood occurrence but may occur at any point across the lifespan. Stereotypical biases and racial stigma experienced by the following special populations are explored, those with differing sexual orientation or gender identity, older adults, refugees and immigrants, people of colour, and Indigenous people. The role that bias and implicit bias play in structural trauma aimed at specific populations is explained. An overview is given of the following specific trauma-related responses, trauma triggers, acute stress disorder, post-traumatic stress disorder, secondary traumatic stress, vicarious traumatization, and compassion fatigue. *The Four Core Assumptions of Trauma-informed Care* as recommended by the Substance Abuse and Mental Health Services Administration (SAMHSA are explored, because they are foundational for providing trauma-responsive care, and consist of realizing, recognizing, responding, and resisting re-traumatization. Healthcare professionals are strongly encouraged to practice in a trauma-responsive and trauma-sensitive manner. Incorporating trauma-informed approaches into the Nursing School curriculum is recommended for the following reasons. Adversity is prevalent in society, and high number of people who access health services have experienced trauma. Student nurses are not currently learning these skills in a comprehensive way in all schools. Student nurses may have a history of trauma, and they are exposed to adverse and stressful events in clinical training. Two Narrative Case Studies are presented. The first shares the story of a Counsellor who developed compassion fatigue, and the second one reveals the complexity of the trigger response. The following learning activities are suggested: connecting with the goodness in life; changing prejudices and stigma; and participating in a trauma-sensitive practice challenge. A self-care strategy that promotes self-compassion is included at the end of the chapter.

Keywords: Adverse childhood experiences (ACEs), Acute stress response, Bias, Caring, Caring pedagogy, Colonization, Compassion, Compassion satisfaction, Compassion fatigue, Empathy, Ethic of care, Gender identity, Historical trauma, Indigenous people, Implicit bias, Implicit bias, Intergenerational trauma, Interpersonal violence (IPV), LGBTQ2S, Narratives, Phenomenology, Post-migration trauma, People of color, Post-traumatic stress disorder (PTSD), Psychological trauma, Residential schools, Racial microaggression, Racial trauma, Resilience, Structural trauma, Systemic racism, Sexual orientation, Secondary traumatic stress (STS), Traumatic stress response, Trauma-responsiveness, Trauma-sensitivity, Trauma, Trauma-informed care, Trauma triggers, Vicarious traumatization, Violent trauma.

LEARNING GUIDE

After completing this chapter, the reader should be able to:

- Briefly be introduced to trauma-informed care.
- Understand that caring is an embedded theme in this book.
- Become aware that the content of this book is supported by evidence, which includes the thematic analysis of narratives, which are a specific form of qualitative, phenomenological study.
- Describe what the ethics of care and trauma-informed care have in common.
- Define trauma, describe the effects of psychological trauma, and be cognizant of trauma's widespread prevalence in society.
- Gain an understanding of specific types of traumas such as historical, intergenerational, violent, structural, and those due to adverse childhood experiences (ACEs).
- Become knowledgeable of the stereotypical biases experienced by specific special populations.
- Gain an awareness that nursing students and practicing nurses must never discriminate for any reason.
- Recognize stereotypical biases toward others through the process of increased self-awareness.
- Learn about specific trauma-related responses, the role of trauma triggers, and traumas associated with working in healthcare.
- Understand The Four Core Assumptions of Trauma-informed Care.
- Be cognizant of the fact that all health professionals should practice in a trauma-responsive and trauma-sensitive manner.
- Identify two essential features of trauma-sensitive approaches that a practitioner should adopt.
- Understand why trauma-informed care should be incorporated into the nursing school curriculum.

- Review two narrative case studies and ensuing thematic analysis. The first one concerns the subject of compassion fatigue, and the other one explores the relationship between a trigger response and past trauma.
- Participate in the following suggested learning activities (*e.g.*, Connecting with the Goodness in Life; Changing Prejudices and Stigma; and Participation in A Trauma-Sensitive Practice Challenge).
- Be encouraged to take part in a self-care strategy that promotes self-compassion.

INTRODUCTION TO THE BOOK

"Be kinder than necessary because everyone you meet is fighting some sort of battle." Sir John Mathew Barrie, Scottish Novelist and Playwright.

According to Haskin (2019), we should assume that every person accessing health services has a history of trauma and that they need kindness, acceptance, and compassion (Fig. **1.1**). It is therefore highly recommended that all healthcare professionals be trained to recognize the symptoms of trauma, the impact it has had on people's lives, and how to practice trauma-informed care (Haskin, 2019; Substance Abuse and Mental Health Services Administration (SAMHSA), 2014; The Institute on Trauma and Trauma-informed Care (ITTIC), 2022).

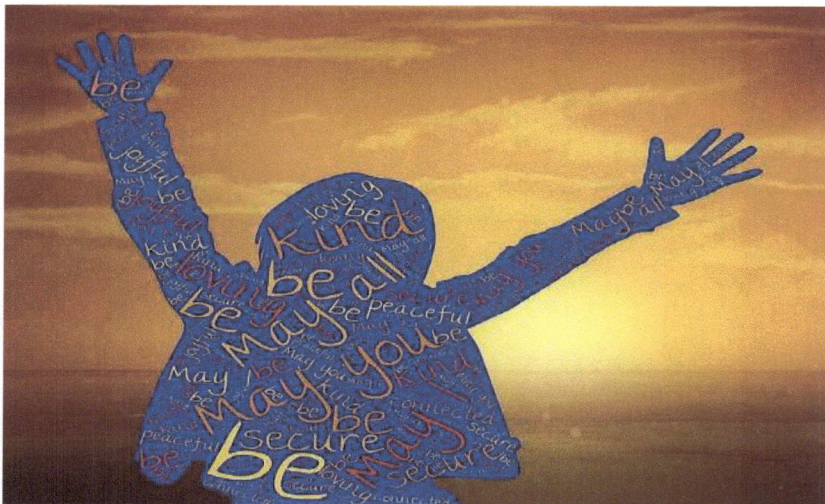

Fig. (1.1). Kindness and Acceptance. Source: www.pixabay.com.

Trauma-informed care endeavours to help people who have experienced adversity and targets change at the organizational and clinical level with the aim of improving client/patient outcomes (Menschner & Maul, 2016). It focuses on prevention, intervention, and treatments that are evidence-based and holistically assist with coping (Knight, 2015; Levenson, 2020; Purkey *et al.*, 2018). Trauma-informed care does not place any blame on the individual who has experienced adversity but focuses on how they have been affected by it. For instance, instead of asking the question, *"What is wrong with you?"* we are advised to use a more suitable, empathetic, and responsive question such as, *"What has happened to you?"* (Young *et al.*, 2019).

A Brief Overview of the Book

The purpose of Chapter One is to explore the many reasons why trauma-informed care is needed in nursing education. The discussion begins by discussing the prevalence of trauma in society, its many forms, and its negative ramifications. Stereotypical biases and racial stigma experienced by special populations are explored, including the role of implicit bias. Trauma-related responses like trauma triggers, acute stress disorder, post-traumatic stress disorder, secondary traumatic stress, vicarious traumatization, and compassion fatigue are discussed. **Crucial components** associated with the delivery of trauma-informed care are introduced, including the importance of being trauma-informed, trauma-responsive, and designing a trauma-sensitive practice, followed by key objectives and assumptions. Integrating trauma-informed approaches into the Nursing School curriculum is highly recommended.

The remainder of the book provides an in-depth overview of the following topics. The key principles of trauma-informed care are emphasized along with tools that are client-centered, person-centered, and resilience-based. Trauma recovery from a positive psychology and post-traumatic growth perspective is recommended. Utilizing a caring pedagogy and fostering resilience, are offered to help offset the secondary traumatic stress and compassion fatigue experienced by student and practicing nurses. Lastly, the benefits of fostering psychological safety, compassion, satisfaction, and joy in work are revealed. All of the chapters include narrative case studies and learning activities to help the reader to actively engage with the subject matter. At the end of each chapter, self-care strategies are suggested as a means to enhance physical and emotional well-being. It is crucially important to also remind the reader that some themes of trauma-informed care explored earlier in the book are reintroduced. However, when that occurs, new information is added to the topic, or it is examined in an alternative way.

Caring as an Embedded Theme

Caring, the ethic of care, and caring pedagogy are key themes in this book. Caring, in general, is thoroughly embedded in the content because it is foundational for nursing practice and a key component of trauma-informed care (Noddings, 2013; SAMSHA, 2014). **Caring** involves being empathetic and compassionate, and treating all the people with respect, fairness, and understanding, and is also concerned with taking action to reduce human suffering (Ray, 2018). The **ethic of care** is a specific component of caring practice that aligns well with trauma-informed care because it is about being aware of and sensing the needs of others, responding to their needs responsibly, while also condemning all exploitation or intentional harm of others (Gilligan, 1982; Slote, 2007: Stephany, 2020). **Caring pedagogy** is student-focused and cultivates an educational environment of engagement, safety, caring relationships, and cultural diversity (Duffy, 2018; Ray, 2018).

QUALITATIVE RESEARCH, PHENOMENOLOGY, NARRATIVES & THE ETHIC OF CARE

Qualitative Research

The content of this book is evidence-based and includes qualitative research into the phenomenological analysis of narratives. Phenomenology is the research methodology, narratives are the methods used for data collection, and the ethic of care is the theoretical foundation for analysis. **Qualitative research** in social sciences focuses on gathering information about people through experiential means. Although there are many methods of qualitative research, key aspects of the process may include the analysis of texts, visual or auditory data, and examining stories (Mihas, 2019). Subgoals associated with some forms of qualitative research theorize a process or to identify contexts or themes and the meaning derived from them (Mihas, 2019).

Phenomenology

Methodology in research refers to the approach used in the study to acquire, categorize, and analyze data (Loiselle & Profetto-McGrath, 2011). The form of qualitative methodology that is used in this book is phenomenology. **Phenomenology** is a theoretical perspective that emphasizes the very substance of lived human experience before any data analysis or theorizing takes place (Mihas, 2019; Morgan & Wise, 2017). Understanding is derived from obtaining a glimpse of how humans live in the present moment and meaning making happens retrospectively (van Manen, 2017).

Narratives

"Share with people who have earned the right to hear your story." Brené Brown, Researcher, Author, and Storyteller

The method for this research is narratives. **Method** refers to the actual way in which data is collected for a study including the sequencing, techniques, and strategies that were utilized (Loiselle & Profetto-McGrath, 2011). **Narratives** are a form of phenomenological inquiry that consists of personal stories. They help us see the world through the unique perspective of others, to understand the essence of their experiences and their personal significance (Morgan & Wise, 2017). Subsequently, this textbook includes many stories as told by people who have either struggled with or experienced trauma. However, considerable details have been altered to protect privacy.

As a nursing instructor, I explain to my students that everyone has a story (Fig. **1.2**). When a client/patient trusts you enough to share their story with you, it is a gift to be cherished and protected because revealing personal aspects of their lives makes them vulnerable. That is why we must always endeavor to earn their trust by ensuring privacy, actively listening, and offering empathy, compassion, and non-judgment.

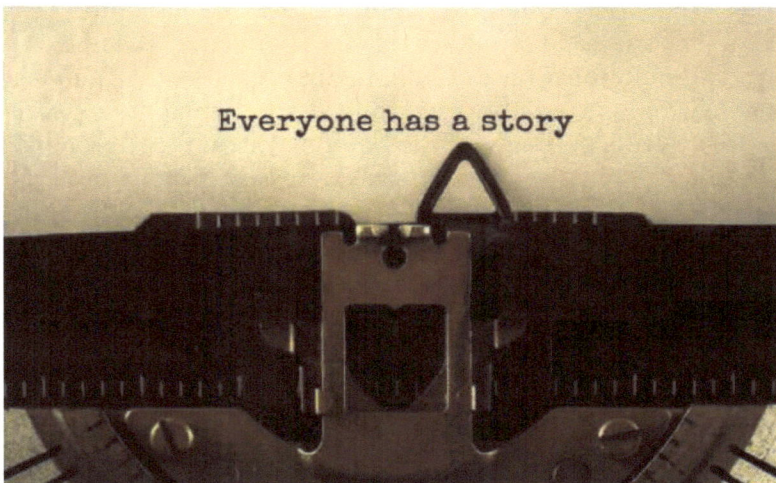

Fig. (1.2). Everyone has a Story. Source: www.pixabay.com.

The Ethic of Care

In research, **theory** is used to generalize and offer explanations of the relationships between the phenomena under study (Loiselle & Profetto-McGrath, 2011). The **ethic of care** is the theoretical basis for analyzing the data derived from the narratives in this book. It is a special feature of nursing ethics that values relationships, context, meaning making, the interconnectedness of all of life, and the self-worth of every person. It does not tolerate discrimination, expects nurses to do what they can to end human suffering, and advocates for those who are marginalized. It insists that unbiased caring be incorporated into everything that nurses do (Noddings, 2013; Stephany, 2020; Watson, 2008).

The ethics of care and trauma-informed care have a great deal in common. For instance, they both fit well in nursing practice because they honor the intrinsic self-worth, autonomy, and choice of each person, and promote practice strategies that support and empower people to heal from suffering. They also acknowledge a person's strengths and abilities to overcome adversity and to change their lives in a positive way.

PSYCHOLOGICAL TRAUMA

According to SAMHSA (2014), **trauma** refers to an event or series of circumstances that are harmful, threatening or a danger to a person's life and has lasting adverse effects on their ability to function on a mental, physical, or spiritual level. When people have been traumatized, they feel disconnected from a sense of belonging, and safety, and may experience an inability to cope with stress (van der Kolk, 2014). **Psychological trauma** refers to a disturbing event that is unexpected and beyond what would normally be anticipated and results in a large array of physical, emotional, and psychological responses (Hordvik, 2019). We are aware that psychological trauma interferes with normal biological homeostasis and has negative effects on many of the body's system functioning and may lead to maladaptive behaviours and psychiatric illnesses (Soloman & Heide, 2005). Evidence indicates that psychological trauma differs from ordinary stress in these specific ways. It is often unexpected, and the person does not feel prepared to deal with it, and there are no actions that the individual can take to prevent it from occurring (Jaffe *et al.*, 2005). Whether a traumatic event will cause emotional suffering in the person depends on the seriousness of the adversity, the person's ability to cope, and the larger meaning attributed to the event by the individual (Jaffe *et al.*, 2005). As Dr. Bessel van der Kolk (2014) explains, trauma is much more than an event that occurred, but an experience that involves the brain, mind, and body, and affects how a person is able to cope with present-day life.

Following a traumatic event, the person may develop adverse reactions right away or the effects may be delayed. When they do occur, physical or psychological symptoms may manifest in numerous ways, such as sleep disturbances, eating disorders, chronic pain, depression, anxiety, panic attacks, irritability, anger, problems with memory, or emotional withdrawal (Jaffe *et al.*, 2005). The person may also be inclined to re-experience the adverse event through nightmares, flashbacks, intrusive thoughts, and detachment (Jaffe *et al.*, 2005). Increased hypervigilance, or overreacting to normal stress is not uncommon, nor is self-medicating with substances to reduce anxiety and alleviate fear. Problems sustaining intimate relationships or social withdrawal are also not uncommon (Jaffe *et al*., 2005).

THE PREVALENCE OF TRAUMA

"Trauma is a fact of life, but it does not have to be a life sentence." Peter A. Levine, Psychotherapist & Author.

Almost everyone experiences some sort of adversity or loss during their lifetime and trauma is more common than most people realize (Haskins, 2019). Research reveals that large numbers of children experience trauma. For example, 25% of children living in the USA have endured physical violence, and 20% report being sexually abused (van der Kolk, 2014). Yet much of the society is still in denial about the frequency of trauma, especially child abuse and neglect, and the long-lasting adverse effects on those who are impacted (Wheeler & Phillips, 2019; van der Kolk, 2014). We also need to be reminded of the fact that adversity can affect anyone at any time in their life regardless of the socioeconomic status, age, or gender (Ravi & Little, 2017; SAMHSA, 2014a; Stephany, 2022). According to Foli and Thompson (2019), the question to ask is not whether a person has experienced or witnessed trauma, but rather when did it occur, what were the circumstances, and how often it occured?

> ### SOMETHING TO REFLECT UPON
>
> **Are you surprised and troubled to hear that trauma is as prevalent as it is in society? How can you ensure that you will be okay when learning about trauma-informed care? How can you protect yourself from feeling overwhelmed or despondent?**

TYPES OF TRAUMA AND TRAUMATIC EXPERIENCES

There are several types of traumas such as historical, intergenerational, violent, structural, and those due to adverse childhood experiences (ACEs) (Burton *et al*., 2019; Suah & Williamson, 2021) (Fig. **1.3**).

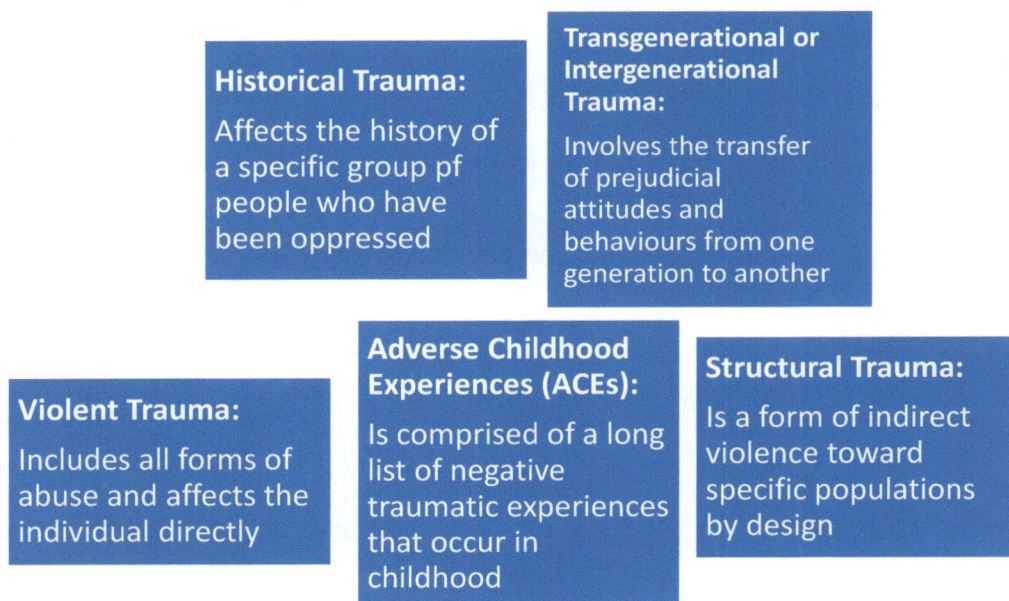

Historical Trauma:

Affects the history of a specific group pf people who have been oppressed

Transgenerational or Intergenerational Trauma:

Involves the transfer of prejudicial attitudes and behaviours from one generation to another

Violent Trauma:

Includes all forms of abuse and affects the individual directly

Adverse Childhood Experiences (ACEs):

Is comprised of a long list of negative traumatic experiences that occur in childhood

Structural Trauma:

Is a form of indirect violence toward specific populations by design

Fig. (1.3). The types of trauma and traumatic experiences (as adapted from Burton *et al.*, 2019; Gaywash & Mordock, 2018; Turney, 2018; Suah & Williamson, 2021; Wynyard *et al.*, 2020).

Historical, Transgenerational & Violent Traumas

Historical trauma consists of adversity and oppression that targets a specific group of people and contributes to systemic racism (Burton *et al.*, 2019). The discrimination often occurs repeatedly across generations and has led to a phenomenon we now refer to as transgenerational trauma (Suah & Williamson 2021). Two examples include slavery in the United States and Residential Schools for Indigenous children in Canada, but numerous other examples exist.

Transgenerational trauma, which is also referred to as **intergenerational trauma,** consists of a transposition of prejudicial attitudes and behaviors from one generation to another (Gaywsh & Mordock, 2018; Suah & Williamson, 2021). Present day experiences are, therefore, interpreted through past experiences that often involve racial or other forms of discrimination. Lack of trust in others, especially strangers, is understandably a key repercussion of this form of trauma (Suah & Williamson, 2021).

Violent trauma includes all forms of abuse and has direct negative consequences for the individual (Burton *et al.*, 2019). Traumatic experiences associated with violence include physical assault, sexual assault, sexual abuse, child neglect, being deprived of basic needs, domestic abuse, other forms of interpersonal violence, elder abuse, being threatened, witnessing violence, exposure to natural disasters, being a victim of war, and all forms of systemic racism or stereotypical biases (Davies *et al.*, 2017; Gerber, 2019; Stephany, 2022).

Intimate partner violence (IPV) is a form of violent trauma that is sexual or physical that may include stalking or purposefully inflicting psychological harm on someone. It could be happening presently or may have occurred in the past. The perpetrator of the abuse is usually known to the victim but is not always a significant partner (Centers for Disease and Prevention (CDP), 2017). IPV causes the person who is affected to feel powerless and isolated. Unfortunately, many IPV survivors also experienced childhood adversity, which decreases their ability to cope and negatively impacts their self-confidence. This often leads to a feeling of disempowerment and an inability to leave the abusive situation Anyikwa, 2016). IPV also results in many negative repercussions, including mental illness and problem substance use (Anyikwa. 2016). Although women are the most identified survivors of IPV, data reveals that members of the LGBTQ community have experienced either equal or higher rates than cisgender heterosexual individuals (Scheer & Poteat, 2021).

Adverse Childhood Experiences (ACEs)

Negative traumatic experiences that occur in childhood are referred to as **adverse childhood experiences (ACEs)** (Fig. **1.4**). Examples of types of ACEs include physical and sexual abuse, neglect, household violence, caregiver mental illness or drug use, parental abandonment, parental death, and parental divorce or separation (Turney, 2018; Wynyard *et al.*, 2020). Other studies have included the following as additional types of ACEs: school bullying, community violence, natural disasters, war, displacement, terrorism, sexual or gender discrimination, sexual harassment, hate crimes, and human trafficking (Grogan & Murphy, 2011; Grossman *et al.*, 2021; Johnson *et al.*, 2013). ACEs are common in children, with approximately 30% of children being exposed to at least one ACE (Turney, 2018). ACEs have both short-term and long-term effects on a child's psychological development and the inability to cope due to brain changes. This alteration in cognitive functioning contributes to emotional deregulation and poor attachment to primary caregivers (Goddard, 2020). When older, many of these children are at risk of resorting to dangerous behaviors such as smoking, substance use, and promiscuity. Research has also revealed that a higher number of ACEs is correlated with a greater number of physical and mental health challenges experienced in adulthood (*e.g.*, heart disease, respiratory problems, chronic lung disease, cancer, liver disease, major depression, anxiety disorders, and post-traumatic stress disorder (PTSD) (Anda *et al.*, 2010; Grossman *et al.*, 2021). Oftentimes in adulthood, a person will hide or bury their history of childhood adversity as a way of coping, or because they feel guilt or shame (Sweeney *et al*., 2018). That is why we should not assume that a person has not been exposed to adversity just because, on the surface, they appear to be okay (Stephany, 2022).

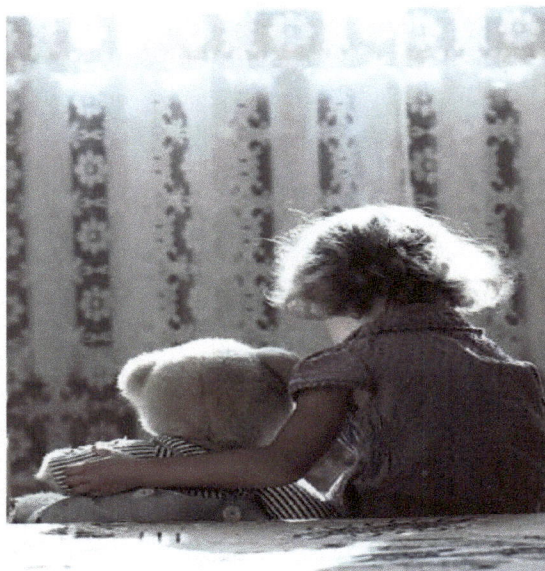

Fig. (1.4). Adverse Childhood Experiences (ACEs). Source: www.pixabay.com.

After learning about the prevalence of adversity and some of its types, you may feel somewhat discouraged, and that is why (Box **1.1**) offers a suggested learning exercise on connecting with the goodness in life.

Box 1.1. Learning activity: connecting with the goodness in life.

A well-known Psychologist and Author, Shauna Shapiro (2020), points out that humans are hardwired to focus on the negative in themselves and others. However, she also asserts that we can learn to focus on positivity. That is why I suggest connecting with the goodness in life by purposely taking a break from the negative and focusing on something that brings you joy. What would that something be for you? Is it taking a walk-in nature, calling a close friend, playing the piano, hugging your child, petting your dog or cat, listening to comforting music, reading something inspiring, watching a funny movie, or being grateful.?

STRUCTURAL   TRAUMAS   EXPERIENCED   BY   SPECIAL POPULATIONS

Structural trauma is a form of indirect violence toward specific populations by design (Burton *et al*., 2019). Grossman *et al*., (2021) make an important point that health professionals have a responsibility to become informed of the facts that many groups of people have been traumatized collectively, either historically, or by past and present systemic oppression and racism. Examples of people who have fallen prey to structural trauma include those with differing gender identity or sexual orientation, ethnic minorities, people of color, people with disabilities, and those of faiths that differ from Christianity (*e.g.*, Judaism and Islamic faiths) (Burton *et al.*, 2019). This is by no means an exhaustive list. There are many other special populations that experience intolerance. However, although it is beyond the scope of this textbook to address all of them, the reader is strongly encouraged to increase their awareness of oppressed groups of people and ways to end discrimination. Nevertheless, the discussion that ensues examines stereotypical biases and targeted acts of adversity towards the following groups: those with differing sexual orientation or gender identity, older adults, refugees and immigrants, people of color, and Indigenous people.

What is Meant by Sexual Orientation & Gender Identity?

Before discussing the trauma experienced by persons with differing sexual orientations or gender identities, it is important to understand what is meant by these and other relevant terms. What is the difference between sex and gender? **Sex** refers to a person's biological designation based on the genitalia that they were born with. **Sexual orientation** refers to the way that a person feels toward people physically, sexually, romantically, or emotionally, and they may be attracted to one or more gender designations (Royal Mental Health Care & Research (RMHCR), 2019). **Heterosexuality** refers to the feelings of a person toward others of the opposite sex and is only one designation of sexual orientation.

Gender is used to describe the way in which a person feels about themselves and may differ from what their biological designation may be. For example, they may feel like a female or, a male or neither (RMHCR, 2019). **Gender identity** refers to a person's individual description of their own personal experience of gender, and their gender identity may be the same or different than that assigned at birth (RMHCR, 2019).

People with sexual orientations or gender identities that differ from being heterosexual or gender identified at birth are often referred to as a set of acronyms (RMHCR), 2019). Although there is a variation of types of abbreviations used to represent members of this population, for the purpose of this discussion, the following acronym will be used, **LGBTQ2S,** which stands for lesbian, gay, bisexual, transgender, queer, and two-spirited. (RMHCR, 2019). Refer to Box (**1.2**) for a description of these and additional terms. The explanations are meant to be inclusive of differing sexual orientations and gender identities and by no means include all diverse communities. The acronyms may also change with time (British Broadcasting Corporation (BBC), 2015). It is, therefore, considered a good practice to be respectful of a person's choices by asking them how they would like to be addressed and inquiring about their preferred pronouns (BBC, 2015).

Box 1.2. The meaning of LGBTQ2S & other relevant terms (as adapted from the BBC, 2015; RMHCR, 2019).

L - Lesbian refers to a woman who is attracted to other women.
G-Gay is a man who is attracted to other men. Some may use the term homosexual.
B-Bisexual is a person who is attracted to both men and women.
T-Transgender or **Trans** is a term that is used by people whose identity differs from the one they were assigned to at birth. It is recommended that the person chooses how they want to be identified.
Q - Queer is a broad term used to include sexual orientation or gender identities within the LGBTQ2S community. Historically this term was used as an insult, so it not always embraced by everyone.
Q - Questioning is used to describe a person who is still exploring their sexuality or gender identity.
2S-Two Spirit is a term used within some Indigenous communities that refers to a person who identifies as a female and male spirit living in the same body.
Asexual is a person who either does not experience physical attraction to other people, or rarely does. But they may still experience an emotional attraction to others.
Gender Fluid is a person whose gender identity and gender expression are not static and can shift with time.

Traumas Experienced by People with Differing Sexual Orientation or Gender Identity

Members of the LGBTQ2S community are known to be exposed to trauma. Even in a society like Canada that legally asserts the rights and privileges of all people, stereotypical biases, stigma, and hatred toward this group prevail and cause harm. For example, youth who identify as LGBTQ2S are known to experience many forms of adversity, such as physical and sexual abuse, interpersonal violence, sexual assault, sexual exploitation, and peer bullying (McCormick *et al.*, 2018). They also experience increased incidences of maltreatment, family and peer rejection, substance use, self-harm, and higher rates of post-traumatic stress disorder (PTSD). The discrimination they experience also often continues into adulthood (McCormick *et al.*, 2018). What is even more troubling is that although young members of this community experience higher than normal rates of all forms of trauma than other youths, they have been largely ignored as a priority population for trauma-informed care (McCormick *et al.*, 2018).

Carabez *et al*., (2015) point out another disturbing fact that nursing as a profession has been reluctant to openly embrace members of this group, and research has demonstrated that many nurses are unaware of patients who are LGBTQ2S or harbour negative views towards them. Furthermore, nurses, in general, lack an understanding of how to care for persons in this community, and nurse educators are also not always trained on how to address their specific health issues (Carabez *et al*., 2015).

Traumas Suffered by Refugees & Immigrants

Displacement due to war, persecution, and violence all over the world in recent years has resulted in significant growth in the number of people who have been exiled from their country of origin. In fact, as of 2019, more than 79 million people were displaced, and 20 million of them became refugees (Shi & Tatebe, 2021). These numbers have increased in 2022 due to the mass exodus of women and children leaving war-torn Ukraine. For people who are refugees, the degree of trauma and adversity that they experience begins prior to being displaced and sometimes continues after stressful migration journeys and settlement in a new country (Shi & Tatebe, 2021).

Although new immigrants are not necessarily exposed to all the hardships experienced by people who are refugees, what they have in common is the distress of leaving their way of life behind, including family and social support, and all of the newly added difficulties that occur once they have migrated. For example, refugees and new immigrants often experience **post-migration trauma** which is due to barriers to access to essential services such as employment opportunities, education, adequate housing, food security, and healthcare (Wylie *et al*., 2021).

It is also crucially important that healthcare professionals be trained to provide trauma-informed care to people who are refugees or new immigrants because they may present with unique physical and psychological trauma that is complex (Wylie *et al*., 2021). Acknowledging cultural differences is an important place to begin, followed by avoiding making assumptions based on how things are done in Western culture. However, Ray (2018) suggests that **transcultural caring** be employed to avoid unintentional harm. In nursing, transcultural caring consists of more than just being sensitive to cultural differences. It involves intentionally and wholeheartedly seeking to understand and respect how a person's behaviors, wants, and needs are influenced by all aspects of their culture (Ray). Furthermore, Wylie *et al*., (2021) also highly recommend that healthcare personnel receive ongoing and updated training in trauma - informed care that is transcultural, mindful, and reflexive and that is tapered to the many diverse needs of those who have recently arrived from another country.

Racial Trauma & People of Color

Racial trauma consists of traumatization that targets ethnicity that is experienced personally or witnessed (Williams *et al.*, 2020). Unfortunately, people of color have historically been subjected to racial trauma. **People of color** in the USA is a term used to describe persons of African descent who were referred to as African American. However, it is now also used in North America to describe groups of people who identify as 'non-white' and includes but is not limited to, Blacks, Latinos, Mexicans, Jamaicans, Chinese, Indigenous people, Asians, Southwest Asians, and Arabs (Perez, 2021; Williams *et al.*, 2020).

An Historical Account of Racial Discrimination Toward Black People of Color

Black people have suffered from structural, historical, and intergenerational trauma due to racism as a direct result of slavery. History reveals that during the 18th Century, ten million Black people were captured and uprooted from their countries of origin and transported to America with the sole purpose of being slaves (Gilda, 2014). They were treated terribly and inhumanely when transported to America, and ten percent did not even survive the long journey due to sickness or other causes of death (Gilda). Upon arrival to America, they were forced to live in barracks with poor shelter, terrible nutrition, little or no medical care, segregated according to sex, and subject to terrible living and working conditions. Even after slavery was legally abolished in 1862, under Jim Crow, many of the states still treated Black and native Indians as inferior human beings, ensured that segregation was enforced, paid them poorly, and forced them to live in impoverished conditions (Gilda).

Discrimination Toward Other People of Color

The terrible historical discrimination endured by Blacks in America must never be minimized or overlooked. However, it is also important to at least mention recent examples of how other people of color have also been traumatized due to acts of racial hatred. For instance, the media has revealed blatant examples of despicable acts of discrimination demonstrated toward Latinos attempting to cross the border in the USA to seek asylum. The Human Rights Watch (HRW) (2022) released alarming statistics that from January 2019 to January 2021, 71,000 asylum seekers were sent back from the US Border to Mexico under the 'Remain in Mexico' agreement between the US and Mexican governments. As a result of this action, many who were involuntarily returned to Mexico were subjected to human trafficking, extremely impoverished conditions, poor nutrition, little or no medical treatment, and some were raped or murdered. As many as 15,000 children were abducted at the border and remained in the US without their parents (HRW).

Present Day Discrimination Toward People of Color

Unfortunately, the trauma experienced by people of color due to racism continues today. The American Psychological Association (APA) (2016) points out that 70 percent of Americans hold stereotypical views toward people who are black. Furthermore, what is also quite alarming is that almost the same percentage of people of color report being discriminated against by white people (APA). In Canada, seven percent of adults admit to being discriminated against during their lifetime, and 79% of them describe prejudice solely due to race (Williams *et al.*, 2020).

Current-day manifestations of racial trauma inflicted upon people of color are rarely due to one single event, are known to be cumulative in nature and result in negative consequences to the person's mental well-being (Williams *et al.*, 2020). For example, everyday incidences of targeted forms of aggression are correlated with an increased risk of anxiety, depression, and problem substance use (Williams *et al.*,). Unfortunately, **racial microaggressions** are commonplace everyday occurrences that are intentional or unintentional, and consist of offensive verbal or behavioral actions that communicate derogatory racial slights or insults toward people of color (Sue *et al.*, 2007). They may occur in the form of insulting words, names or labels, dismissive looks, racial jokes, or slurs (Sue *et al.*, Williams *et al.*,).

I regret that the occurrences of trauma experienced due to racial discrimination toward people of color that were explored in this current discussion have not been extensive and have excluded many other groups. This was not done because of insensitivity or indifference, but due to the limited breadth of this book. Therefore, the reader is strongly encouraged to conduct their own research into other examples that exist.

Traumas Experienced by Older Adults

Since its origins, trauma-informed care has focused primarily on the treatment of children and youth. One group of people that are often overlooked are older adults, even though elder abuse has been identified as a global issue of concern (Ernst & Maschi, 2018). **Elder abuse** consists of one or more acts, or a lack of helpful action, that causes harm or distress to an older adult, that may occur within any relationship where there is an expectation of trust (World Health Organization, 2017, as cited in Ernst & Maschi, 2018, p. 354). Some forms of elder abuse include physical, psychological, and financial abuse and intentional neglect by caregivers (Ernst & Maschi).

Not all circumstances fit the category of elder abuse. Other situations are deemed to be traumatizing that exist outside of abuse because experience is subjective, and individual factors determine how an older adult will respond to adversity. Nevertheless, there is significant evidence to indicate that multiple traumas do occur over the course of a person's lifetime, and an accumulation of adverse events can result in considerable distress (Ramsey-Klawsnik & Miller, 2017). For instance, as a person ages, many close relatives and friends die and the loss of a spouse has been identified by numerous seniors as quite stressful (Kusmaul & Anderson, 2018). Some of the following events are also associated with negative outcomes for older adults: loss of ability to live independently, loss of driver's license, forced relocation, being placed in a nursing home, financial worries, being diagnosed with a new physical disability, being diagnosed with a form of dementia, suffering from a chronic illness, being treated with indifference because of age, and lack of proper care. For many, loss of independence has been deemed to be quite devastating because one's sense of autonomy, dignity, and self-esteem is impacted (Kusmaul & Anderson). Other negative consequences associated with loss include increased depression, a sense of uncertainty about the future, loss of personal pride in one's achievements, and a loss of hope. Therefore, it is highly recommended that healthcare professionals apply the principles of trauma-informed and person-centered strategies when planning care for older adults to assist them in productive ways to adapt to loss and change in their lives and to prevent further re-traumatization (Kusmaul & Anderson; Ramsey-Klawsnik & Miller).

Indigenous People & Trauma

Indigenous people are descendants from various areas all around the world who have lived or currently reside in areas spanning from the Arctic Pole to the South Pacific seas (United Nations Permanent Forum on Indigenous Issues (UNPFII), n.d.). **Indigenous** refers to people who consider themselves to be related to, or historically connected to, "First Peoples" whose civilizations predate a time before invasion or colonization by others (Allan & Smylie, 2015, p. 3). Indigenous people have also been referred to as "distinct social and cultural groups that share collective ancestral ties to lands and natural resources where they live, occupy, or from which they have been displaced" (The World Bank, 2022, par. 1).

The United Nations have chosen not to adopt an official definition of the term Indigenous and prefers that individuals self-identify as indigenous either personally or be identified by members of the specific community that they belong to (UNPFII, n.d.). Some people prefer to be called by their unique associations; for example, in Canada, First Nations, Inuit, and Metis are some of those designations (MacDonald & Steenback, 2015). It is always best to ask a person who may identify as Indigenous what their preferred designation is so we can show respect by calling them by their name of choice.

The Impact of Colonization & Intergenerational Trauma on Indigenous People

Colonization refers to the way in which foreign nations invade other nations, force their values and ways of living on their people, exploit their resources, and inflict other forms of harm (MacDonald & Steenbeek, 2015). Due to colonization, most indigenous people have either experienced past trauma or are currently affected by trauma (Linklater, 2014). In Canada, the purpose of colonization by European Nations was to force indigenous people to assimilate into Western society and negatively impact their lives in the following ways. They were forced to live on reserves, which resulted in the suppression of their ability to openly share their culture, beliefs, and customs, or to live off the land. They were also often forbidden to follow their spiritual practices or to speak their native language (MacDonald & Steenbeek). Linklater (2014) summarizes the negative result of colonization in the following manner. "Over 500 years of contact between the original peoples of the Americas and settler nations has produced displacement and disconnection . . . the root of injury has been caused by colonial violence" (p. 20).

Intergenerational Trauma & Canadian Residential Schools

Intergenerational trauma is also prevalent amongst Indigenous people and, as previously pointed out, happens when the negative repercussions of an original and historical trauma are passed on to the next generation or subsequent generations (Gaywsh & Mordoch, 2018). Intergenerational trauma contributes to learned, fear-based ways of being and mistrust of others that are difficult to change. MacDonald and Steenbeek (2015) point out that many indigenous people all over the globe continue to experience the repercussions of historical trauma due to colonization in the form of poorer determinants of health, substandard education, and living in impoverished conditions.

A Canadian example of intergenerational trauma is evident in the devastating effects of the residential school system, which was established by the government in the late 1800s and continued for more than a century, with the last residential school closed in 1996 (Barker *et al.*, 2018). **Residential schools** were boarding schools created by the Canadian government and operated by people of the Christian faith to forcibly remove native children from their families, with the goal of destroying the "Indian," in the child (Barker *et al.*,). In these residential schools, native children received substandard education, were underfed, and purposefully exposed to diseases like smallpox. They were forbidden to speak their native languages and suffered physical, sexual, and emotional abuse. Many died. Furthermore, those who survived the residential school system and later became parents were known to live in poverty and lacked food security. There is also an overrepresentation to this day of Indigenous families in the child welfare and foster care system (Barker *et al.*,).

Systemic Racism and its Negative Impact on Indigenous Health

Systemic racism is harmful and consists of actions, practices, and policies that perpetrate unjust prejudicial attitudes that target specific racial, ethnic, or other special populations (Stephany, 2020). Matthews (2017) reveals that systemic racism toward Indigenous people continues today and negatively impacts their overall health due to a lack of fair access to health services that is perpetuated by government and policymakers. According to Paradies (2018), racism toward Indigenous people is correlated with poorer health outcomes, including mental illness, obesity, and cardiovascular disease. This author attributes the lack of willingness of Indigenous people to readily access healthcare services, to a fear of being judged, being treated unfairly, or having their concerns ignored. Many of these assumptions are based on actual experiences. Some have reported that they firmly believe that they are treated in a discriminatory manner because of their appearance and designation as Indigenous (Fonseca, 2020). They also report that they find this treatment to be traumatizing.

EMBRACING DIVERSITY & SELF-AWARENESS TO COMBAT IMPLICIT BIAS

"Don't hate what you don't understand." John Lennon, an English Singer, Songwriter, and Peace Activist.

The Role of Bias & Implicit Bias in Inflicting Harm

We have just explored many examples of **structural trauma** intentionally inflicted upon select groups of people. It is, therefore, crucially important to gain an understanding that some of the origins of such harmful behaviors lie in bias and implicit bias. Hagiwara *et al.*, (2020) point out that **bias** consists of stigma, stereotypes, and discriminatory behaviours, and **implicit bias** involves prejudicial attitudes and beliefs directed at a specific group of people (p. 1457). These prejudicial views are often acquired automatically when people unconsciously adopt ideas held by others that they assume to be true, like those taught to them by parents, educators, religious leaders, or social media (Hagiwara, *et al.*,; Narayan,

2019). All forms of biases are also attributed to limited knowledge or exposure to different people, cultures, or beliefs (Hagiwara *et al.*,).

Unfortunately, caregivers, including nurses, sometimes contribute to the problem because they harbour and act on stereotypical views toward specific populations while administering care (Narayan, 2019). To purposefully avoid intolerance towards others, nurses are strongly encouraged to make it their intention to whole heartedly embrace diversity, but what does that entail? To **embrace diversity** is to be willing to accept ways of living and believing that may differ from your own (Stephany, 2020). You do not need to completely understand all differences, or necessarily agree with others, but you need to make a conscious effort to avoid harming them through stigmatization and stereotypical acts. According to the Canadian Nurses Association (CNA) (2017) *Code of Ethics*, nurses are not ethically or professionally permitted to discriminate for any reason.

The Role of Self-awareness

"Everything that irritates us about others can lead us to an understanding of ourselves." Carl Gustav Jung, Swiss Psychiatrist & Psychotherapist.

Making a conscious effort to become self-aware is a known strategy that may assist in modifying any untoward attitudes or stereotypes toward other groups (Stephany, 2020) (Fig. **1.5**). **Self-awareness** involves the process of purposefully examining the motives behind our actions. It begins by pausing, taking a step back, and mindfully looking at our own behaviour (Stephany, 2020).

Actions that facilitate increased self-awareness include those in Box (**1.3**) that require you to closely examine your thinking and behaving.

Changing Inherent Biases Requires Action

"No one is born hating another person because of the color of his skin, or his background, or his religion. People must learn to hate, and if they can learn to hate, they can be taught to love, for love comes more naturally to the human heart than its opposite." Nelson Mandela, Antiapartheid Activist and Former President of South Africa.

Although increased self-awareness may serve the purpose of bringing our inherent biases to the surface, it is not enough. Once we are aware of them, we must make a conscious effort not to allow those views to negatively affect the care we

provide, for an exercise on how to change prejudices and stigma, refer to Box (**1.4**).

Fig. (1.5). Self-awareness. Source: www.pixabay.com.

Box 1.3. Strategies for increasing self-awareness: examining the motives behind our actions (as adapted from Stephany, 2020).

- Ask yourself why you are behaving the way that you are.
- Seek feedback from others on how you are acting.
- Consider reflective journaling.
- Make the effort to listen to opinions or values that differ from our own.

Box 1.4. Learning activity: changing prejudices & stigma.

Goleman (2005) explains that the roots of personal prejudice run deep because they are acquired early on in life and learned, and that makes them difficult to eradicate completely, but the following three strategies are known to help and are worth considering.

1-Sometimes, what is needed is for other people to speak up when they see acts of discrimination happening, like vulgar and hurtful language and offensive jokes (Goleman, 2005).

2-Another beneficial tool is to teach people how to understand and empathize with another person's experiences, and the best way to facilitate understanding is to listen to other people's stories (Goleman, 2005). Listening to another person's story helps us to see past their life decisions and circumstances and to see them as another fellow human being who is vulnerable and just like you in many ways.

3-Rakel (2018) makes another powerful suggestion. They advise that we make a choice to be present on purpose, without judgment. This involves paying full and undivided attention to the person you are caring for, as though they are the only one in the world who matters, and it is this form of human connection that fosters healing.

QUESTIONS TO PONDER FOR FURTHER REFLECTION

1-Can you make a commitment to speak up when you hear or see someone treating or talking about others in a disrespectful way? If not, why not?

2-What about your own attitudes toward specific populations? Are you aware that you have them? Are you acting on them unconsciously?

3-What strategies that we have not suggested can you take to change your personal views?

SPECIFIC TRAUMA-RELATED RESPONSES

"The effects of unresolved trauma can be devastating. It can affect our habits and outlook on life, leading to addictions and poor decision-making. It can take a toll on our family life and interpersonal relationships. It can trigger real physical pain, symptoms, and disease, and it can lead to a range of self-destructive behaviors." Peter A. Levine, Psychologist & Author

Human beings experience many specific trauma-related responses, adverse effects, or reactions due to trauma that include the following: the traumatic stress response, acute stress disorder, physical problems, mental illness, substance use, relationship difficulties, and trauma triggers.

The Traumatic Stress Response

When someone experiences a traumatic event, a **traumatic stress response** may ensue, which is a specific but normal neuropsychological reaction (American Psychological Association (APA), 2019; Wilson, 2011). This response is inherent, old, and instinctual and involves the amygdala part of the brain that causes a quick emotional reaction and a slower cognitive rational response. For example, when a person feels threatened, a stress response is activated that triggers a reaction to either escape from or eliminate that source of distress (Christopher, 2004). Symptoms associated with traumatic stress may include some or all of the following: being sad, anxious, angry, sleep disturbances, intrusive thoughts, bad dreams, memories of the incident, and avoiding situations that are similar (APA). Usually, these symptoms diminish with time. However, although a traumatic stress response can be normal, sometimes, the symptoms remain or worsen, and the reaction then becomes problematic (APA; Christopher). What happens is that the stressor activates a sequala of neurophysiological responses that alter function in the cortical, subcortical, and autonomic circuits of the brain (Pal & Elbers, 2018). Although this form of alteration in brain function may have historically served to protect the person from situations that have the potential to threaten their survival, in the present day, this degree of response to non-life-threatening stressors can lead to physical, emotional, or psychological disturbances, and decreased ability to cope (Pal & Elbers).

Acute Stress Disorder

An **acute distress disorder** develops when emotional reactions to a stressor linger over time and result in persistent post-traumatic disturbing symptoms that interfere with a person's everyday life. Some or all of the following disturbing symptoms may persist: anxiety, anger, problems with sleep, intrusive thoughts, re-experiencing the event, bad dreams, flashbacks, avoiding situations that remind the person of the incident, and relationship difficulties (APA, 2019; Christopher, 2004; Wilson *et al.*, 2011).

With acute stress disorder occurring, the persisting distressing symptoms develop due to an alteration in mental function. For instance, trauma leaves a strong impression on the vulnerable areas of the brain (*e.g.*, hypothalamic-pituitary, adrenal axis, amygdala, hippocampus, and prefrontal cortex), which impairs the person's ability to react appropriately and creates a template for how the person will react or respond to future stressors (Wilson *et al.*, 2011). The individual is no longer able to *via* adequately determine the degree of a perceived or actual danger and will tend to react quite extremely to a minimal danger. They are easily triggered, experience hyperarousal to external cues, and may resort to instinctual responses to a perceived threat in dramatic ways that activate a fight, flight or freeze reaction (Levine, 2010; van der Kolk, 2014).

Physical Problems Associated with Trauma

According to Swartz (2019), the challenges experienced by people who are traumatized are complex and multifactored and often negatively affect a person's health and well-being. For example, trauma has been linked to serious medical issues such as cardiovascular disease, diabetes, hypertension, and chronic pain (Haskins, 2019). Sometimes, a person will experience **somatization** due to trauma, which is an emotional response that surfaces as physical symptoms in the body. Headaches, stomach aches, fatigue and other bodily discomforts are examples of a somatic response. Many people who have these types of symptoms are not fully aware of the connection between their trauma and a physical ailment (SAMHSA, 2014b). However, SAMHSA warns that everyone who has experienced trauma and presents with physical complaints must still be properly assessed by a medical professional to rule out an actual physical cause for their symptoms before assuming they are somatic.

Trauma, Mental Illness & Substance Use

Trauma is associated with an increased risk for mental illnesses such as depression, anxiety, and PTSD (Gerber, 2019; Felitti *et al.*, 2019; Levine, 2010). Adults with childhood trauma are also known to have earlier onset of mental illness and poorer outcomes than those without a history of adversity (Felitti *et al.*,). Trauma has also been linked to substance use. For instance, Rogers *et al.*, (2021) conducted a longitudinal study and found that exposure to ACEs was linked to increased substance use in adolescence and adulthood, and in those with a higher number of ACEs, the degree of substance use was exacerbated. Javeri and Artigas (2018) explained the connection between trauma and substance use. They point out that the impact of the trauma can be cumulative and may result in more extensive emotional responses to future traumas. This, in conjunction with a decreased ability to cope with stress, puts the person at increased risk for using substances to self-medicate to alleviate some of their distressing symptoms (Javero & Artigas, 2018).

Trauma and Its Impact on Relationships

SAMHSA (2014b) points out that although a good support network can somewhat protect a person who has been traumatized from developing adverse responses, their interpersonal relationships can still be negatively impacted. Two of the most common behaviors exhibited by a traumatized individual that causes difficulty in their relationships consist of unhealthy interpersonal dependence or aloofness (SAMHSA, 2014b). They either over-rely on the people who support them, which can be quite taxing for their helpers, or they purposefully push them away, which interferes with connection and intimacy (SAMHSA). When the traumatized individual avoids personal connection, fear and a lack of trust are usually at the core of their response. (SAMHSA). Persons who have been traumatized are also often easily angered, which may cause further difficulty in their relationships and contribute to problems with attendance and performance at school or work (van der Kolk, 2014). Peer support and professional counselling are, therefore, highly recommended to assist traumatized person in improving their interpersonal relationships (SAMHSA).

THE ROLE OF TRAUMA TRIGGERS

"Triggers are like little psychic explosions that crash through avoidance and bring the dissociated, avoided trauma suddenly, unexpectedly, back into consciousness." Carol Spring, Author, Trainer & Trauma Survivor.

A **trauma trigger** refers to a perceptual stimulus involving the senses that cause a link to a previous traumatic experience (Foli & Thompson, 2019). The actual trigger can be anything that causes an emotional connection to the memory of the adverse event and is personal in nature (Cori, 2008). It may be a sound, smell, or visual stimulus that brings the person back to a situation that hurt them, and once a person is triggered, they relive the same feelings and behaviors that occurred when the actual event transpired (Cori). The following Case Study tells the story of what happened to Sandeep when she was unexpectedly triggered (Box **1.5**).

NARRATIVE CASE STUDY ONE: IDENTIFICATION OF THEMES & ANALYSIS

Three key themes were identified from this story.

Theme # 1: When Sandeep became triggered by the moldy smell of the Hotel Room, she did not immediately recognize why. She had blocked out the memory of what occurred in the past because it was painful for her.

Theme # 1 Analysis: There are reasons why someone may inadvertently suppress an unwanted memory. According to Hu *et al.*, (2017), forgetting may serve as a defense and a way to avoid recalling something that was traumatizing. However, when an object, place or situation inadvertently triggers memory retrieval of the incident, it may elicit a flood of physical or emotional responses.

Box 1.5. Narrative case study one: when a trigger results in an unexpected emotional response.

Sandeep is a very successful therapist who specializes in providing counselling to people who suffer from anxiety and depression. Sandeep regularly attends conferences to ensure that she is kept up to date with best practices in Counselling. Last Winter, Sandeep registered for an out-of-town conference in Toronto featuring the latest research in Cognitive Behavioral Therapy (CBT). Sandeep arrived a day early for the scheduled conference so she could purposefully do some sightseeing and shopping. She checked into the Hotel and proceeded to her Room. When she got to her Hotel Room, she noticed that the room smelt kind of musty and moldy. She looked around to see if there was any visible mold and could not see any. Then something quite unexpected happened. Sandeep began experiencing chest tightness and shortness of breath and broke out into a cold sweat. She tried to do some deep breathing to calm herself down, but it didn't work. In fact, she felt panic-stricken, like the whole room was spinning and closing in on her. Sandeep was self-aware enough to realize that she was experiencing a full-blown panic attack and she instinctually knew she had to get out of that place right away. She bolted out of the room with her cell phone in her hand, found a quiet corridor, sat on the floor because she felt dizzy, and called her husband, who was also a trained counsellor. Sandeep was relieved when he picked up the phone. Noting that Sandeep was quite upset, her husband asked her what was going on. Sandeep described in detail what had just happened to her. Her husband proceeded to reassure Sandeep that she was safe and assisted her with deep breathing exercises and some mindfulness techniques. After about a half hour transpired Sandeep' symptoms had completely subsided, and she finally felt normal again. Her husband then advised that she go to the Front Desk and ask for a new room that was not moldy. Once she felt a bit better, she proceeded to do what he advised and was checked into a newer wing of the Hotel. When Sandeep entered the new room, she was relieved that it was fresh smelling and new. She attended the conference the next day and did not experience any more unusual symptoms. However, once she got back home, and at the direct advice of her husband, Sandeep made an appointment to see a Counsellor. After a long therapy session, Sandeep became aware for the first time why she experienced a panic attack when she entered the mold-smelling room. Her therapist helped her to go back into her history to look for clues as to why she was triggered by a moldy smell. Sandeep recalled when she was only ten years old, her only other sibling and her father both died suddenly. Following these deaths, her mother was devastated by her loss, had a serious reactive depression, and was hospitalized for nine months. Sandeep was placed into the care of an elderly relative, who was quite good to her, but lived in an old house. Sandeep remembered that the bedroom that she slept in was cold, dark, and smelt quite moldy. Sandeep recalled how she would cry every night in that old musty room before falling asleep. At that time in her life, she felt despondent and hopeless because she was grieving and was desperately afraid that her mother would never get better and come home to take care of her. It was a sad time for Sandeep. The moldy smell in the Hotel Room triggered her, and she became overwhelmed with fear without knowing why. Sandeep had blocked out the memory of that time in her life because it was too traumatic for her. Now that she was aware of her trauma history, she could begin her journey to heal.

Theme # 2: The moldy smell of the Hotel Room triggered a visceral fear response in Sandeep, followed by a panic attack.

Theme # 2 Analysis: Psychological trauma occurs due to an event, experiences, or circumstances that a person perceives as frightening, threatening or harmful and can leave a lasting imprint in the person's brain that may last a lifetime (Levine, 1997). The memory of that trauma can resurface through a trigger reaction, that activates a sequence of psychic defenses and even physical ones like fight, flight, or freeze (Levine, 1997). The reaction is often quite profound and not related to any actual or imminent threat of harm but is nevertheless quite distressing for the person experiencing it (Cori, 2008).

Theme # 3: Sandeep's experience, although quite stressful, launched her into recovery from a suppressed trauma.

Theme # 3 Analysis: Research demonstrates that healing from trauma is a threefold process with safety as the first stage, remembering what happened as the second phase, and forming a reconnection with the goodness of life as the third step (Herman, 2015). When Sandeep became aware of her history of trauma through a trigger reaction, the first step she took, as advised by her husband, was to remove herself from the stimulus so she could feel safe. The second step, as facilitated by a therapist, was to remember the painful experiences that occurred when she was a child. The third stage will be for her to take further steps to heal, which may involve more therapy.

QUESTIONS FOR FURTHER DISCUSSION

1 What stood out for you about this story?

2-What did you learn that you may not have been aware of before?

3-Were you surprised to discover that something that happened so long ago could still cause someone to react emotionally and physically?

4-As a student nurse, how would you respond if a client/patient you were caring for had a panic attack because of a trigger reminding them of a previous trauma?

5-When caring for a client who has experienced trauma, caregivers do not necessarily know how to be or what to say. Can you think of actions that may make them feel accepted? Have an open discussion about what you have learned so far that either helps or hinders when caring for others. Feel free to share stories if you feel safe to do so.

TRAUMAS ASSOCIATED WITH WORKING IN HEALTHCARE

There are several conditions that are trauma-related that are known to occur in student nurses, practicing nurses, and other people employed in a healthcare setting (Jenkins *et al.*, 2022; Mottaghi & Poursheikhali, 2020). Some examples include post-traumatic stress disorder, secondary traumatic stress, vicarious traumatization, and compassion fatigue. Although these conditions differ in some ways, they are all related to exposure to trauma.

Post-traumatic Stress Disorder

Direct exposure to a traumatic event or a series of stressful situations can result in **post-traumatic stress disorder (PTSD)**. Some of the symptoms associated with PTSD include reliving the incident in dreams or flashbacks, experiencing fearful thoughts, anger, irritability, depression, avoiding situations that resemble trauma, and an inability to cope (Jenkins *et al.*, 2022). What is quite alarming is that during the COVID-19 pandemic, healthcare workers, including nurses, reported high levels of PTSD symptoms, including anxiety and depression and the severity of symptoms was noted to be significantly higher than pre-pandemic levels (Johnson *et al.*, 2020). For example, estimates of PTSD symptomology among health professionals working during the pandemic were higher than those in the general population and significantly higher when compared to other stressful circumstances associated with working as a healthcare professional (Johnson *et al.*, 2020).

Secondary Traumatic Stress

A key work-related condition that negatively affects the health of nurses is **secondary traumatic stress (STS)** (Mottaghi & Poursheikhali, 2020). Personal exposure to trauma is not necessary for STS to develop. In fact, it most often occurs after direct contact with and repetitious exposure to those who have experienced adversity or manifests after viewing, hearing about, or being exposed to traumatic events. Some of the symptoms associated with STS are fear, feelings of helplessness, and difficulty forgetting the memory of the situation (Mottaghi & Poursheikhali).

Vicarious Traumatization

Nursing is a caring profession and the importance of establishing a trusting relationship with clients and caring for them is a known expectation associated with nursing practice. However, sometimes, the ability to act in caring ways is eroded due to the traumatic nature of the work and may result in the development of vicarious traumatization (Isobel & Thomas, 2021). **Vicarious traumatization** consists of a distressing emotional response after directly witnessing trauma or hearing the stories of people who have had adverse experiences (Clark *et al.*, 2022). Vicarious traumatization is like secondary traumatic stress in that the cause and sequelae of symptoms are quite similar for both conditions. Vicarious

Traumatization can also be considered a possible sub-category of PTSD (Schiff & Lane, 2019). It can also result in serious cognitive changes in a nurse's self-esteem and may impede their ability to form or maintain trusting relationships (Kennedy & Booth, 2022). Because it contributes to decreased job satisfaction and a diminished ability to offer empathy, vicarious traumatization is also closely related to compassion fatigue.

Compassion Fatigue

Mottaghi and Poursheikhali, (2020) point out that in addition to caring, empathy and compassion are also hallmarks associated with the profession of nursing. **Empathy** is the ability to identify with all experiences of another person and to understand what they have gone through. **Compassion** specifically identifies with the suffering of another person, and there is a public expectation that nurses act with compassion (Mottaghi & Poursheikhali). Nurses who care for us often do feel good about the work they do which is referred to as **compassion satisfaction** (Schiff & Lane, 2019). However, **compassion fatigue (CF)** has the opposite effect. It occurs due to exposure to other people's suffering, is acute in onset, and results in the caregiver becoming emotionally exhausted. It subsequently interferes with their ability to act in empathetic ways as a means to avoid further psychological trauma (Kearney & Weininger, 2011; Schiff & Lane, 2019). It is, however, crucially important to point out that the caregiver does not stop being empathetic because they no longer care but because they care too much (Mottaghi & Poursheikhali). Note that although secondary traumatic stress and compassion fatigue are similar in some ways, STS occurs over time, and CF develops quite acutely.

Compassion fatigue not only negatively affects the nurse's professional life but also adversely impacts them on a personal level, physically and emotionally. Nurses report feeling extremely exhausted, experiencing frequent headaches, anxiety, and sadness, and loneliness (Gustafsson & Hemberg, 2022). In the following case study, we will explore and analyze the experiences of Michael, who gave up his career as a counsellor because of compassion fatigue (Refer to Box **1.6**).

NARRATIVE CASE STUDY TWO: IDENTIFICATION OF THEMES & ANALYSIS

Two key themes were identified from this story.

Theme # 1: Michael experienced compassion fatigue and lost all interest in listening to the sad stories of the youth he was working with. He subsequently took a break from his job as a Youth Counsellor.

Box 1.6. Narrative case study two: when feeling too much empathy causes harm to a caregiver.

Michael worked as a Youth Counsellor in the community, offering private and group therapy to troubled children and teens. Michael loved his job and decided to become a therapist because of his own life experience. For instance, when he was thirteen years old, Michael got into trouble with the Law for stealing a car, and it was a caring Social Worker mandated by the Juvenile court system that helped him turn his life around. However, it wasn't an easy journey to become a Counsellor. It involved years of training and Michael worked really hard to get to where he was today. For many years, the work that he did was quite fulfilling for Michael. He felt he was making a positive difference in the lives of the troubled youth he worked with. But after 10 years of doing this work, Michael noticed that he was becoming increasingly sad about the stories he was listening to, day after day, and he began to notice that he was no longer able to emotionally disconnect from his work when he got home. Michael started to feel sad or angry most of the time. His wife pointed out that he was no longer the same person she had married and was very concerned about him. Michael informed his wife that he suspected that he was developing the symptoms of a condition he had learned about in his training called compassion fatigue. He went on to explain to her that although he tried to ignore what he was feeling, it was not working and he admitted to her that he could not bear to hear another sad story. She convinced Michael to seek medical attention. On the advice of his doctor, Michael took a six-month medical leave from his job to heal. He went to counselling and was reminded of the importance of care for the caregiver. Michael's therapist pointed out that ever since Michael became a Counsellor, in addition to his professional work, he had also been offering free help to everyone close to him. He advised Michael to stop trying to help everyone and set boundaries as a form of emotional self-preservation. Michael listened and felt a huge relief after letting that obligation go. Michael was also reminded by this therapist and wife that his own personal happiness was necessary to offset the trying circumstances of his work.

Theme # 1 Analysis: Taking a break from constant exposure to the sadness associated with his work was a needed action for Michael's emotional well-being. Sometimes, we need to admit to ourselves that there is a problem before we can look for solutions. Prioritizing one's emotional needs, taking measures toward a healthier lifestyle, setting aside time to reflect, and reaching out to others for support can all be used to combat or heal compassion fatigue (Gustafsson & Hemberg, 2022). Seeking professional help is also beneficial, but often, caregivers can be somewhat reluctant to reach out for help. As Shapiro (2020) so poignantly points out, it takes courage to prioritize our well-being, especially when we are so used to care for others and putting their needs first.

Theme # 2: Michael realized that he learned something valuable from his experience with compassion fatigue. He learned the importance of taking steps to take better care of himself.

Theme # 2 Analysis: Research conducted by Gustafsson and Hemberg (2022) has revealed that although compassion fatigue can create stress for the caregiver, it also offers an opportunity for valuable learning to take place. That learning often begins in the form of prioritizing self-compassion and self-care but may also result in additional benefits. For example, a nurse in Gustafsson and Hemberg's study revealed that compassion fatigue humbled her, forced her to take better care of herself, and not to feel guilty when she made her self-care a priority. Others reported enjoying aspects of everyday life that they had been ignoring.

SOME KEY COMPONENTS OF TRAUMA-INFORMED CARE

Trauma-informed care acknowledges the long-term effects associated with trauma with the goal of helping people who have experienced adversity (Stokes *et al.*, 2017). It offers hope and facilitates healing from deep emotional wounds that will not easily dissipate without the right type of treatment (Knight, 2015; Young *et al.*, 2019) (Fig. **1.6**). Because this whole textbook explores various aspects of trauma-informed care in depth, only a few components of this crucially important therapeutic premise will be presented here. They consist of the importance of being trauma-informed, trauma-responsive, and designing a trauma-sensitive practice, followed by the key objectives and assumptions of trauma-informed care.

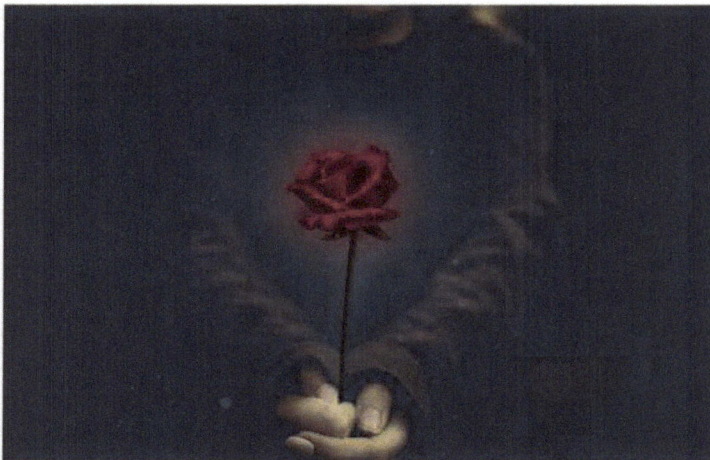

Fig. (1.6). Healing from trauma. Source: www.pixabay.com.

The Importance of Being Trauma-Informed and Trauma-Responsive

It is essential that caregivers become educated in trauma-informed and trauma-sensitive practices. To be **trauma-informed** involves the ability to recognize the ways that various forms of adversity have negatively impacted the lives of people (Cannon *et al.*, 2020; Carello & Butler, 2015). **Trauma-responsiveness** is concerned with every aspect of the delivery of services once a person has interfaced with a healthcare setting, with the goal of preventing unintentional harm (Goddard, 2020). It consists of the ability to be empathetic and understanding with someone when faced with reactive behaviors linked to past adversity (Stephany, 2020).

Creating a Trauma-Sensitive Practice

Being **trauma-sensitive** in clinical practice consists of being aware and responsive to a person's history of adversity or interpersonal violence (Ravi & Little, 2017). Although many community services have contact with people who have experienced trauma, professionals who work in healthcare have the most frequent contact with these individuals, and that is why they need to be trained in trauma-sensitive practices (Davies *et al.*, 2017). According to Davies *et al.*, (2017), two essential features of trauma-sensitive approaches that a practitioner should practice are to communicate messages that convey safety, and to conduct a self-assessment to ensure that they are practicing with understanding. Specific ways to implement these approaches are presented in Box (**1.7**) & Box (**1.8**). A learning exercise for classroom discussion is included in Box (**1.9**).

Box 1.7. Trauma-sensitive caregiver messages that covey safety (as adapted from Davies *et al.*, 2017).

Consider communicating these messages to clients/patients seeking assistance.
1-We are aware that people who we care for, including our staff, may have experienced some sort of trauma or violence.
2-We are skilled to support you in a safe, non-judgmental way.
3-It is okay for you to talk about your experiences with us.
4-The symptoms or feelings you have are a normal response to what you have gone through.
5-Nothing is wrong with you.
6-We are here to help.

Box 1.8. Self-assessment questions for caregivers to adopt that ensure understanding (as adapted from Davies *et al.*, 2017).

Ask yourself these questions to assess your level of understanding.
1-Do our clients/patients feel physically and emotionally safe?
2-Does everyone act in a caring, respectful, and professional way?
3-After assessing and ascertaining direct or indirect cues displayed by the person, is it okay to talk about abuse or trauma?
4- If I do talk about violence, will I ensure it will be handled carefully and skilfully?
5-Are all the people who work here sensitive when they ask about traumatic experiences?
6-Do the people and staff practicing here listen to what the client/patient wants when making decisions on their behalf?
7- Do people in this work setting like working here and with the rest of the team?

Box 1.9. Learning activity: a trauma-sensitive practice challenge.

After reading the suggested questions for caregivers to ask and self-assessment queries for them to adopt to assess for understanding, do you think there should be additional items added to either list? Why or why not? Feel free to research the literature or to draw from lived experiences when participating in this learning activity.

Two Key Objectives of Trauma-Informed Care

Although trauma-informed care is multi-faceted in its approach it focusses on two key objectives. One targets organizational change and the second aims to affect clinical practice (Menschner & Maul, 2016). At the organizational level, the approach focusses on recruiting workers who are trauma-informed; training others already working in health care; and preventing secondary traumatic stress in staff (Menschner & Maul). At the clinical practice level staff training is conducted to ensure that assessment and screening of people occur in a safe, respectful, and dignified manner; that clients/patients are included in the planning of their own care; and that any additional treatment that is needed is co-ordinated with appropriate community support services (Menschner & Maul).

THE FOUR CORE ASSUMPTIONS OF TRAUMA-INFORMED CARE

The Four Core Assumptions of Trauma-informed Care are essential and foundational for providing trauma-responsive care and consist of realize, recognize, respond, and resist re-traumatization (SAMHSA, 2014) (Fig. **1.7**).

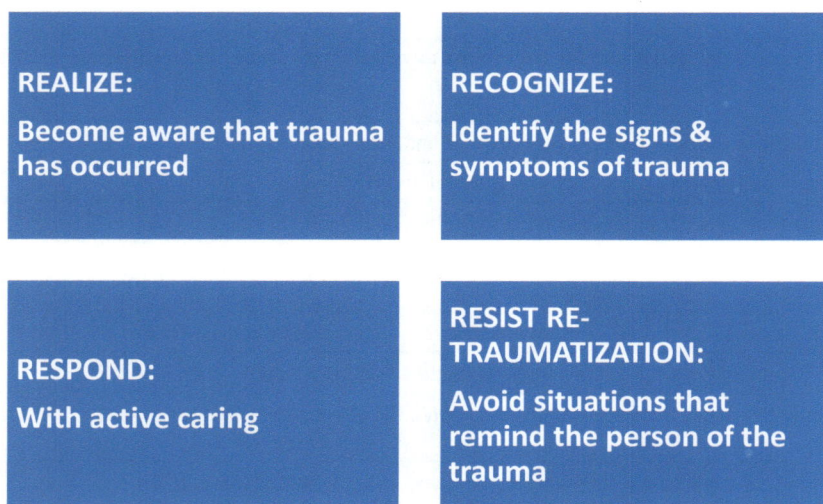

REALIZE:
Become aware that trauma has occurred

RECOGNIZE:
Identify the signs & symptoms of trauma

RESPOND:
With active caring

RESIST RE-TRAUMATIZATION:
Avoid situations that remind the person of the trauma

Fig. (1.7). The Four Core Assumption of Trauma Informed Care (as adapted from SAMHSA, 2014).

Realize consists of being aware that trauma is prevalent and the effects of experiencing adversity are long-term and negatively impact the person mentally, physically, emotionally, and socially (Goddard, 2020). For example, trauma not only results in widespread harmful repercussions for those who have experienced it, it also hurts people closest to them and their caregivers, like family members, teachers, early childhood care workers, and health care professionals (Goddard, 2020; SAMHSA, 2014).

Recognize is about the identification of the signs and symptoms of trauma and may involve training healthcare professionals to be trauma-sensitive (SAMSHA, 2014). This could involve teaching caregivers to ask the right questions in a supportive and non-judgmental way, such as, "Has your living situation changed in any way?" and *"Has anything stressful., sad, or scary happened to you or your child?"* (Goddard, 2020, p. 148). If trauma is suspected, healthcare professionals are encouraged to express genuine concern, and to communicate that the effects of adversity manifest in different ways for everyone. For example, children may present with eating problems, difficulty sleeping, exhibit emotional aggression, or difficulty with school (Goddard, 2020).

Respond consists of active caring in the form of taking action that may include referral to trauma-based community support (SAMSHA, 2014). The types of services that are required vary but may include, assessment, screening, support, and professional referrals for specific interventions (*e.g.*, family, or individual counselling, cognitive behavioral therapy, and other recommended treatment modalities) (Goddard, 2020).

Grossman *et al.*, (2021) point out a difficult truth, that many health care services, or personnel sometimes inadvertently contribute to re-traumatization. **Resisting re-traumatization** is therefore crucially important and involves a plan of action to avoid exposing people to situations that remind them of a particular adversity or event. For example, people with a history of trauma may exhibit a reluctance to undress or be touched physically or feel anxious when alone with a caregiver. It is therefore imperative that all health professionals be trained to identify the signs of trauma triggers, and how to respond with sensitivity when the client becomes anxious or fearful (Goddard, *et al.*, 2021; SAMHSA, 2014).

WHY TRAUMA INFORMED CARE IS NEEDED IN NURSING EDUCATION

"Nurses are a unique kind. They have this insatiable need to care for others, which is both their biggest strength and fatal flaw." Jean Watson, American Nurse, Professor, and Care Theorist

Trauma-informed care is needed in Nursing School schools and should be considered as part of the curriculum for the following reasons. Trauma is prevalent in society and high numbers of people who access health services have experienced adversity. Student nurses are not currently learning these skills in a comprehensive way in all schools, they are a risk group for trauma, and they are exposed to adverse events in clinical training (Fig. **1.8**). The ensuing discussion offers explanations that will hopefully legitimatize the validity of these assertions.

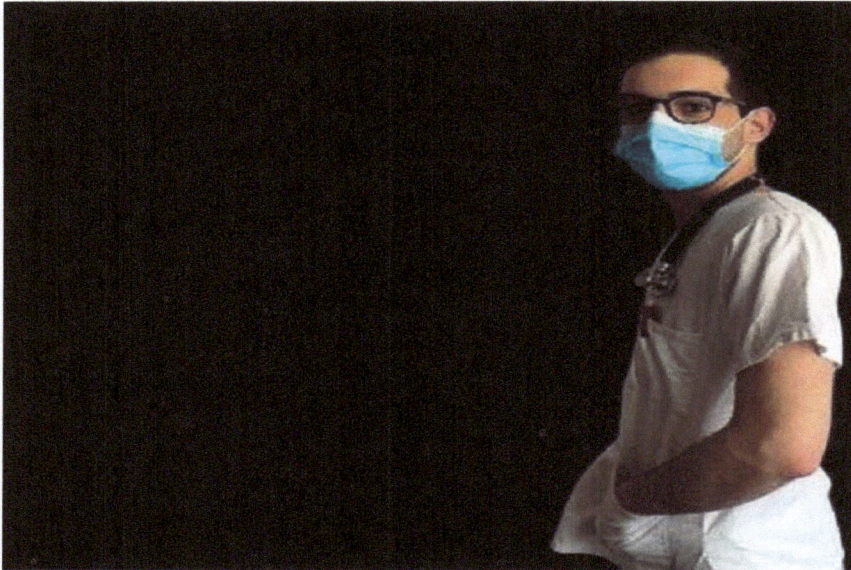

Fig. (1.8). Nursing student. Source: www.pixabay.com.

Student Nurses & Inadequate Preparation in Trauma-informed Care

Nurses as a group are known for their capacity to care. However, caring is not always an easy task and may require additional skills when looking after people who have experienced trauma (Goddard *et al.*, 2021). Furthermore, knowledge related to trauma-informed care is still quite limited in nursing, and when education in trauma-informed care is instigated, it has largely focused on practicing nurses and not taught to undergraduate nurses on a broad scale (Burton *et al.*, 2019; Cannon *et al.*, 2020; Goddard *et al.*, 2021; Stokes *et al.*, 2017; Turner & Harder, 2018; Yang *et al.*, 2019). Therefore, Pfeiffer and Grabbe (2022) recommend that in order not to re-traumatize clients/patients, all student nurses should be taught trauma-informed skills that are trauma-sensitive, strength-based, and resilience-based.

Student Nurses & A Personal History of Trauma

There is evidence that some student nurses have a history of trauma before they begin nursing school. They are often referred to as wounded healers who choose to enter a caring profession because they themselves have suffered and want to help others (Ng *et al.*, 2020; Wolf, 2019). For instance, the rates of adverse childhood experiences (ACEs) in student nurses and other healthcare professionals entering training are likely at least equal to, or greater than, that of the general population (Girouard & Bailey, 2017; Hendrick *et al.*, 2021). A study by McKee-Lopez *et al.*, (2019) found the rates of ACEs in student nurses to be higher than first realized and noted that roughly 23% of nursing students reported experiencing four or more types of ACEs, and 72% admitted to experiencing at least one. An **ACE score** refers to the degree of exposure to different types of traumas in childhood. Additional research has shown that student nurses with higher ACE scores do not perform as well academically as those without a history of trauma (Hendrick *et al.*, 2021). Student nurses with higher ACE scores also suffer from increased depression, anxiety, and stress, and may be triggered when caring for people who have been traumatized (Hendrick *et al.*,).

Student Nurses & Clinical Training & Exposure to Trauma & Death

Nursing students encounter situations in their training that may traumatize them. For instance, they take care of people who have experienced adversity or abuse and may become re-traumatized when triggered (Bosse *et al.*, 2021; Goddard *et al.*, 2021; Wolf, 2019; Zhai & Du, 2020). They are also in danger of being further distressed when caring for those who are very ill, injured or dying. In fact, both student and practicing nurses find caring for the severely ill, or dying client/patient to be emotionally upsetting, and find the death of a child to be quite devastating to deal with (Foli & Thompson, 2019; Wedgeworth, 2016). In fact, although being confronted with death and dying is often inevitable when working in healthcare, student nurses still find it difficult to deal with. For instance, not being adequately supported during their initial exposure to death can result in unresolved issues for student nurses that are cognitive, emotional, and clinically related (Anderson *et al.*, 2015). In one study, both practicing nurses and student nurses expressed feelings of distress and inadequate coping when their early encounters with death were deemed difficult and unresolved (Anderson *et al.*, 2015). This, in turn, negatively impacted the quality of care provided, decreased overall satisfaction with work, and resulted in higher attrition rates for students (Anderson *et al.*, 2015). It is therefore recommended that student nurses not only be taught the skills to care for the dying, but also better supported to deal more effectively with their own ensuing anxiety and sadness related to this experience (Cavaye & Watts, 2014; Gurdogan *et al.*, 2019).

The Learning Environment & Increased Emotional Stress Due to COVID-19

Student Nurses generally experience higher levels of anxiety than other college students. Some of the reasons include fierce competition to get into nursing, the extent of course difficulty when they are in a program, and the pressure of working long clinical shifts (Wedgeworth, 2016). Due to the COVID-19 pandemic and the current landscape of healthcare delivery, nursing students admit that they have experienced additional emotional distress (Asian & Pekince, 2021). Examples of their concerns include worrying about caring for the very ill or becoming sick themselves, being less confident in the clinical setting; feeling inadequately supported by some instructors, and experiencing communication difficulties with other health professionals (Asian & Pekince, 2021). A more disturbing fact is that student nurses' exposure to chronic stress in the clinical setting due to COVID-19 has resulted in reports of complicated forms of grief, anxiety, and depression (Goddard *et al.*, 2021).

Positive Outcomes Associated with Implementing Trauma-informed Care into Nursing School

Teaching trauma-informed care to student nurses has been shown to be helpful (Bosse *et al.*, 2021; Goddard *et al.*, 2021). For example, when trauma-informed strategies were intentionally incorporated into nursing school, the risk factors for secondary traumatic stress in students were reduced, and student nurses reported an enhanced experience of social, emotional, and academic safety (Bosse *et al.*,). Furthermore, nursing students are more likely to stay in their program, graduate, and remain as practitioners in the field of nursing if they receive the following supports, being trained to care for persons with a history of trauma; receiving support for past trauma and adverse experiences that happen in training; and being taught in a psychologically safe learning environment (Christopher *et al.*, 2020; Foli & Thompson, 2019; Goddard *et al.*, 2021; Wynyard *et al.*, 2020).

Nursing Faculty also Need Support

It is crucially important to emphasize that nursing Instructors may also require support in doing their job, especially when they suspect that a student may be traumatized. For example, they will need to learn how to set respectful and professional boundaries concerning the self-disclosure of students' trauma history and should not be expected to act as counselors (Foli & Thompson, 2019). Therefore, ideally, instructors should receive formal training in how to recognize when a student is experiencing secondary trauma or re-traumatization and where to refer the student for professional help and support (Pfeiffer & Grabbe, 2022).

SELF-CARE STRATEGY: LEARNING SELF-COMPASSION

"A moment of self-compassion can change your entire day. A string of such moments can change the course of your life." Christopher Germer, Clinical Psychologist

Many nurses are very hard on themselves and resort to self-degradation and negative self-talk and research reveals that this is harmful to their overall mental health (Hofner *et al.*, 2020). Subsequently, it is highly recommended that nurses and student nurses learn the art of self-compassion to protect their mental wellness. Self-compassion begins with acknowledging our needs and demonstrating the same empathy and care for ourselves as we offer others. When we prioritize our wellbeing, we are acknowledging that our needs do matter. However, some of us may feel that prioritizing our well-being is selfish. Forrest (2003) refutes that assumption and explains that self-care and selfishness are not same, and that practicing self-compassion can actually make us better caregivers. They explain that self-care is actually benevolent and unselfish, because when we are kind to ourselves, we are more likely to have the needed energy to be more understanding and empathetic with others (Forrest).

Self-Compassion Challenge

1-What would it be like for you to move away from trying to be perfect all the time and embrace the fact that you are human?

2-Can you make it your intention to give yourself a break? Try it. It is very freeing.

Note: Any suggested strategies are not intended to be a substitute for medical or psychological advice from a trained professional. The reader is therefore encouraged to seek medical or other professional help in any matters related to their physical or emotional health.

CONCLUSION

- The purpose of Chapter One was to explore the reasons why trauma-informed care is needed in nursing education.
- We learned that the goal of trauma-informed care is to help people who have experienced trauma and targets change at the organizational and clinical level, with the aim of improving client/patient outcomes.
- Caring, the ethic of care, and caring pedagogy are key themes in this book. Caring in general is thoroughly embedded in the content because it is foundational for nursing practice and a key component of trauma-informed care.

- We were informed that narratives are used as a specific form of qualitative, phenomenological study, that derives knowledge from actual life experiences as told by people living through them.
- The ethic of care was deemed to be the theoretical premise for data analysis. It is a special feature of nursing ethics that values relationships, context, meaning making, the interconnectedness of all of life, and the self-worth of every person.
- The ethic of care aligns well with trauma-informed care in nursing practice because they both honor the intrinsic self-worth, autonomy, and choice of each person, and promote practice strategies that empower people to heal from adversity.
- Trauma was defined as an event or series of circumstances that are harmful, threatening or a danger to a person's life, and has lasting adverse effects on their ability to function.
- Psychological trauma refers to a disturbing event that is unexpected and beyond what would normally be anticipated, and results in a large array of physical, emotional, and psychological responses.
- It was brought to our attention that trauma is prevalent in society, is widespread, can affect anyone, and may occur at any point across the life span.
- Several types of traumas were described. Historical trauma affects the history of a specific group of people who have been oppressed. Transgenerational trauma involves the transfer of prejudicial attitudes from one generation to another. Violent trauma includes all forms of abuse and affects the person directly. Adverse childhood experiences (ACEs) consist of a long list of negative traumatic experiences that occur in childhood, and structural trauma is indirect violence aimed at specific populations by design.
- The number of groups of people who have fallen prey to structural trauma is quite extensive. This Chapter specifically drew attention to targeted acts of stigma and adversity toward these groups of people, those with differing sexual orientation or gender identity, older adults, refugees and immigrants, people of colour, and Indigenous people. The reader was also strongly encouraged to become aware of other oppressed groups of people and ways to end discrimination.
- We became aware that some of the origins of harmful behaviors perpetrated toward specific populations lies in bias and implicit bias. Embracing diversity and increasing self-awareness were recommended to combat stigma.
- Nurses were reminded that they are not ethically or professionally permitted to discriminate for any reason.
- The following specific trauma related responses were explored, the traumatic stress response, an acute stress disorder, physical problems, mental illness, substance use, relationship difficulties, and trauma triggers.

- There are several conditions that are trauma related that are known to occur in health professionals, and although these conditions differ in some ways, they are all related to exposure to adversity. Some examples include post-traumatic stress disorder, secondary traumatic stress, vicarious traumatization, and compassion fatigue.
- Nursing is a caring profession. However, sometimes the ability to act compassionately is eroded due to the traumatic nature of the work and may result in the development of secondary traumatic stress, vicarious traumatization, or compassion fatigue.
- Trauma-informed care has two primary objectives. One targets organizational change and the other affects clinical practice.
- *The Four Core Assumptions of Trauma-informed Care* were deemed essential and foundational for providing trauma-responsive care and consist of realize, recognize, respond, and resist re-traumatization. To realize is to be aware that trauma has occurred. To recognize involves identifying the signs and symptoms of trauma. Responding consists of actively caring, and resist-re-traumatization consists of avoiding situations that cause the person to be triggered.
- Professionals working in health care need ensure that they are practicing in a trauma-responsive and trauma-sensitive manner. The following two essential features of trauma-sensitive approaches were subsequently recommended, how to convey messages that enhance safety, and to how to conduct a self-assessment that communicates understanding.
- Two Narrative Case Studies were presented. The first one revealed the complexity of a trigger response, and that it can occur after a long time has transpired since the event, and how it can elicit a profound visceral fear response.
- The second Narrative Case Study demonstrated how compassion fatigue (CF), or the inability to respond empathetically, develops over time, and can be precipitated by over exposure to sad stories. We also learned that recovery from CF often begins with prioritizing one's emotional needs.
- The following rationale for why trauma-informed care should be incorporated into Nursing School curriculum was given. Trauma is prevalent in society and high numbers of people who access health services have experienced adversity. Student nurses are not currently learning these skills in a comprehensive way in all schools, they are a risk group for trauma, and they are exposed to traumatic events in clinical training.
- Three Learning Activities are suggested (*e.g.*, Connecting with the Goodness in Life; Changing Prejudices & Stigma; and Participation in A Trauma-Sensitive Practice Challenge).
- The chapter ended with a recommended self-care strategy that promotes self-compassion.

RECOMMENDED READINGS

Foli, K., and Thompson, J. R. (2019). *The influence of psychological trauma in nursing.* Sigma Theta Tau International.

Levine, P. A., (2010). *In an unspoken voice: How the body releases trauma and restores goodness.* North Atlantic Books.

Linklater, R. (2014). *Decolonizing trauma work: Indigenous stories and strategies.* Fernwood Publishing.

Shapiro, S. (2020). *Good morning, I love you: Mindfulness and self-compassion practices to rewire your brain.* Sounds True Inc.

REFERENCES

Allan, B & Smylie, J (2015) Available from: https://www.wellesleyinstitute.com/wp-content/uploads/2015/02/Summary-First-Peoples-Second-Class-Treatment-Final.pdf

American Psychological Association (APA) (2016) Available from: https: //www.apa. org/news /press/ releases/ stress/2015/ impact-of- discrimination. pdf

American Psychological Association (APA) (2019) *How to cope with traumatic stress* Available from: https://www.apa.org/topics/trauma/.stress

Anda, R F, Butchard, A, Felitti, V J & Brown, D W (2010) Building a framework for global surveillance of the public health implications of adverse childhood experiences. *American Journal of Preventive Medicine,* 39, 93-8.

Anderson, NE, Kent, B & Owens, RG (2015) Experiencing patient death in clinical practice: Nurses' recollections of their earliest memorable patient death. *Int J Nurs Stud,* 52, 695-704. [http://dx.doi.org/10.1016/j.ijnurstu.2014.12.005] [PMID: 25577307]

Anyikwa, VA (2016) Trauma-informed approaches to survivors of intimate partner violence. *J Evid Inf Soc Work,* 13, 484-91. [http://dx.doi.org/10.1080/23761407.2016.1166824] [PMID: 27142906]

Aslan, H & Pekince, H (2021) Nursing students' views on the COVID☐19 pandemic and their percieved stress levels. *Perspect Psychiatr Care,* 57, 695-701. [http://dx.doi.org/10.1111/ppc.12597] [PMID: 32808314]

Barker, B, Sedgemore, K, Tourangeau, M, Lagimodiere, L, Milloy, J, Dong, H, Hayashi, K, Shoveller, J, Kerr, T & DeBeck, K (2019) Intergenerational trauma: The relationship between residential schools and the child welfare system among young people who use drugs in Vancouver, Canada. *J Adolesc Health,* 65, 248-54.https://www.rrh.org.au/journal/article/6411 [http://dx.doi.org/10.1016/j.jadohealth.2019.01.022] [PMID: 30948272]

Bosse, JD, Clark, KD & Arnold, S (2021) Implementing trauma-informed educational practices in undergraduate mental health nursing education. *J Nurs Educ,* 60, 707-11. [http://dx.doi.org/10.3928/01484834-20211103-02] [PMID: 34870506]

British Broadcasting Corporation (BBC) We know what LGBT means but here's what LGBTQQIAAP stands for,2015 Available from: https://www.bbc.com/news/newsbeat-33278165

Brooks, R & Goldstein, S (2003) *The power of resilience: Achieving balance, confidence, and personal strength in your life.* McGraw Hill.

Burton, CW, Williams, JR & Anderson, J (2019) Trauma-informed education in baccalaureate nursing

curricula in the United States: Applying the American Association of Colleges of Nursing Essentials. *J Forensic Nurs*, 15, 214-21.
[http://dx.doi.org/10.1097/JFN.0000000000000263] [PMID: 31764525]

Mateo, CM & Williams, DR (2020) Addressing bias and reducing discrimination: The professional responsibilities of health care providers. *Acad Med*, 95, S5-S10.
[http://dx.doi.org/10.1097/ACM.0000000000003683]

Canadian Nurses Association (CNA) (2017) *CNA code of ethics for registered nurses.* Available from: https://cna.informz.ca/cna/data/images/Code_of_Ethics_2017_Edition_Secure_Interactive.pdf

Cannon, LM, Coolidge, EM, LeGierse, J, Moskowitz, Y, Buckley, C, Chapin, E, Warren, M & Kuzma, EK (2020) Trauma-informed education: Creating and pilot testing a nursing curriculum on trauma-informed care. *Nurse Educ Today*, 85, 104256.
[http://dx.doi.org/10.1016/j.nedt.2019.104256] [PMID: 31759240]

Carabez, R, Pellegrini, M, Mankovitz, A, Eliason, M, Ciano, M & Scott, M (2015) "Never in all my years . . ." Nurses' education about LGBT health. *J Prof Nurs*, 31, 323-9.
[http://dx.doi.org/10.1016/j.profnurs.2015.01.003] [PMID: 26194964]

Carello, J & Butler, LD (2015) Practicing what we teach: Trauma-informed educational practice. *J Teach Soc Work*, 35, 262-78.
[http://dx.doi.org/10.1080/08841233.2015.1030059]

Cavaye, J & Watts, J H (2014) An integrated literature review of death education in pre-registration nursing curricula: Key themes. 2014
[http://dx.doi.org/10.1155/2014/564619]

Centers for Disease Control and Prevention (CDC) (2017) *Intimate partner violence: definitions.* Available from: https://www.cdc.gov/violenceprevention/intimatepartnerviolence/definition.html

Christopher, M (2004) A broader view of trauma: A biopsychosocial-evolutionary view of the role of the traumatic stress response in the emergence of pathology and/or growth. *Clin Psychol Rev*, 24, 75-98.
[http://dx.doi.org/10.1016/j.cpr.2003.12.003] [PMID: 14992807]

Christopher, R, de Tantillo, L & Watson, J (2020) Academic caring pedagogy, presence, and Communitas in nursing education during the COVID-19 pandemic. *Nurs Outlook,* 68, 822-9.
[http://dx.doi.org/10.1016/j.outlook.2020.08.006] [PMID: 32981671]

Clark, N, Slemon, A & Jenkins, E (2022) Trauma, violence, and mental health uma, violence, and mental he. *A concise introduction to mental health in Canada,* Canadian Scholars. 126-41.

Cori, JL (2008) *Healing for trauma: A survivors guide to understanding your signs and symptoms and reclaiming your life.* Marlowe & Company.

Davies, JA, Todahl, J & Reichard, AE (2017) Creating a trauma-sensitive practice: A health care response to interpersonal violence. *Am J Lifestyle Med*, 11, 451-65.
[http://dx.doi.org/10.1177/1559827615609546] [PMID: 30202371]

Duffy, JR (2018) *Quality caring in nursing and health systems: Implications for clinicians, educators, and leaders* Springer Publishing Company.
[http://dx.doi.org/10.1891/9780826181251]

Ernst, JS & Maschi, T (2018) Trauma-informed care and elder abuse: A synergistic alliance. *J Elder Abuse Negl*, 30, 354-67.
[http://dx.doi.org/10.1080/08946566.2018.1510353] [PMID: 30132733]

Felitti, VJ, Anda, RF, Nordenberg, D, Williamson, DF, Spitz, AM, Edwards, V, Koss, MP & Marks, JS (2019) Relationship of childhood abuse and household dysfunction to many of the leading causes of death in adults: The adverse childhood experiences (ACE) study. *Am J Prev Med*, 56, 774-86.
[http://dx.doi.org/10.1016/j.amepre.2019.04.001] [PMID: 31104722]

Foli, K & Thompson, JR (2019) *The influence of psychological trauma in nursing.* Sigma Theta Tau

International.

Fonseca, S (2020) Institutional racism in Canada: Indigenous lived realities. *The Society. Sociology & Criminology Undergraduate Review,* 5, 50-60.

Forrest, MS (2003) *A short course in kindness: A little book on the importance of love and the relative unimportance of just about everything else.* L. M. Press.

Gaywsh, R & Mordoch, E (2018) Situating intergenerational trauma in the educational journey. *in education,* 24, 3-23.
[http://dx.doi.org/10.37119/ojs2018.v24i2.386]

Gerber, MR (2019). *Trauma-informed healthcare approaches: A guide for primary care.* Springer.
[http://dx.doi.org/10.1007/978-3-030-04342-1]

Graff, G (2014) The intergenerational trauma of slavery and its aftermath. *J Psychohist,* 41, 181-97.
[PMID: 25630191]

Gilligan, C (1982) *In a different voice: Psychological theory and women's development.* Harvard University Press.

Girouard, S & Bailey, N (2017) ACEs implications for nurses, nursing education, and nursing practice. *Acad Pediatr,* 17, S16-7.
[http://dx.doi.org/10.1016/j.acap.2016.09.008] [PMID: 28865650]

Goddard, A (2021) Adverse childhood experiences and trauma-informed care. *J Pediatr Health Care,* 35, 145-55.
[http://dx.doi.org/10.1016/j.pedhc.2020.09.001] [PMID: 33129624]

Goddard, A, Jones, RW, Esposito, D & Janicek, E (2021) Trauma informed education in nursing: A call for action. *Nurse Educ Today,* 101, 104880.
[http://dx.doi.org/10.1016/j.nedt.2021.104880] [PMID: 33798984]

Goleman, D (2005) *Emotional intelligence: Why it matters more than IQ.* Bantam Dell.

Grogan, S & Murphy, KP (2011) Anticipatory stress response in PTSD: Extreme stress in children. *J Child Adolesc Psychiatr Nurs,* 24, 58-71.
[http://dx.doi.org/10.1111/j.1744-6171.2010.00266.x] [PMID: 21272115]

Grossman, S, Cooper, Z, Buxton, H, Hendrickson, S, Lewis-O'Connor, A, Stevens, J, Wong, LY & Bonne, S (2021) Trauma-informed care: recognizing and resisting re-traumatization in health care. *Trauma Surg Acute Care Open,* 6, e000815.
[http://dx.doi.org/10.1136/tsaco-2021-000815] [PMID: 34993351]

Gurdogan, EP, Kınıcı, E & Aksoy, B (2019) The relationship between death anxiety and attitudes toward the care of dying patient in nursing students. *Psychol Health Med,* 24, 843-52.
[http://dx.doi.org/10.1080/13548506.2019.1576914] [PMID: 30727771]

Gustafsson, T & Hemberg, J (2022) Compassion fatigue as bruises in the soul: A qualitative study on nurses. *Nurs Ethics,* 29, 157-70.
[http://dx.doi.org/10.1177/09697330211003215] [PMID: 34282669]

Hagiwara, N, Kron, FW, Scerbo, MW & Watson, GS (2020) A call for grounding implicit bias training in clinical and translational frameworks. *Lancet,* 395, 1457-60.
[http://dx.doi.org/10.1016/S0140-6736(20)30846-1] [PMID: 32359460]

Haskins, J (2019) *What if we treated every patient as though they had lived through trauma?.* Available from: https://www.aamc.org/news-insights/what-if-we-treated-every-patient-though-they-had-lived-through-trauma

Hedrick, J, Bennett, V, Carpenter, J, Dercher, L, Grandstaff, D, Gosch, K, Grier, L, Meek, V, Poskin, M, Shotton, E & Waterman, J (2021) A descriptive study of adverse childhood experiences and depression, anxiety, and stress among undergraduate nursing students. *J Prof Nurs,* 37, 291-7.
[http://dx.doi.org/10.1016/j.profnurs.2021.01.007] [PMID: 33867083]

Herman, J (2015) *Trauma and recovery: The aftermath of violence – From domestic abuse to political terror.* Basic Books.

Hofmeyer, A, Taylor, R & Kennedy, K (2020) Knowledge for nurses to better care for themselves so they can better care for others during the Covid-19 pandemic and beyond. *Nurse Educ Today,* 94, 104503.
[http://dx.doi.org/10.1016/j.nedt.2020.104503] [PMID: 32980179]

Hordvik, E (2019) What is psychological trauma? Methods of treatment.*Childhood trauma* Routledge 23-30.
[http://dx.doi.org/10.4324/9780429461637-3]

Hu, X, Bergström, ZM, Gagnepain, P & Anderson, MC (2017) Suppressing unwanted memories reduces their unwanted influences. *Curr Dir Psychol Sci,* 26, 197-206.
[http://dx.doi.org/10.1177/0963721417689881] [PMID: 28458471]

Human Rights Watch (HRW) (2022) Available from: https://www.hrw.org/news/2022/02/04/us-borde--programs-huge-toll-children

Institute on Trauma and Trauma-informed Care (ITTIC) (2022) *What is Trauma-informed care?.* Available from: https://socialwork.buffalo.edu/social-research/institutes-centers/institute-on-trauma-and--rauma-informed-care/what-is-trauma-informed-care.html

Isobel, S & Thomas, M (2022) Vicarious trauma and nursing: An integrative review. *Int J Ment Health Nurs,* 31, 247-59.
[http://dx.doi.org/10.1111/inm.12953] [PMID: 34799962]

Jaffe, J, Segal, J & Dumke, LF (2005) Available from: https: //www. help guide. org/mental /emotional_ psych ological_ trauma.htm

Jarero, I & Artigas, L (2018) AIP model-based acute trauma and ongoing traumatic stress theoretical conceptualization. *Iberoamerican Journal of Psychotraumatology and Dissociation,* 10, 1-10.

Jenkins, E, Slemon, A, Bilsker, D & Goldner, EM (2022) *A concise introduction to mental health in Canada* Canadian Scholars.

Johnson, SB, Riley, AW, Granger, DA & Riis, J (2013) The science of early life toxic stress for pediatric practice and advocacy. *Pediatrics,* 131, 319-27.
[http://dx.doi.org/10.1542/peds.2012-0469] [PMID: 23339224]

Johnson, SU, Ebrahimi, OV & Hoffart, A (2020) PTSD symptoms among health workers and public service providers during the COVID-19 outbreak. *PLoS One,* 15, e0241032.
[http://dx.doi.org/10.1371/journal.pone.0241032] [PMID: 33085716]

Kearney, M & Weininger, R (2011) Whole person self-care: Self-care from the inside out. In: Hutchinson, T.A., (Ed.), *Whole person care: A new paradigm for the 21st century* Springer Science & Business Media 109-25.
[http://dx.doi.org/10.1007/978-1-4419-9440-0_10]

Kennedy, S & Booth, R (2022) Vicarious trauma in nursing professionals: A concept analysis. *Nurs Forum,* 57, 893-7.
[http://dx.doi.org/10.1111/nuf.12734]

Knight, C (2015) Trauma-informed social work practice: Practice considerations and challenges. *Clin Soc Work J,* 43, 25-37.
[http://dx.doi.org/10.1007/s10615-014-0481-6]

Kusmaul, N & Anderson, K (2018) Applying a trauma-informed perspective to loss and change in the lives of older adults. *Soc Work Health Care,* 57, 355-75.
[http://dx.doi.org/10.1080/00981389.2018.1447531] [PMID: 29522384]

Levenson, J (2020) Translating trauma-informed principles into social work practice. *Soc Work,* 65, 288-98.
[http://dx.doi.org/10.1093/sw/swaa020] [PMID: 32676655]

Levine, PA (1997) *Waking the tiger: Healing trauma.* North Atlantic Books.

Levine, PA (2010) *In an unspoken voice: How the body releases trauma and restores goodness.* North Atlantic Books.

Linklater, R (2011) Decolonizing trauma work: Indigenous stories and strategies. Fernwood.

MacDonald, C & Steenbeek, A (2015) The impact of colonization and Western assimilation on the health and wellbeing of Canadian Aboriginal people. *International Journal of Regional and Local History,* 10, 32-46. [http://dx.doi.org/10.1179/2051453015Z.00000000023]

Matthews, R (2017) The cultural erosion of Indigenous people in health care. *CMAJ,* 189, E78-9. [http://dx.doi.org/10.1503/cmaj.160167] [PMID: 27620632]

McCormick, A, Scheyd, K & Terrazas, S (2018) Trauma-informed care and LGBTQ youth: Considerations for advancing practice with youth with trauma experiences. *Fam Soc,* 99, 160-9. [http://dx.doi.org/10.1177/1044389418768550]

McKee-Lopez, G, Robbins, L, Provencio-Vasquez, E & Olvera, H (2019) The relationship of childhood adversity on burnout and depression among BSN students. *J Prof Nurs,* 35, 112-9. [http://dx.doi.org/10.1016/j.profnurs.2018.09.008] [PMID: 30902402]

Menschner, C & Maul, A (2016) *Issue Brief: Key ingredients for successful trauma-informed care implementation* Available from: https://www.samhsa.gov/sites/default/files/programs_campaigns/ childrens_mental_health/atc-whitepaper-040616.pdf

Mihas, P (2019) *Qualitative data analysis.* Oxford Research Encyclopedias.

Morgan, M S & Wise, M N (2017) Narrative science and narrative knowing: Introduction to special issue on narrative science. *Studies in History and Philosophy of Science* Elsevier Ltd 1-5.

Motta, RW (2008) Secondary trauma. *Int J Emerg Ment Health,* 10, 291-8. [PMID: 19278145]

Mottaghi, S, Poursheikhali, H & Shameli, L (2020) Empathy, compassion fatigue, guilt and secondary traumatic stress in nurses. *Nurs Ethics,* 27, 494-504. [http://dx.doi.org/10.1177/0969733019851548] [PMID: 31284826]

Narayan, MC (2019) CE: Addressing implicit bias in nursing: A review. *Am J Nurs,* 119, 36-43. [http://dx.doi.org/10.1097/01.NAJ.0000569340.27659.5a] [PMID: 31180913]

Ng, QX, De Deyn, MLZQ, Lim, DY, Chan, HW & Yeo, WS (2020) The wounded healer: A narrative review of the mental health effects of the COVID-19 pandemic on healthcare workers. *Asian J Psychiatr,* 54, 102258. [http://dx.doi.org/10.1016/j.ajp.2020.102258] [PMID: 32603985]

 Noddings, N (2013) *Caring: A relational approach to ethics and moral education.* University of California Press.

Pal, R & Elbers, J (2018) Neuroplasticity: The other side of the coin. *Pediatr Neurol,* 84, 3-4. [http://dx.doi.org/10.1016/j.pediatrneurol.2018.03.009] [PMID: 29685608]

Paradies, Y (2018) Racism and Indigenous health. *Glob Public Health.* [http://dx.doi.org/10.1093/acrefore/9780190632366.013.86]

Perez, E (2021) *Diversity's child: people of color and the politics of identity.* University of Chicago Press. [http://dx.doi.org/10.7208/chicago/9780226799933.001.0001]

Pfeiffer, K & Grabbe, L (2022) An approach to trauma-informed education in prelicensure nursing curricula. *Nurs Forum,* 57, 658-64. [http://dx.doi.org/10.1111/nuf.12726]

Purkey, E, Patel, R & Phillips, SP (2018) Trauma-informed care: Better care for everyone. *Can Fam Physician,* 64, 170-2.https://www.cfp.ca/content/cfp/64/3/170.full.pdf [PMID: 29540379]

Rakel, D (2018) *The Compassionate connection: The healing power of empathy and mindful listening.* W. W. Norton Company Ltd..

Ramsey-Klawsnik, H & Miller, E (2017) Polyvictimization in later life: Trauma-informed best practices. *J Elder Abuse Negl,* 29, 339-50.
[http://dx.doi.org/10.1080/08946566.2017.1388017]

Raso, R, Fitzpatrick, JJ & Masick, K (2021) Nurses' intent to leave their position and the profession during the COVID-19 pandemic. *J Nurs Adm,* 51, 488-94.
[http://dx.doi.org/10.1097/NNA.0000000000001052] [PMID: 34519700]

Ravi, A & Little, V (2017) Curbside consultation: Providing trauma-informed care. *Am Fam Physician,* 95, 655-7. https://www.aafp.org/afp/2017/0515/p655.html
[PMID: 28671409]

Ray, MA (2018) *Transcultural caring dynamics in nursing and health care.* F. A. Davis Company.

Rogers, CJ, Forster, M, Grigsby, TJ, Albers, L, Morales, C & Unger, JB (2021) The impact of childhood trauma on substance use trajectories from adolescence to adulthood: Findings from a longitudinal Hispanic cohort study. *Child Abuse Negl,* 120, 105200.
[http://dx.doi.org/10.1016/j.chiabu.2021.105200] [PMID: 34252647]

Royal Mental Health Care & Research (RMHCR) (2019) Available from: https://www.theroyal.ca/resource-library/lgbtq2s-what-does-it-mean#:~:text=Sexual%20orientations%20and%20gender%20identities,Questioning%2C%20and%20Two%2DSpirit

Scheer, JR & Poteat, VP (2021) Trauma-informed care and health among LGBTQ intimate partner violence survivors. *J Interpers Violence,* 36, 6670-92.
[http://dx.doi.org/10.1177/0886260518820688] [PMID: 30596315]

Waegemakers Schiff, J & Lane, AM (2019) PTSD symptoms, vicarious traumatization, and burnout in front line workers in the homeless sector. *Community Ment Health J,* 55, 454-62.
[http://dx.doi.org/10.1007/s10597-018-00364-7] [PMID: 30684127]

Shapiro, S (2020) *Good morning, I love you: Mindfulness & self-compassion practices to rewire your brain.* Sounds True Inc..

Shi, M, Stey, A & Tatebe, LC (2021) Recognizing and breaking the cycle of trauma and violence among resettled refugees. *Curr Trauma Rep,* 7, 83-91.
[http://dx.doi.org/10.1007/s40719-021-00217-x] [PMID: 34804764]

Slote, M (2007) *The ethics of care and empathy.* Routledge.
[http://dx.doi.org/10.4324/9780203945735]

Solomon, EP & Heide, KM (2005) The biology of trauma: Implications for treatment. *J Interpers Violence,* 20, 51-60.
[http://dx.doi.org/10.1177/0886260504268119] [PMID: 15618561]

Stephany, K (2020) *The ethic of care: A moral compass for Canadian Nursing practice* Bentham Science Publishers Pte. Ltd..

Stephany, K (2022) *Cultivating empathy: Inspiring health Professionals to communicate more effectively.* Bentham Science Publishers Pte. Ltd.
[http://dx.doi.org/10.2174/97898150364801220101]

Stokes, Y, Jacob, JD, Gifford, W, Squires, J & Vandyk, A (2017) Exploring nurses' knowledge and experiences related to trauma-informed care. *Glob Qual Nurs Res,* 4.
[http://dx.doi.org/10.1177/2333393617734510] [PMID: 29085862]

Substance Abuse and Mental Health Services Administration (SAMHSA) (2014) Available from: https://www.refugees.org/wp-content/uploads/2022/02/sma14-4816.pdf

Suah, A & Williams, B (2021) How should clinicians address a patient's experience of transgenereational trauma? *AMA J Ethics,* 23, E440-5.
[http://dx.doi.org/10.1001/amajethics.2021.440] [PMID: 34212844]

Substance Abuse and Mental Health Services Administration (SAMHSA) (2014a) Available from: http://store.samhsa.gov/shin/content//SMA14-4884/SMA14-4884.pdf

Substance Abuse and Mental Health Services Administration (SAMHSA) (2014b) *Trauma-Informed Care in Behavioral Health Services* Available from: https://store.samhsa.gov/sites/default/files/d7/priv/sma14-4816.pdf

Sue, DW, Capodilupo, CM, Torino, GC, Bucceri, JM, Holder, AMB, Nadal, KL & Esquilin, M (2007) Racial microaggressions in everyday life: Implications for clinical practice. *Am Psychol,* 62, 271-86.
[http://dx.doi.org/10.1037/0003-066X.62.4.271] [PMID: 17516773]

Swartz, R (2022) Re-stor(y)ing Trauma. *International Journal of Social Work Values and Ethics,* 19, 28-36.
[http://dx.doi.org/10.55521/10-019-107]

Sweeney, A, Filson, B, Kennedy, A, Collinson, L & Gillard, S (2018) A paradigm shift: Relationships in trauma-informed mental health services. *BJPsych Adv,* 24, 319-33.
[http://dx.doi.org/10.1192/bja.2018.29] [PMID: 30174829]

Turney, K (2018) Adverse childhood experiences among children of incarcerated parents. *Child Youth Serv Rev,* 89, 218-25.
[http://dx.doi.org/10.1016/j.childyouth.2018.04.033]

Turner, S & Harder, N (2018) Psychological safe environment: A concept analysis. *Clin Simul Nurs,* 18, 47-55.
[http://dx.doi.org/10.1016/j.ecns.2018.02.004]

United Nations n.d. Available from: https: //www .un.o rg/ esa/ socd ev/ unpfii / docu ments/5se ssion _fact sh eet1 .pdf

van der Kolk, B (2014) *The body keeps score: Brain, mind, and body in the healing of trauma.* Viking Penguin.

van Manen, M (2017) Phenomenology in its original sense. *Qual Health Res,* 27, 810-25.
[http://dx.doi.org/10.1177/1049732317699381] [PMID: 28682720]

Watson, J (2008) *Nursing: The philosophy and science of caring.* University Press of Colorado.

Wedgeworth, M (2016) Anxiety and education: An examination of anxiety across a nursing program. *J Nurs Educ Pract,* 6, 23-6.
[http://dx.doi.org/10.5430/jnep.v6n10p23]

Wheeler, K (2018) A call for trauma competencies in nursing education. *Journal of the American Psychiatric Nurses Association,* 24, 20-2.
[http://dx.doi.org/10.1177/1078390317745080]

Wheeler, K & Phillips, K E (2019) The development of trauma and resilience competencies for nursing education. *J Am Psychiatr Nurses Assoc,* 27, 322-33.
[http://dx.doi.org/10.1177/1078390319878779]

Williams, MT, Davis, AK, Xin, Y, Sepeda, ND, Grigas, PC, Sinnott, S & Haeny, AM (2021) People of color in North America report improvements in racial trauma and mental health symptoms following psychedelic experiences. *Drugs Educ Prev Policy,* 28, 215-26.
[http://dx.doi.org/10.1080/09687637.2020.1854688] [PMID: 34349358]

Wilson, KR, Hansen, DJ & Li, M (2011) The traumatic stress response in child maltreatment and resultant neuropsychological effects. *Aggress Violent Behav,* 16, 87-97.
[http://dx.doi.org/10.1016/j.avb.2010.12.007]

Wolf, ZR (2019) Wounded healers, second victims, caring environments. In: Wolf, Z.R., (Ed.), *Int J Hum*

Caring, 23, 272-4.
[http://dx.doi.org/10.20467/1091-5710.23.4.272]

World Bank (2022) *Indigenous peoples overview* Available from: https: //www. world bank .or g/en/ topi c/i ndig enousp eople s

Wylie, L, Van Meyel, R, Harder, H, Sukhera, J, Luc, C, Ganjavi, H, Elfakhani, M & Wardrop, N (2018) Assessing trauma in a transcultural context: Challenges in mental health care with immigrants and refugees. *Public Health Rev,* 39, 22.
[http://dx.doi.org/10.1186/s40985-018-0102-y] [PMID: 30151315]

Wynard, T, Benes, S & Lorson, K (2020) Trauma-sensitive practices in health education. *J Phys Educ Recreat Dance,* 91, 22-9.
[http://dx.doi.org/10.1080/07303084.2020.1811622]

Li, Y, Cannon, LM, Coolidge, EM, Darling-Fisher, CS, Pardee, M & Kuzma, EK (2019) Current state of trauma-informed education in the health sciences: *Lessons for nursing. J Nurs Educ,* 58, 93-101.
[http://dx.doi.org/10.3928/01484834-20190122-06] [PMID: 30721309]

Young, J, Taylor, J, Paterson, B, Smith, I & McComish, S (2019) Trauma-informed practice: A paradigm shift in the education of mental health nurses. *Ment Health Pract,* 22, 14-9.
[http://dx.doi.org/10.7748/mhp.2019.e1359]

Zhai, Y & Du, X (2020) Letter to the Editor: Addressing collegiate mental health amid the COVID-19 pandemic. *Psychiatric Research,.*
[http://dx.doi.org/10.1016/j.psychres.2020.113003]

CHAPTER 2

The Six Guiding Principles of Trauma-Informed Care

Abstract: A principle-based approach to trauma-informed care is effective in promoting healing and chapter two explores the crucial aspects of each of *The Six Guiding Principles of Trauma Informed Care* as recommended by the Substance Abuse and Mental Health Services Administration (SAMHSA). They consist of safety; trustworthiness and transparency; peer support; collaboration and mutuality; empowerment, voice, and choice; and cultural, historical, and gender issues. The discussion begins by describing the physical, social, and psychological aspects of safety. They include the location of the health facility, the atmosphere of the healthcare clinic, staff attitudes, ensuring that health professionals are kept emotionally safe, and avoiding re-traumatization. It is pointed out that people who have been intentionally harmed by others do not easily trust. Therefore, trust must be earned through compassionate connection, and by protecting a person's privacy. Transparency is highly recommended and occurs when a person is fully informed about all aspects of the plan of care. Peer support is the help received from others who have lived through similar experiences and facilitates healing. Collaboration and mutuality are suggested to create a shared environment where there is an assumption that everyone, including the client/patient, will be involved in decision-making. Empowerment, voice, and choice when consistently applied foster an environment that utilizes a person's strengths to help them overcome adversity, gives them an opportunity to be listened to, and to make their own choices. The power of empathy and other-focused listening, and the importance of addressing cultural, historical, and gender issues are emphasized. Poor health outcomes experienced by people of the LGBTQ2S community are highly correlated with stigma. Nurses are identified as harbouring prejudicial attitudes toward members of this population, and educational efforts are strongly suggested to change these behaviours. Cultural humility is recommended as an effective way to counteract racism and power difficulties through empowerment, excellence in care, and an atmosphere of mutual respect. Self-awareness and self-reflection are recommended to incorporate cultural humility into practice. Two Narrative Case Studies are reviewed. The first one emphasizes the importance of safely conducting a client assessment, and the second one explores how peer support helps a bereaved child. Participation in these four learning activities is advised, strategies that enhance the environmental safety of a healthcare facility; when breaching confidentiality is necessary; situations that promote or impede trust; and actively communicating other-focused listening. The Chapter ends with a self-care strategy that encourages nurses to participate in mindfulness techniques to enhance the overall well-being.

Keywords: Cultural sensitivity, Cultural awareness, Cultural safety, Cultural humility, Confidentiality, Collaboration, Choice, Empathy, Empowerment, Gender issues, Mutuality, Microaggressions, Mindfulness, Other-focused listening, Physical safety, Psychological safety, Peer support, Resisting re-traumatization, Reflective journalling, Social safety, Safety, Self-awareness, Self-reflection, Strength-based approach, Secondary traumatic stress disorder (STS), Trustworthiness, Trauma-informed care, Transparency, Unconditional positive regard, Voice.

LEARNING GUIDE

After completing this chapter, the reader should be able to:

- Identify, *The Six Guiding Principles of Trauma Informed Care.*
- Gain an understanding of why safety is a priority, and be introduced to the physical, social, and psychological aspects associated with safety.
- Revisit strategies to avoid re-traumatization.
- Review ways to keep staff emotionally safe.
- Learn how to use non-verbal and verbal communication techniques that foster trustworthiness.
- Be informed of the importance of protecting privacy.
- Explore key elements that foster transparency such as promise-keeping, explaining expectations, and ensuring confidentiality.
- Understand when breaching confidentiality is necessary.
- Recognize the benefits of peer support.
- Learn why collaboration and mutuality are needed when providing trauma-informed services.
- Describe how empowerment, voice, and choice are interrelated and why they matter.
- Learn how to effectively ask questions, create a safe place for people to tell their stories, how be empathetic, and be an other-focused listener.
- Be cognizant of the importance of addressing cultural, historical, and gender issues.
- Become aware that many of the health challenges experienced by members of the LGBTQ2S community are due to stigma, and the unfortunate truth that many nurses harbour prejudicial attitudes toward members of this group.
- Learn how cultural humility can counteract racism and power struggles.
- Review two narrative case studies and ensuing thematic analysis. The first is about safely conducting an assessment. The second one explores how peer support helps a bereaved child.

- Participate in the following Suggested Learning Activities (*e.g.*, Strategies that Enhance the Environmental Safety of a Healthcare Facility; when breaching confidentiality is necessary; situations that promote or impede trust; and actively communicating other-focused listening).
- Consider participating in a self-care strategy that promotes mindfulness to enhance coping.

Introduction to Chapter Two & The Six Guiding Principles to Trauma Informed Care

"Walk gently in the lives of others. Not all wounds are visible." Author Unknown

Psychological wounds related to adversity are not always apparent because people do a fairly good job of intentionally, or unconsciously suppressing them as a way to cope (Fig. **2.1**). Yet, when trauma does occur in the life of an individual, it negatively affects their self-identity, their worldview, and their core beliefs. A principle-based approach to trauma-informed care is effective in promoting healing by reducing re-traumatization, decreasing suffering, supporting autonomy, enhancing coping, and fostering empowerment (Doncliff, 2020). *The Six Guiding Principles of Trauma Informed Care* are therefore highly recommended by the Substance Abuse and Mental Health Services (SAMHSA) (2014) as valuable tools for caring for people who have been subjected to traumatic experiences. These principles consist of safety; trustworthiness and transparency; peer support; collaboration and mutuality; empowerment, voice, and choice; and cultural, historical, and gender issues (Fig. **2.2**). All these values are beneficial, and their focus occasionally overlaps because they are interrelated. However, they are not meant to be prescriptive in nature but are generalized across various settings, with the aim of creating an environment that has the overall physical and emotional welfare of the person in mind (Doncliffe, 2020; Institute on Trauma and Trauma-informed Care (ITTIC), 2022). How each of these six principles are operationalized in practice, is the key focus of Chapter 2.

The following questions have been proposed for you to keep in mind as you review all of the guiding principles of trauma-informed care, as a way to ascertain whether or not they are being applied in your particular healthcare setting (Box **2.1**). It does not matter what your initial answer is for all, or any of these questions. Just keep them in mind as you read through this Chapter because key components related to them will be presented.

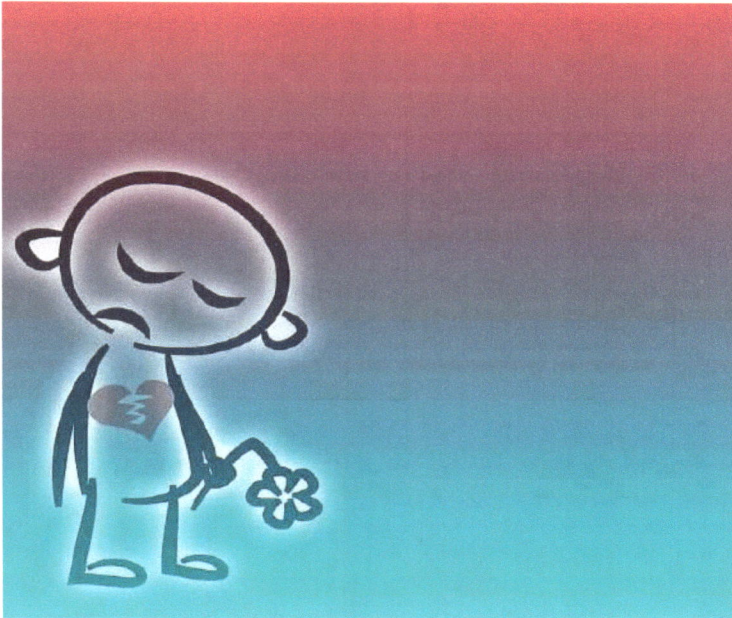

Fig. (2.1). Emotional Pain Can Often Be Hidden. Source: www.pixabay.com.

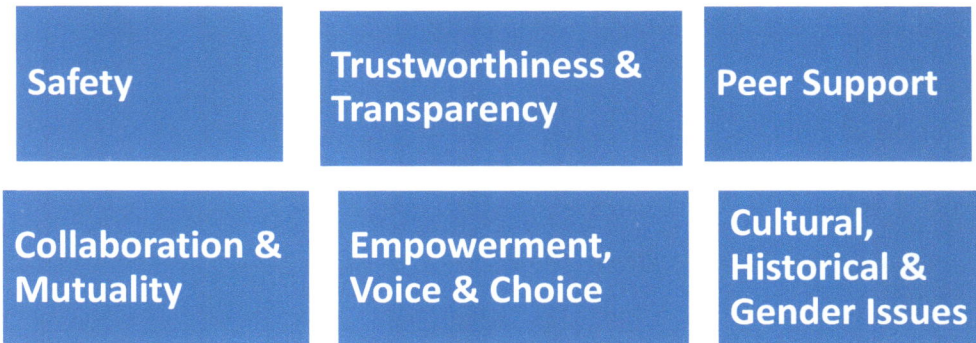

Safety	Trustworthiness & Transparency	Peer Support
Collaboration & Mutuality	Empowerment, Voice & Choice	Cultural, Historical & Gender Issues

Fig. (2.2). The six guiding principles of trauma informed care (SAMHSA, 2014).

Box 2.1. Questions to assess if the six guiding principles of TIC are being considered in your healthcare setting (as adapted from Collin-Vézina *et al.*, 2022; Isobel, 2015; ITTIC, 2022; Knight, 2019; Stephany, 2020).

1-Is the health clinic located in a protected area?
2-Do the caregivers ensure that emotional safety occurs through non-judgment, empathy, and validation?
3-Are they trustworthy? For example, will they protect a person's right to confidentiality, and do they care enough to genuinely want to help?
4-Is peer support offered as an avenue to recovery and healing?

(Box 2.1) cont.....

5-Is collaboration, or including what the individual wants, an integral part of care?
6-What about mutuality and the fact that healing is best facilitated in a shared environment?
7-Are the health professionals trained to empower a person who has experienced trauma? Do they even know what that entails? Are they aware that the person is not just a victim of their circumstances, but an autonomous human being capable of developing resilience, and making their own choices?
8-Do the people who work in the setting consider cultural, historical or gender issues when planning and implementing care?

SAFETY

We begin our discussion with safety because it is a priority when caring for someone who has experienced trauma. Safety is comprised of many diverse components, physical, social, and psychological in nature, that include the location of the health facility, the atmosphere of the clinic, and the attitude of the people who work there (Knight, 2019).

Physical Safety is Important

Physical safety consists of an absence of harm or injury in one's environment. People who have experienced violence need to feel secure when they are being treated for health-related issues, because if they feel unsafe in any way, they may become anxious and even reluctant to attend a clinic (ITTIC, 2022). According to Menschner and Maul (2016), creating a safe physical environment will increase the probability that the person will consent to treatment, and they are more likely to return for further care in the future. Refer to Box (**2.2**) to explore specific ways to enhance a physically safe healthcare environment Box (**2.3**) presents a learning activity to explore other ways to enhance physical safety.

Box 2.2. Cultivate a physically safe healthcare environment (as adapted from Knight, 2019; Menschner and Maul, 2016).

1-Areas both outside and inside of the healthcare facility need to be open and well-lit, such as parking lots, entrances, restrooms, and exits.
2-Are there security personnel both inside and outside of the clinic, and are these people trained in how to treat people who have experienced past trauma?
3-Are the waiting rooms comfortable and reasonably free of loud noises or music?
4-Is privacy respected during the assessment?
5-Do examining rooms have easy access to exist so that the person does not feel trapped in any way?

Box 2.3. Learning activity: explore additional strategies that may enhance the environmental safety of a healthcare facility.

In small groups spend time identifying other methods that a healthcare facility can adopt to make their environment more physically safe. Feel free to search the academic literature for ideas. After you have completed your session in groups, join the rest of the class to present your ideas for discussion and consideration.

Social Safety

The expectation of **social safety** in a trauma-informed practice is that the person seeking help will be protected from emotional harm or injury. It consists of an atmosphere that is welcoming, respectful, and supportive (Menschner and Maul, 2016). Specific strategies to foster social safety in a health setting should include a welcoming, friendly atmosphere when a person first arrives, followed by ensuring that all forms of communication are clearly articulated, and compassionate in nature (Menschner and Maul). Survivors of trauma are quite sensitive to non-verbal communication, especially if it is intimidating. That is why being rushed or having one's concerns ignored, can damage the rapport between the client/patient and the caregiver (Purkey *et al.*, 2018). When possible pre-set appointments should be kept, and if they need to be changed, sufficient explanation for the changes should be given to maintain trust (Menschner and Maul).

Facilitating the Psychological Safety of Clients/Patients

"Oh, the comfort, the inexpressible comfort of feeling safe with a person, having neither to weigh thoughts or measure words but to pour them all out, just as they are, chaff and grain together, knowing that a faithful hand will take and sift them, keep what is worth keeping, and then with a breath of kindness, blow the rest away." George Eliot, British & Victorian Author.

In trauma-informed care, **psychological safety** is achieved when a person feels safe from being harmed emotionally (Wilson *et al.*, 2013) (Fig. **2.3**). A psychologically safe environment is extremely important because someone who has experienced trauma, does not easily trust strangers or people in positions of authority. For instance, if a healthcare professional speaks, or acts in an insensitive or condescending manner, the person may inadvertently react physically in the form of outrage or respond emotionally with anger or sadness (Wilson *et al.*,).

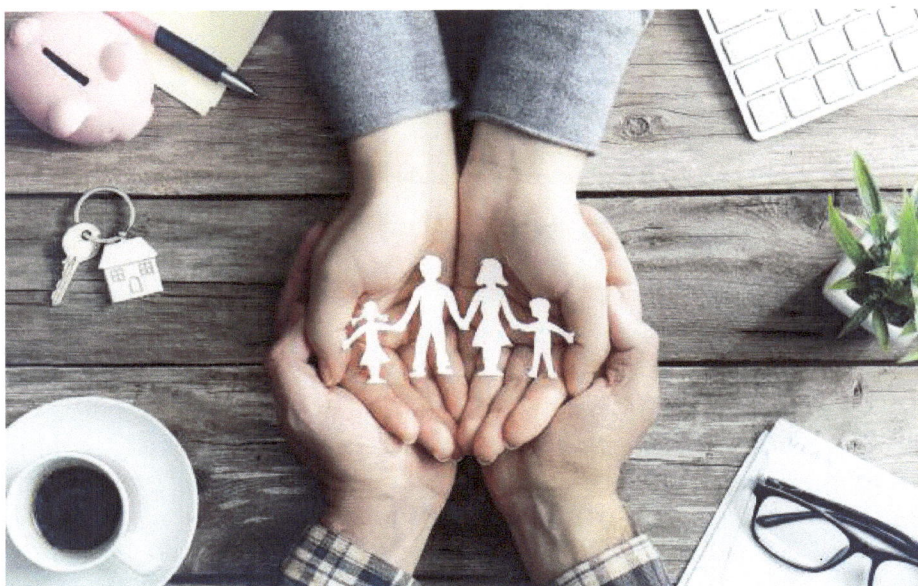

Fig. (2.3). The Feeling of Being Psychologically Safe. Source: www.pixabay.com.

Creating a safe place in the relationship between caregiver and client during an intake or an initial encounter should occur through specific steps, such as informing the person of all expectations, explaining everything that is about to occur, and avoiding unpredictable surprises (Levenson, 2020; Szczygiel, 2018). The caregiver's way of being must be genuine and nonthreatening. Shaming or judging should be avoided (Levenson).

How to Avoid Re-traumatization

Resisting re-traumatization is crucially important and involves a plan of action to avoid exposing people to situations that remind them of a particular adversity or event (SAMHSA, 2014). For example, even if a health clinic's policy demands a full history, the caregiver who is doing the intake must be careful to avoid asking too many intrusive questions, especially at a first meeting, because it may trigger the person to recall a previous traumatizing experience (Levenson, 2020). If the person does get triggered, a sequence of responses may follow which will most likely impede the caregiver's ability to complete the assessment. What is recommended is to avoid eliciting details of a past traumatic experience. Alternatively, it is best to acknowledge that trauma has occurred but discourage open sharing of actual events or experiences. Ask them to focus on sharing their feelings. The following Case Study explores how a mental health nurse was able conduct an initial client assessment in a safe manner. Refer to Box (**2.4**).

Box 2.4. Narrative case study one: safely conducting a client assessment.

Susan is a mental health nurse, and she was assigned to care for a new patient named John, who was just admitted to an Acute Adolescent Psychiatry Unit at the hospital where she worked. John was diagnosed with major depression and substance use. He was admitted to the hospital because he had recently relapsed and started using again, and he wanted to come clean. Susan proceeded to conduct an intake interview as part of her assessment. Before entering the examining room, Susan took a moment to take a deep breath so she could be mindful of her body language, and to ensure that she was completely present. She then walked into the room and introduced herself to John.

"Hello John, I am your nurse, and I am here to take your history. I will be asking you a few questions. I want you to know that this is a safe place, that I care about you, and want to help. If at any time, you feel you need a break, you just let me know, and if you start feeling upset about any part of the assessment we can also stop or change the focus. Is that okay with you?"

Right after Susan's brief introduction John seemed anxious and interrupted her before she could speak again.

"Sure, I guess it's okay. But you need to know that I had really bad stuff happen to me when I was a kid, lots, and lots of bad stuff, and that is why I do drugs, not that it is an excuse, but really awful stuff happened."

Susan noticed that John was upset, fighting back tears, looking down, and avoiding eye contact. Sensing that he was embarrassed, Susan chose her words carefully and spoke softly and kindly.

"I am so deeply sorry to hear that you had painful experiences when growing up. I do not need to hear any details about what happened because I do not want to remind you of things that may upset you and make you feel scared. I just want you to know that I am here to help you and I will not judge you."

Looking puzzled, but sensing that Susan might be genuine, John started telling her more of his story.

"Everything is my fault, I think. I was put in foster care when my mom died. I was only six and I acted out because I missed my mom. The foster parents were mean to me, and I was beaten every time I did something they didn't like. I think I deserved it. I won't like, talk about actual stuff they did to me, because you said I shouldn't. But it was not good. I waited until I was old enough to fight back and that made things way worse, so I ran away. I've been homeless since I was 13 and I did bad stuff to survive. The drugs helped me forget some of that stuff, but they also really messed with my head. I was off them for a while but started using again. I really want to come clean and change things. I am not even sure why I am telling you all of this."

Once again, Susan chose her words cautiously.

"Maybe you are telling me because you feel safe. I am sorry to hear that you think what happened to you was your fault. You need to be reminded that you were a child, you had lost your Mom, and that was very difficult for you. Even if you acted out, being beaten was wrong and should not have happened. You do not need to feel guilty or blame yourself for that."

John paused for a little bit, looked at Susan in a puzzling way and then tested her.

"Why are you being so nice to me? I don't think I am a good person and I do not think I deserve to be treated nicely."

John was visibly crying now so Susan waited for him to process his thoughts before she spoke.

(Box 2.4) cont.....

"You seem sad and that is okay. I cannot imagine how difficult things were for you growing up. I get that you do not think you are a good person, but that is not necessarily the truth. We are all human and make some mistakes, but that does not necessarily mean we are bad people. Tell me a little bit about you. Tell me something that you think you do well or what you are proud of."
With only a little bit of hesitancy, John began to share some good stuff about himself, although he was still crying.
"Well, you know, I am a good friend to some other kids on the street. I look out for the younger ones because the vultures are always trying to take advantage of them. When I can, I share my food with them and help them find a shelter to sleep in so they can get off the street for a while. Sometimes they listen, but other times they don't. I just try my best to help them when I can."
Susan responded.
"John, I need you to know that what you do for others is very caring and that makes you a good person. A bad person would not care about those kids and try to help. You have a kind heart John. You need to try to own that part of you."
John made eye contact, wiped away his tears, and smiled just a little bit.
"Thanks."
Sensing that an initial rapport and some trust had been achieved, Susan proceeded to conduct the rest of her assessment and John willingly cooperated. She also offered John something to eat and drink when he informed her that he had not eaten for two days. When Susan served him a sandwich and juice, he seemed incredibly grateful.

NARRATIVE CASE STUDY ONE: IDENTIFICATION OF THEMES & ANALYSIS

Four key themes were identified from this story.

Theme # 1: Before conducting the assessment and during the process, Susan made a conscious effort to convey safety by being present and building trust and rapport.

Theme # 1 Analysis: There were several specific actions taken by Susan that communicated safety. For example, before entering the examining room, Susan took a take a deep breath, was mindful of her body language, and ensured that she was completely present. At the onset of the assessment, Susan also introduced her patient to the process in a non-intimidating way and ensured that she acted in a caring manner during the whole process. Susan's actions were consistent with best practices and fostering safety in a practice setting. For example, what is highly recommended is to adopt a caring demeanor, demonstrate genuine compassion, and offer clear expectations, and for the caregiver to allow time for trust to develop before discussing any painful information (Levenson 2020).

Theme # 2: Because he felt safe, John willingly shared his past experiences with his nurse without fear of being judged, and what he experienced and felt was subsequently validated.

Theme # 2 Analysis: Too often, people who have been traumatized have experienced being ignored or judged. That is why validation is so important. **Validation** consists of being able to communicate that you fully accept and want to understand, another person's experience. It is a form of empathy that legitimately acknowledges their feelings (Pedneult, 2022). Susan was also aware that shame is quite often associated with childhood traumatic experiences, and helping John get in touch with some of his strengths could assist him in stepping away from the victim stance and moving forward.

Theme # 3: Susan used a strengths-based approach to help John stop blaming himself and focus more on the positive.

Theme # 3 Analysis: A **strength-based approach** to trauma-informed care helps by emphasizing a person's abilities and what they have learned from their experiences, rather than primarily focusing on their deficits or mistakes.

Theme # 4: By not judging John, Susan offered him unconditional positive regard, which in turn helped him to feel accepted and worthy.

Theme # 4 Analysis: Non-judgment fosters healing, and non-judgment is demonstrated through unconditional positive regard. **Unconditional positive regard** consists of the action of caring for someone without any conditions. The person does not need to be perfect to deserve care. If they misbehave or have done something in the past that they feel is wrong, you still care for and about them without restrictions, because they are human beings worthy of being cherished (Rogers, 1980).

QUESTIONS FOR FURTHER DISCUSSION

1-What else did you notice about this story?

2-What did you learn that you may not have been aware of before?

3-If you were Susan, is there anything you would have done differently?

Measures that Help to Keep Caregivers Psychologically Safe

People accessing services are not the only ones who need to be kept psychologically safe. People employed in these settings also require protection from emotional harm. According to Isobel and Edwards (2017) harm also occurs to clinicians who work with people who have been traumatized, but this fact is not always acknowledged or addressed. For example, they can develop **secondary traumatic stress disorder (STS)**. STS consists of distress due to being exposed to the traumatic experiences of another person, like hearing their sad accounts or stories. This condition may result in disturbing thoughts, chronic fatigue, emotional disengagement, absenteeism, and physical ailments, and contributes to burnout (Menschner & Maul, 2016; Mottaghi & Poursheikhali, 2020).

In order to prevent STS, Isobel and Edwards (2017) highly recommend that healthcare personnel and other staff be taught how to interact with people who have experienced trauma in a way that avoids exploring details of the adversity. Additional measures include hiring staff that are already trained to work with people who have been traumatized and offering mandatory training to those without these skills. Staff should also be encouraged to pursue self-care through increased physical fitness, meditation, scheduling mental health days, and practicing mindfulness. Management could ideally consider, promote, and respect reflective dialogue between staff and their supervisors (Menschner and Maul (2016).

> ### SOMETHING TO REFLECT UPON
>
> What would you do if you felt triggered about a previous trauma while hearing someone else's story? How would you make sure that you were okay? Would you be willing to make your own psychological well-being a priority?

TRUSTWORTHINESS & TRANSPARENCY

Trustworthiness

Trust and safety are closely aligned because if we want to foster trust, we must ensure that safety occurs first (Knight, 2015) (Fig. **2.4**). However, trust may not necessarily occur quickly between the caregiver and the client/patient, especially when the person we are caring for has been in an abusive relationship (Szczygiel, 2018). Therefore, Knight (2015) recommended that helping professionals not to take rejection personally. If it does occur, it is beneficial to be reminded that difficulties that do arise, likely stem from the person's past, and not because of what is occurring presently.

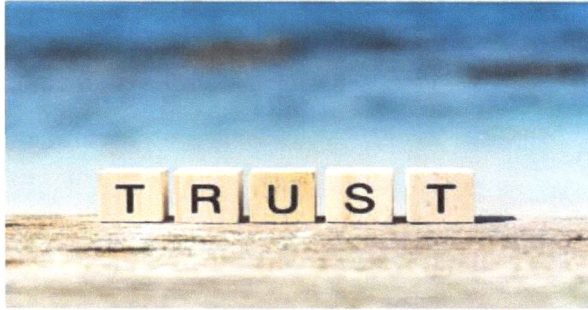

Fig. (2.4). Trust. Source: www.pixabay.com.

The Way that You Communicate Matters

"What you do speaks so loud that I cannot hear what you are saying." Ralph Waldo Emerson, American Essayist, Lecturer and Philosopher.

The best way to establish trust between caregiver and client/patient is to politely present yourself and identify your role. Even if you have treated the person in the past, they may not recognize you so you should re-introduce yourself (Fleishman *et al.*, 2019). The way you communicate is also important. Rakel, (2018) speaks about the importance of compassionate connection. He reminds us that our nonverbal communication can reveal a great deal about our attitude, and a person will more readily forgive us if we inadvertently say the wrong thing, as long as the tone of our voice and our nonverbal signals convey that we care. For example, research has indicated that being at the same level as the client/patient is important, is as being attentive, actively listening, not interrupting them when they speak, and not being distracted (Rakel, 2018). Being rushed with the interview, abruptly changing the subject, and not allowing the person time to respond has the opposite effect. Ensuring that the person is close to an exit is also important because many trauma survivors may have been in past situations where they were unable to escape violence or abuse (Fleishman *et al.*,).

Protect Personal Privacy

Trauma-informed care that fosters trust must include efforts to protect a person's privacy. When conducting an assessment or taking a history, additional people may be in the room which may include staff, other patients/clients, or the person's family or friends. However, a person who has experienced trauma may not want other people present but may not feel confident enough to ask for them to leave. That is why it is best if you ask the client/patient in private, without others listening, if they want to be alone. It is also a good idea to make an effort to abide by their wishes (Fleishman *et al.*, 2019).

Be Cautious with Physical Touch

Fleishman *et al.*, (2019) emphasize that because inappropriate touching may be a part of a person's past trauma, a caregiver should always ask for permission before touching someone. Sometimes you may be required to touch them for the purposes of physical assessment or to provide care. However, it is highly recommended that you clearly explain why you need to touch them and articulate in detail everything that is about to happen. If they require time or ask for a person of another gender to examine them, you need to be patient with them and open to arranging for someone more suitable to take over their care. If you refuse to consider their wishes an automatic frightful response such as fight, flight, or freeze may inadvertently occur (Fleishman, 2019). Dr. van der Kolk (2014) further warns to proceed cautiously because, for someone who has been violated, a certain touch may trigger a limbic response that causes them to react as though they are back in that frightening situation.

Transparency

Transparency consists of openness in providing information about the care that is provided and ensuring that there are no hidden agendas (Isobel, 2015). A lack of transparency in the form of unwarranted surprises, misleading information, or not keeping our promises, is often viewed as a betrayal of trust (Dowdell, 2022). Three key elements that foster transparency include promise keeping, explaining expectations, and safeguarding confidentiality.

Keeping Promises & Clearly Explaining Explanations

Promising keeping in trauma-informed care consists of ensuring that we deliver the service we have promised in a timely manner, and that we follow through with the commitments that we make (Kusmaul,*et al.*, 2019). It also entails not making false assurances that you cannot deliver, such as saying that everything will be okay when that may not be the case. **Clear expectations** consist of being honest and upfront about what the person can reasonably expect concerning all aspects of assessment and treatment (Knight, 2019). For example, they should be made aware of what services are available and their limitations, when and where they are offered, and the environment where they are located (Wolf *et al.*, 2014). Depending on a specific set of circumstances, each and every one of those parameters has the potential to either calm the person or make them anxious. For example, measures like full and clear informed consent, information manuals or leaflets handed out on a first meeting, and careful explanations of all expectations given by a skilled and empathetic staff member, are forms of transparency that contribute to safety and trust. Furthermore, when caregivers are truthful and forthcoming with the services that will be provided and their limitations, persons are more willing to return for further treatment (Wolf *et al*., 2014). The opposite is also true. A lack of transparency can often scare them away.

Protecting Confidentiality

In nursing, **confidentiality** concerns protecting and safeguarding all pertinent aspects of the privacy of a client/patient's history, care, and treatment (Canadian Nurses Association (CNA), 2017). Examples of how a nurse should proceed to protect information pertaining to persons in their care include the following. Restrict who is informed of client information to other members of the team who are providing direct care for the client/patient. Disclosure of health information should only be on an as-needed basis. Preserve anonymity when feasible, respect privacy, and safeguard security when using information technology (CNA, 2017, p. 30).

Limits to Confidentiality

A client/patient needs to be explicitly informed of the limits of confidentiality. However, they need to be reassured that their information will be protected and not revealed to outsiders unless required by extenuating circumstances or the law (Knight, 2019). For nurses, the specific guidelines for what client/patient specific information can be disclosed, and with whom, are usually decided upon through professional regulatory bodies at the Governmental level and depends on the country you are employed in. In Canada, confidentiality guidelines for nurses are enforced by professional Colleges or Associations that are obligated to obey laws set at the provincial, federal, and territorial levels (Canadian Nurses Protective Society (CNPS), 2022). For example, in rare situations, a nurse may be required to share confidential information with persons outside the care team to warn others of intended possible danger or harm (CNPS, 2022). Box (**2.5**) suggests a dynamic learning activity to explore when breaching privacy may be required and how you would plan to assist your client/patient in understanding why this may be required.

Is it Ever Okay to Lie to a Client/Patient?

It is ever ethically okay for a health professional to lie, or to withhold information from a client/patient, even if it is for their good? An example is refusing to inform a mentally competent adult of their terminal diagnosis at the request of a family member. Although the idea may appear to be appealing on the surface because it may be in the person's best interests, it is not ethically permissible to withhold crucially important medical information from a mentally competent person, at the request of someone else. The reason is that to do so constitutes a breach of trust, is unprofessional, and violates their rights and freedoms (Stephany, 2020). A cognitively capable person has a right to be fully informed of their diagnosis, prognosis, and treatment options (CNA, 2017; Stephany, 2020). Lanphier (2021) agrees and asserts that transparency in trauma-informed care must also avoid lying to a client/patient, even if it is intended to avoid triggering them.

Box 2.5. Learning activity: when breaching confidentiality is necessary.

Part I:
Break out into groups and have each group research one of the following questions concerning when breaching privacy may be required. Ensure that you follow directives as determined by your country's laws and your nursing regulatory body. When you are done with Part I and Part II, share your findings with the rest of the class.
1-Are you allowed to share information with the person's family without their permission?
2- Is it okay to disclose information about your client/patient to the police? If not, why not? If required to share information with police, what is the legal process for doing so?
3-What do you do if you are subpoenaed to give evidence concerning your client/patient? What is the proper legal protocol and what is your legal obligation as a witness?
4-Find out what the law requires you to report and to whom, concerning each of the following situations concerning a client/patient (*e.g.*, arrives with a gunshot wound or stabbing; diagnosed with a sexually transmittable disease; admission of committing violence toward a minor; admission of committing a sexual assault; threatening to self-harm; or threatening to harm another person).
Part II:
Discuss how you as a nurse would proceed to tell a client/patient who has experienced trauma, that their information will need to be shared, why it must be disclosed, and with whom. For example, how do you inform them in a manner that somehow maintains their trust?

What is, therefore, recommended is that a transparent discussion occurs with the person but with a degree of sensitivity and care (Lanphier, 2021). However, in a situation when the person has been designated mentally incompetent to make their own choices, you are obliged to inform the person who has been legally designated to decide for them. The conversation with the designate should ideally address what specific information the client/patient would like to be informed of, and what they wish to be kept secret. A highly scrutinized informed decision-making process avoids intentional deception and honors autonomy (CNA; Lanphier).

Additional Situations that Impede Trust

When do we not keep our promises, mistrust occurs, and it can often be difficult to get trust back once it has been violated. Some situations that impede trust include, canceling an appointment without explanation; not feeling comfortable in a caregiver's presence because their demeanor is unfriendly; the caregiver taking too much of a personal interest in them; physical touching without warning or permission; the health professional asking too many questions in a short period of time; being gay and not trusting others especially when the person may be from a country where being gay is illegal (Kusmaul *et al.*, 2019; Fleishman *et al.*, 2019) Box (**2.6**) contains a learning strategy to explore further options that either facilitate or hinder trust.

Box 2.6. Learning activity: explore other situations that promote or impede trust.

Have an open discussion about actions implemented by a caregiver, that have not already been shared in this Chapter, that may encourage or erode trust when caring for someone who has experienced trauma.

PEER SUPPORT

"It's important that we share our experiences with other people. Your story will heal you and your story will heal somebody else. When you tell your story you free yourself and give other people permission to acknowledge their own story." Iyanla Vanzant, American Inspirational Speaker, Author & Life Coach.

Peer support in mental health has been described in the literature as the help and encouragement received from others who have lived through similar experiences (Shalalaby & Agyapong, 2020). The reason why people value peer support is that they feel a connection to others who have gone through similar trials, and it also affords them the opportunity to normalize their experience as a part of their life's journey (Gillard, 2019).

Peer Support Following Tragic Loss

I have a saying, *"Trust someone who has gone through it,"* and as a practising Psychologist, I witnessed firsthand the power of peer support in helping people to deal with a tragic personal loss. For example, in a traditional Grief Support Bereavement Group, there are typically participants attending who are at varying stages of their journey. Some in attendance may have experienced a recent tragedy, others may have lost a loved one a little while ago, or may have been grieving for quite some time. What often occurs is that new attendee with recent loss feel overwhelmed by their heartache, yet they are listened to by a compassionate audience who understands their pain. That same person also receives a glitter of light when they hear stories of how others have been able to survive after their loss, and eventually move forward with living their lives again. It is quite an inspiring demonstration of human beings exchanging hope.

The Value of Peer Support Groups After Trauma: It is All About Trust

People who have experienced trauma have learned through negative experiences in many of their past relationships, not to confide in strangers, and unfortunately, they often view healthcare professionals as outsiders. Therefore, peer support groups for people who have been traumatized are appealing simply because they typically consist of other trauma survivors, who are perceived as more reliable and trustworthy (Collin-Vézina *et al.*, 2022). These trauma-informed specific peer support groups do not strive to fix the person's problems but offer people hope. The person's trauma history is listened to and validated, but they also learn that they are much more than what has happened to them. In time they even gain an understanding that they have attained strength, endurance and resilience from surviving their adversity (Dowdell, 2022).

Peer Grief Support for Helping Bereaved Children

Although trauma may occur at any point in time during the course of a lifetime, adverse childhood experiences (ACEs) have both short-term and long-term effects on the child's physical and psychological well-being (Rajaraman *et al.*, 2022). Aside from the long list of extenuating circumstances that contribute to ACEs, there are life experiences that are sometimes assumed not to be as traumatic for children, because they are related to everyday life. Yet, these circumstances still cause considerable distress for children. They include the death of a loved one, parents getting divorced or being jailed, being placed into foster care, or being adopted into another family (Ferow, 2019). Children who go through these situations are thrust into grief and may have a difficult time coping due to their young age and lack of life experience. They are at risk of developing serious emotional and psychiatric issues and unresolved guilt is also problematic. Types of interventions that prove beneficial, depending on the child's stage of development include, motivational interviewing, interventions that involve a parent or parental guardian, or group therapy, particularly peer grief support (Ferow, 2019).

Evidence has confirmed that peer support is helpful for bereaved children (Metal & Barnes, 2011). For example, Stylianou and Zembylas (2018) conducted research into an educational effort that taught school children how to offer peer support to grieving children. In their study, they trained childhood peers who had not experienced a serious loss to try and understand what the suffering children were going through. What was discovered was that the grieving children were helped and those who offered support were able to genuinely be empathetic, even though they themselves had not suffered.

Grieving children also shared with their peers what was not helpful like, being told to stop crying, that their loved one is in a better place now, or to just forget about what happened. Depending on the nature of the relationship that they had with the deceased, some of them wanted to remember their loved one and the good experiences they shared, especially if the person who died had been sick for a long time before dying (Stylianou & Zembylas, 2018). The following case study explores how a young girl was assisted through peer group support after the sudden death of her mother. Refer to Box (**2.7**).

Box 2.7. Narrative case study two: peer support and childhood bereavement.

Simran was only eight years old when her mother was suddenly killed in a tragic car accident. Simran was an only child, and her mother was a single parent. After her mother's tragic death, Simran went to live with her mother's sister, Sandeep, who was single with no children of her own, and lived in a different city. Prior to going to live with her, Simran had not spent very much time with her Aunt. There were also so many other changes in Simran's life when she moved away. She had to leave everything familiar behind. There was a new school and a new teacher. Simran did not know anyone there and she was too grief-stricken to try and make new friends. Simran, who was normally quite an engaged child, also changed into someone different. When not at school, Simran spent most of her time in her room alone. She seemed to have difficulty with schoolwork even though she had previously been a good student, and she was visibly sad most of the time. In fact, Sandeep would sometimes hear her niece crying herself to sleep at night, and when she tried to comfort her, she felt she failed because she could not get Simran to stop crying. Sandeep became very worried about her niece and arranged through her family doctor to have Simran referred to a Child Psychologist for Grief Counselling. After just three therapy sessions, the psychologist confided in Sandeep that talk therapy was not working because Simran was not willing to participate. She suggested play therapy, but Simran was not interested. She therefore recommended that Simran attend a peer group for children who had lost a parent or sibling. Sandeep was reluctant to join the group at first, but after coaching from her Aunt she agreed to give it a try.
For the first three peer group sessions, Simran refused to participate. She sat and listened to the other children in the group, most of whom were a little bit older than her. Although she did not actively get involved with the process straight away, Simran did tell her Aunt Sandeep that she didn't mind attending. In the fourth session, something amazing happened. Simran asked if she could speak. Everyone waited in anticipation. She didn't say very much but the message she relayed was quite profound.
"I am here because my Mom was killed in a bad accident. I thought I did something wrong and that was why she died. Maybe I didn't clean my room enough or do better at school. After my Mom died I also felt really bad when I enjoyed stuff like riding my bike, coloring, or watching TV. My Mom could not be here to have fun anymore, so maybe I should not have fun."
Simran paused for a few moments while she fought back the tears. As part of the group rules, the Facilitator and other peer members of the group stayed silent and allowed Simran to process her thoughts and feelings before she was ready to speak again.
"I like coming here because I listen to you, your stories and that you hurt just like me. I am still really sad, but you have told me that it is okay to be sad and cry. I am not happy like I was before, but that is okay too. I don't always think everything is my fault anymore, but I really miss my Mom so very much."
Simran was really sobbing now. Another little girl, Karen, who had lost a younger sibling to cancer six months ago, got out of her seat, and after receiving a non-verbal nod of approval from the Facilitator, approached Simran.

(Box 2.7) cont.....

"Simran, is it okay if I give you a hug."
Simran nodded and Karen went over to her and just gently held her in her arms. Simran did not resist, and they both just stayed there embracing for a while.
That session turned things around for Simran. Simran was still grieving, but with time she started to pay a little more attention to what was going on around her. She even noticed that her Aunt Sandeep was also sad a lot of the time, because she missed Simran's Mom too. Simran was also getting kind of attached to Sandeep and no longer felt like she was betraying her Mom if she liked her Aunt. Simran asked the Group Facilitator if her Aunt could join the group. The Facilitator told Simran that she would have her Aunt join them on special times when parents or guardians were asked to attend.

NARRATIVE CASE STUDY TWO: IDENTIFICATION OF THEMES & ANALYSIS

Three key themes were identified from this story.

Theme # 1: Simran was clearly not coping after the death of her mother. She also refused to respond to the individual Grief Counselling offered to her by a Child Psychologist.

Theme # 1 Analysis: Even though formal one-to-one therapy may be recommended as a way to assist a grieving child, Rajaraman *et al.,* (2022) point out that there are barriers to that process. A key obstacle is the reluctance of the child to readily trust a Counsellor who is both a stranger and an adult. Another impediment is that very young children often do not find individual therapy to be engaging. Oftentimes something else is needed.

Theme # 2: Simran was eventually able to willingly share her feelings with other grieving children in her peer support group, because they also were suffering, and she felt safe and understood.

Theme # 2 Analysis: A peer-group support setting can help improve grieving children's feelings of loneliness and isolation and may help them to cope. In the study conducted by Metel and Barnes (2011), when questioned as to why they felt that a peer support environment was helpful, the overall resounding message from the children was that being able to socially interact with other children who were also grieving, helped them to feel less alone in their experience. Even relatively young children feel free to talk about their feelings and experiences with other suffering children because their hurtful experience of loss unites them in some inexplicable way (Stylianou & Zembylas, 2018).

Theme # 3: This story revealed that involving others who are part of the family system is sometimes warranted in bereavement therapy.

Theme # 3 Analysis: With the passage of time, Simran got closer to her Aunt Sandeep and noticed that she was also grieving the loss of her sister. She then asked if her Aunt could join the Group Counselling session. That was a wise request. For example, Cohen *et al.*, (2017) recommend that co-joint child-parent or child-guardian therapy sessions can help the adult caregiver with their traumatic grief, by enhancing safety, reducing traumatic symptoms, and teaching new parenting skills.

QUESTIONS FOR FURTHER DISCUSSION

1-How much can peer support really help? Are there limitations to what can be achieved?

2-Empathy seems to be the key to trust between children in a peer support program designed to help children who are grieving. Do you think we should be teaching children how to be empathetic with others or are children naturally empathetic in nature? Why or why not? Support your views with evidence.

3-Research demonstrates that bereaved adolescents report feeling isolated and not having that much in common with peers, after experiencing a serious loss (Ferow, 2019). How should the plan for helping them be similar or different when compared to younger youth? Make sure you back up your ideas with evidence.

COLLABORATION AND MUTUALITY

In trauma-informed care, healing occurs best in a shared environment where collaboration and mutuality are practiced together (Collin-Vézina *et al.*, 2022). **Collaboration** involves an unwritten contract between a client/patient and caregiver where the person's preferences and cultural perspectives are seriously considered in their plan of care. Whereas **mutuality** consists of clear lines of communication between the caregiver and the person seeking treatment (Doncliff, 2020; Knight, 2019).

Equal Partners & Working Together Toward a Common Goal

Dowdell (2022) strongly asserts that collaboration and mutuality can only occur when the people who are seeking assistance, and those who are providing the services, are treated as equal partners in the planning and implementation of care (Fig. **2.5**).

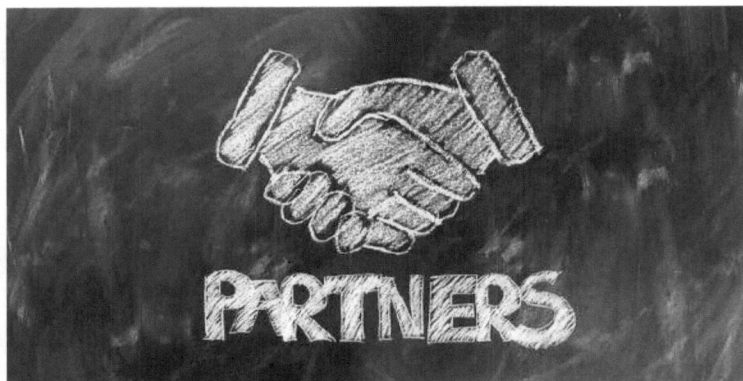

Fig. (2.5). Partners in care. Source: www.pixabay.com.

In fact, the opinions and wishes of the client/patient should be honored because they often know what is best for them. Wolf *et al.*, (2014) so poignantly state that it is about fostering an environment of doing *"with"* rather than doing *"for"* and getting the client/patient to be in charge. Everyone works together toward common objectives, which include giving the consumer of services a starring role in planning, type of service, goals to set, sequencing of treatment, and evaluation of the care after it is provided (Wolf *et al.*,). However, not all health professionals are willing participants in such a mutual endeavor. Some social workers, medical personnel, and nurses have traditionally made decisions for the client/patient without their input, because they think they know best (Wolf *et al.*, 2014). Even with good intentions this goes against the notion of mutual co-operation.

Don't Give Advice or Make False Reassurances

According to Levenson (2020), collaboration works better when the Healthcare professional avoids giving advice. Advice giving is not a very therapeutic measure, because it is disempowering. If they follow your suggestions and they succeed, they give the credit to you, but if they fail, they will blame you. Therefore, although it can be tempting to just tell them what to do, especially if they persistently ask for your guidance after making bad choices, you must resist because it will not help them in recovery (Levenson, 2020).

False reassurances that everything will be okay are another mistake. This happens, not because of a lack of willingness to help, but due to a caregiver's lack of comfort, or not being able to offer quick remedies, to what is perceived as complex problems. Despite good intentions, offering misleading reassurances communicate insensitivity, and a total lack of understanding, and more importantly, erodes trust.

EMPOWERMENT, VOICE & CHOICE

"It's not always necessary to be strong to feel strong. Incredible change happens in your life when you decide to take control of what you do have power over instead of craving control over what you don't" Jon Krakauer, American Writer & Author.

Empowerment, voice, and choice are closely aligned with collaboration and mutuality. They are also central components to the implementation of trauma-informed care for the following reasons. Empowerment utilizes the person's strengths to enable them to develop and implement their own plan for treatment. Voice and choice honour their autonomy by making sure their desires are listened to, and their right to make their own decisions are respected (Doncliffe, 2020; Menschner & Maul, 2016).

Empowerment Builds Confidence

Empowerment is a multifaceted strategy that assists the individual to realize that they have the skills, confidence, ability, and fortitude to pursue and achieve their goals (Bulanda and Johnson, 2016; Levenson, 2020) (Fig. **2.6**). People who have experienced trauma often feel that they have lost control of many aspects of their lives, and empowerment gives them back a sense of control by focusing on their strengths instead of their problems (Collin-Vézina, 2020).

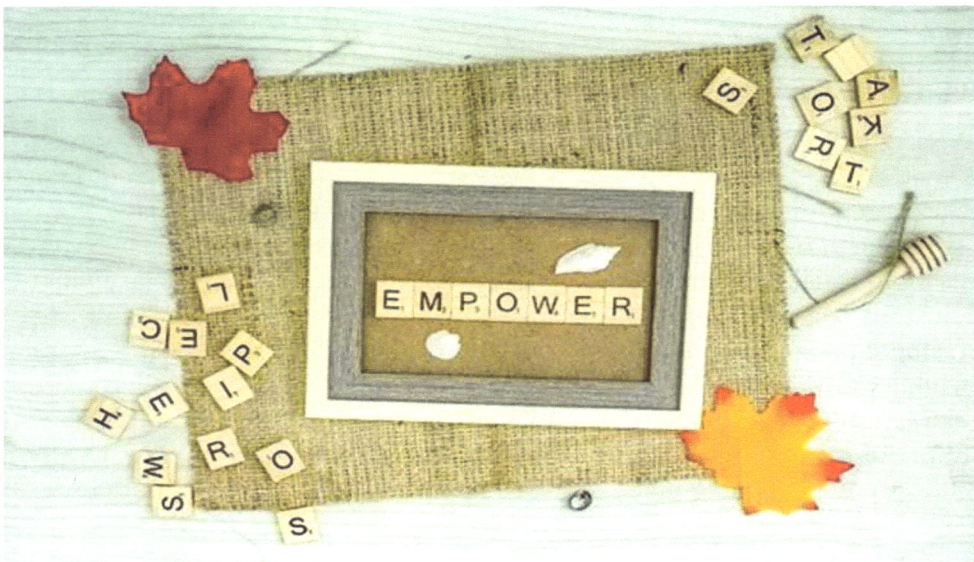

Fig. (2.6). Empowerment. Source: www.pixabay.com.

Do Your Best to Avoid Power Struggles

People who have experienced trauma often feel a loss of control over aspects of their lives. Others have made decisions for them, and many of them have been betrayed by those in positions of authority (Levenson, 2020). They may even expect or want the healthcare professional to make choices for them because they are used to passively obeying orders (Levenson, 2020). As caregivers, it is our duty to do what we can to empower them to be self-determined. We, therefore, aim to neutralize power struggles between us and them. Ways that can be achieved are through role modelling shared power, encouraging open discussions, avoiding any dynamic that is coercive, and clearly communicating that they are equal partners in their care.

Be Aware of Language Usage

When conversing directly with others or referring to them indirectly in a conversation, the words that we use to describe them matter. Therefore, it behooves us to do what we can to avoid all disparaging labels. Some caregivers have used hurtful terms like, *"junkie" "loser"* or *"drug addict."* Respectful language in comparison, avoids defining people by their life situation. Words should be chosen that address the person in a respectful manner. Even when the person has made less than favourable life choices, it is much better and less offensive, to describe the person's behaviour with non-blaming language. For example, in comparison to labels you can choose to say something like, *"she is using substances"* or *"they are in recovery"* or *"they have made some unfortunate choices in the past."* Phrases like these are descriptive but not insulting or hurtful (Levenson, 2020).

Avoid Microaggressions

The use of **microaggressions** is another way to cause harm. They consist of casual innuendos that may be intentional or unintentional and are belittling, insulting, uncaring, or inconsiderate. Examples include drawing biased and false conclusions based on a presenting situation. For instance, concluding that if you are a single parent, you must be promiscuous; that if you are homeless, you are a drug addict or too lazy to get a job; or everyone who is Indigenous has a drinking problem. Many other harmful examples exist, but it is important to remember that all forms of microaggression are unacceptable, and although the perpetrator may be unaware that they are being disrespectful, the hurt they inflict is felt by those who are targeted.

Encourage Them to Move Past Victimization

We know that many forms of trauma and abuse can cause a person to feel helpless and hopeless. That is why, as healthcare professionals, it is our responsibility to do our very best to assist those who have experienced trauma to understand that they are much more than what has happened to them. Conveying the message that it takes a great deal of determination and fortitude to endure and survive, serious adversity is a good beginning (Purkey *et al.*, 2018). We can also point out some of the noble character traits they have developed as a direct result of surviving trauma, like perseverance, kindness, strength, and resilience. However, you need to be prepared for an outburst of emotion because when a person who has been traumatized views their strengths for the very first time, it can be quite an emotionally moving experience for them. It may cause them to express a wide range of feelings that may include anger and sadness. Your role as a caregiver in these situations is to be fully present with them, be willing to allow them to sort through what they are feeling, and help them to see that this may be the beginning of something good.

Empowerment Programs that Target Teenaged Youth

Empowerment programs that target teenaged youth should avoid solely focusing on rehabilitation or just keeping the youth out of trouble because these actions do not necessarily produce long or lasting results (Bulanda & Johnson, 2016). What has proved to be more successful is fostering the youths' participation in decision-making in conjunction with supportive adults in an environment of shared power. Although there are few standardized models for youth programs that specifically focus on empowerment, a review of the literature by Bulanda and Johnson (2016) revealed the following key components to success (Box **2.8**).

Box 2.8. The key components of youth programs that foster empowerment (as adapted from Bulanda & Johnson, 2016, pp. 308 – 309).

- The staff who participate in the program need training on the prevalence, symptoms, and effects of trauma.
- Youth should ideally be assessed through a strength-based viewpoint that honours their voice and their right to make their own choices.
- Programs need to ensure physical and psychological safety and avoid re-traumatization.
- Activities must ideally be created to increase self-esteem, foster coping, encourage teamwork, and help the youth develop a social conscience and want to affect positive change in the lives of others.
- For disadvantaged youth, providing opportunities to get involved with social action gives them an opportunity to be part of something that improves the lives of others.

VOICE & CHOICE

Honouring a person's voice and choice are key components of trauma-informed care because they create a safe space for people to voice their concerns, desires and hopes, and directly involve them in decisions concerning the treatment and care they receive.

Include Clients/Patients in their Plan of Care & in Informed Decision-Making

Honouring voice and choice respectfully treat the person who is reaching out for support as a worthy recipient of those services, totally and transparently involves them in the planning of treatment and honours their ability to make decisions for themselves. A strategy that works well includes recruiting and training people with lived trauma experience to work with trauma survivors (Menschner & Maul, 2016; Stephany, 2020).

Involving client/patients in informed decision-making is essential because people reaching out for help need to be fully informed of the proposed treatment and its benefits and given the opportunity to either accept, refuse, or request an alteration to any proposed plan (Purkey *et al.*, 2018). Professional helpers also need to make sure that the treatment that is offered is not mandated or forced on them. Sometimes, the person is not quite ready for a change. They may require some time to think about it before taking the first step. We also know that if they are not a willing participant, very little will be accomplished if treatment is mandated. They are more likely to not attend appointments and refuse to alter unacceptable behaviours even when promising to do so (Purkey *et al.*,).

Three Ways to Effectively Ask Questions

When we ask rather than advise, we personify a coaching role, honour the person's autonomy, and communicate the message that they are in the driver's seat on their journey toward personal healing (Levenson, 2020). Asking questions is a beneficial means to assist clients/patients in setting their own realistic and achievable goals, and ideally should be followed by the co-development of a doable plan of action on how to reach those targets. This enables them to be the drivers in charge of their own recovery (Levenson).

First Rule

What is the best way to ask questions? Frist and foremost, let go of your to-do list and the things you intend on accomplishing. When working with persons who suffer from mental illness, I instruct my students not to take their history in an overly structured manner, but rather seek to gather everything they need in an informal conversation that begins with wanting to get to know them. I remind my students that many of these people have been betrayed in the past and they do not trust easily for very valid reasons. They are subsequently more willing to trust you and tell you the truth if you are genuinely interested in them.

Second Rule

Do not interrupt the person when they are in the midst of expressing their ideas or telling their story, especially just because you feel the urge to ask another question. Interruption, although it may be well intended, can cause them to lose track of what they want to share, may undermine the importance of their ideas, or cause them to feel that what they have to say is not that important to you(Rakel, 2018). Alternatively, if what you want to ask is needed, make a note of it and ask a question when the opportunity arises and the timing is right.

Third Rule

Make it your goal to ask questions for the following valid reasons. You need to know how to better plan their care, you want to be empathetic or you need to clarify that the message that they shared with you is what they intended to convey. In this manner, you are not only gathering data, but seeking to understand, which communicates empathy and that you value what they have to say.

Create a Safe Place for People to Tell Their Stories

It is not uncommon for people who have experienced violence, especially women, to remain silent because of the shame associated with what they have gone through (Porter, 2016). Sometimes, they are unwilling to disclose what has happened to them for fear of retaliation from the perpetrator or not wanting to be judged by you (Rakel, 2018). Yet, there are negative physical consequences associated with the suppression of traumatic experiences. It may cause chronic stress on the autonomic nervous system, resulting in an on-going secretion of cortisol, which decreases immunity and contributes to other health problems, including depression. The opposite is also true. Sharing one's story allows the repressed thoughts to surface, which is often the starting point for healing to commence. That is why it is important for people who have experienced trauma to be heard by someone who does not judge them and is willing to listen (Rakel).

Pursue Empathy & Other-focussed Listening

"Listen with curiosity. Speak with honesty. Act with integrity. The greatest problem with communication is that we don't listen to understand. We listen to reply." Roy T. Bennett, Author of the Book, *The Light in the Heart.*

What a traumatized client/patient needs most from a caregiver is empathy. **Empathy** is the capacity to try and understand the essence of another person's experience and to literally imagine what it must be like to be them. Rosenberg (2003) points out that empathy can only occur when we deliberately set aside all preconceived assumptions or judgments of the other person, and being empathetic requires something of us that is not always easy to achieve. It obliges us to seek to truly understand, not just with our minds, but also with our hearts (Rosenberg).

Rakel (2018) suggests that as caregivers, we learn how to participate in a special form of attentiveness called **other-focused listening**. This type of attention demands more of us than ordinary listening. It requires us to be fully present and to listen deeply and compassionately to what the other person is sharing while providing an environment of nurturing care, acceptance, and non-judgment.

Rakel (2018) has several suggestions on how to be other-focused when attending to someone. He proposes adopting a curious approach to the process, with no hidden agenda. We need to be genuinely interested in them as a fellow human being. When at all possible, we are to refrain from thinking about other things. Remaining quiet and paying attention to everything that we are observing, including body language and voice tone, is crucially imperative to the process. We must resist the temptation to verbally fill in the silence, because moments of solitude allow the person time to reflect, to sort through what they are feeling, and an opportunity for you to try and understand (Rakel, 2018). For a Learning Activity to explore additional ways to communicate other-focused listening, refer to Box (**2.9**).

Box 2.9. Learning activity: ways to actively communicate other-focused listening (as adapted from Rakel, 2018).

Other-focused listening is more than ordinary listening. It requires us to be fully present. However, giving someone our full attention is often not that easy to do, especially in today's climate of social media interruptions, and other distractions. As a white board activity, preferably in groups, identify non-verbal and verbal activities that actively communicate that you are other-focused when listening to your client/patient.

CULTURAL, HISTORICAL & GENDER ISSUES

The last listed sub-category of *The Six Guiding Principles of Trauma Informed Care* concerns cultural, historical, and gender issues (SAMHSA, 2014). It requires practitioners to do their very best to demonstrate cultural and historical understanding, and to be respectful concerning the multidimensional components of gender identity and sexuality (Dowdell, 2022).

Cultural & Historical Understanding

When working in healthcare we may need to be cognizant of the fact people who are from minority groups experience higher rates of trauma than non-minorities, and trauma is seldom experienced outside of a cultural/social context (Ranjbar *et al.*, 2020). For many people from marginalized groups, or those who may be newcomers to their community, being seen as an outsider and characterized as not fitting in with expected societal norms, contributes to their trauma. This is in addition to other forms of stress, such as open racial discrimination, living in less-than-ideal housing in impoverished conditions, and having contacts with the criminal justice system (Ranjbar *et al.*,).

In trauma-informed care, a person's unique individuality is closely associated with their race, culture, ethnicity, religion, and ways of living. Therefore, to be authentically interested in them involves wanting to get to know as much as possible about what the person perceives to be important. For some people, getting to know them may also include learning about some of the tragedies and adversities experienced by their ancestors, in the form of historical trauma (Dowdell, 2022). **Historical trauma** consists of a traumatic event or series of circumstances shared by a group of people. It increases their likelihood of developing physical ailments, makes them more prone to developing less than ideal parenting skills, may contribute to mistrust, and makes subsequent generations more susceptible to mental illnesses (Patel & Nagata, 2021). For example, historical trauma can often lead to intergenerational transmission of negative impacts of the trauma and the shame associated with it. That is why sensitivity to any group of people who have been stigmatized or marginalized should be a requirement of any or all trauma-informed interventions aimed at assisting them (Purkey *et al.*, 2018). For example, it is vitally important for a caregiver to avoid acting in an authoritarian role. What is more beneficial is to directly ask the person what it is that they require, including culturally preferred approaches to their treatment and care. In this manner, the healing journey is undertaken in a co-operative relationship of mutual understanding and care (Ranjbar *et al.*, 2020).

Discrimination Due to Sexual Orientation or Gender Identity

Although many different acronyms exist to refer to persons with different sexual orientations, other than heterosexuality or gender identity that differs from birth, the following two are commonly used in the literature. LGBT or LGBTQ2S. LGBT refers to lesbian, gay, bisexual, and transgender. LGBTQ2S also includes those sub-groups but has added queer and two-spirited to the list. Chapter One includes a description of each of these designations. In the ensuing discussion, the acronym that is presented, is the one used in the literature that is cited, and not meant to exclude any member of this community.

Members of these populations are known to experience significant trauma. For example, they report excessive rates of victimization, rejection from family and peers, and intimate relationship violence (McCormick *et al.*, 2018). LGBT youth experience physical and sexual abuse, peer bullying, homelessness, and substance use, and are targeted for sexual exploitation at higher rates than other teens. They are also two to three times more likely to attempt suicide (Carabez *et al.*, 2015; Mc Cormick, 2018).

According to Meyer (2013), many poor health outcomes experienced by members of the LGBT population can be directly attributed to stigma, prejudice, and stress. Yet, this group has been largely ignored as a priority for trauma-informed care. What is even more distressing is that many health professionals, including nurses, lack proper training in addressing LGBT health care needs and have been known to harbour negative views of them (Carabez *et al.*, 2015; McCormick *et al.*, 2018).

Nurses, A Lack of Education & Stigma

A lack of education among nurses is a known contributor to the stigmatization of members of this group. For instance, research into a large sample of nurses conducted by Carabez *et al.*, (2015) into the training of nurses on LGBT health in the San Francisco Bay area revealed the following results. Almost 80% of nurses reported that they did not receive any training on inclusivity, and some indicated that their educational exposure to this subject only consisted of a one-hour lecture. Nurses who were interviewed as a part of this study admitted that when they cared for people who were LGBT, they resorted to microaggressions in the form of derogatory language and making fun of them. The authors of this research assert that some of these problems can be rectified through educational efforts that target student nurses and promote inclusivity, and subsequently recommended some of the following strategies. Refer to Box (**2.10**).

Box 2.10. Ways to educate student nurses about inclusivity & LGBT people (as adapted from Carabez *et al.***, 2018, pp. 328-329).**

-Incorporate culturally competent and patient-focused educational efforts into nursing school training.
-Make use of existing on-line educational tools that foster inclusivity that are already readily available (*e.g.*, case studies, on-line modules, webinars, readings, and assignments).
-Refer student nurses to on-line links that feature LGBT subjects and inclusivity.
-Invite guest speakers to address LGBT health.
-Incorporate interactive experiences in simulation that emphasize competent care for members of this group.
-Consider offering a Certificate course in expertise in this area.
-Have upfront and open discussion forums concerning how to deal with discomfort in caring for persons in the clinical setting who are LGBT.

QUESTIONS TO PONDER FOR FURTHER REFLECTION

1-Can you think of additional strategies that may prove beneficial in teaching nurses and student nurses how to be more tolerant, inclusive, and accepting of persons from the LGBTQ2S population?

2-Would you be willing to stand up to someone who resorts to making fun of someone from this group? If yes, how would you approach doing that in a manner that would help to change their attitude?

Cultural Competence, Cultural Awareness & Cultural Sensitivity

Cultural competence has been traditionally used as a tool to assist health professionals, including nurses, to attain the necessary skills to practice inclusivity when caring for diverse populations (Burkhardt *et al.*, 2015). Cultural awareness, cultural sensitivity, cultural safety, and cultural humility are all components of cultural competency. **Cultural awareness** consists of the desire to want to understand the beliefs and values of people from differing cultures. **Cultural sensitivity** moves beyond cultural awareness by incorporating a person's cultural beliefs into practice (Burkhardt *et al.*, 2015). **Cultural safety** addresses power imbalances that exist in health care and aims to foster an environment that is free of racial stigma and other forms of discrimination (Foster, 2017).

Humility & Cultural Humility

Humility consists of human character traits that are void of arrogance, that entail refusing to act with an attitude of superiority or making the false assumption that we know what is best for others. It also requires adopting an attitude of interest in others and what they know and being willing to admit when we are wrong or do not know. Ranjbar *et al*., (2020) advise that we adopt humility as a way of being, and that we demonstrate it in every encounter with another human being.

Cultural humility, as a specific aspect of general humility, embraces what cultural safety sets out to achieve but does so in a more personal and all-encompassing way. For example, **cultural humility** aims to effectively counteract racism and power difficulties through intentional actions of empowerment and excellence in care. This is accomplished through an atmosphere of mutual respect as an adopted way of living and being into our professional persona (Foronda *et al*., 2016). Cultural humility also accepts that true understanding of others may not always be attainable, but what is within our reach is our capacity to identify with the humanness of the other, our equal standing as people deserving of respect, and a genuine willingness to appreciate where the other person is coming from (Foronda *et al*., 2020; Ranjbar *et al*., 2020; Stephany, 2020).

How do we, as health professionals, achieve cultural humility when administering trauma-informed care? Gottlieb (2021) challenges us to be aware that a person's sense of identity shapes what they regard to be normal or healthy and may differ from what we assert to be true for us. Bearing their best interests in mind requires us to prioritize their views in care planning. Failure to act in this manner impedes trust, results in non-adherence to any advised plan of care and renders our efforts fruitless. Ranjbar *et al*., (2020) also advise that we demonstrate humility in every encounter.

The Role of Self-Awareness, Self-Reflection in Fostering Cultural Humility

Self-awareness is a useful tool in helping us to become more culturally humble. Sometimes, we act without thinking and our words or actions may not always be kind. They may even be hurtful. If we want to understand what motivates us to act or be a certain way, and if we want to change undesirable prejudices or biases, we need to become more self-aware. **Self-awareness** consists of purposefully wanting to understand the motives behind our assumptions and behaviors (Stephany, 2020). It involves looking at yourself as an outsider, viewing what you do or say, to understand why. **Self-reflection** enhances self-awareness because it forces you to take deliberate action to truthfully examine why you think and act the way that you do. It often involves **reflective journalling**, where you freely write about your values, beliefs, and attitudes to discover hidden aspects of your personality, including those that may be impeding your ability to change (Ray, 2018). There are many positive personal benefits from reflective journalling aside from increasing self-awareness. They expose personal character traits that no longer serve you, enhance your peace of mind, contribute to self-growth and your ability to better care for yourself and others (Ray).

SELF-CARE STRATEGY: THE BENEFITS OF MINDFULNESS FOR CAREGIVERS

According to Rakel (2018), **mindfulness** consists of being fully present and aware and in the moment, as though it is the only time that matters. It often also involves observing your thoughts, feelings, and sensations. Some personal benefits of mindfulness include peacefulness, noticing aspects of life that you may not have been aware of before, feeling kinder towards yourself, and feeling compassionate toward other people (Rakel).

There are also benefits to you as a health professional. Lomas *et al.*, (2017) conducted a systematic review of the impact of mindfulness on the well-being of healthcare professionals and concluded that it helped reduce distress, anxiety, and depression. Results from another study that involved a large meta-analysis of randomized controlled trials were conducted by Spinelli *et al.*, (2019). It reviewed mindfulness and its benefits for those training or working in healthcare. The results revealed that mindfulness improved the person's overall sense of wellness and their ability to handle stress and helped to alleviate insomnia.

Mindfulness Challenge

I encourage you to seriously consider introducing mindfulness into your life in some small way. The following are useful suggestions.

1-To stay present, take a few minutes when alone to deep breathe and be aware of your breath.

2-When performing any activity, give it your full attention. Purposefully look at a particular object in your environment as though you are seeing it for the first time. Take note of what you may not have been aware of before.

3-Sit quietly somewhere in nature and observe creatures participating in their daily tasks without making elaborate goals for themselves. What can you learn from them?

4-Make a concentrated effort to accept all parts of yourself, flaws included, without judgment.

5-Challenge yourself to also view and accept others who annoy you, without judgment.

6-When and if you are ready, consider taking up mindfulness meditation or yoga. They are more demanding of your time and commitment but rewarding.

Note: Any suggested strategies are not intended to be a substitute for medical or psychological advice from a trained professional. The reader is, therefore, encouraged to seek medical or other professional help in any matters related to their physical or emotional health.

CONCLUSION

- The purpose of Chapter Two was to explore the crucial aspects of each of *The Six Guiding Principles of Trauma Informed Care* as suggested by (SAMHSA) (2014). They include safety, trustworthiness and transparency; peer support; collaboration and mutuality; empowerment, voice, and choice; and cultural, historical, and gender issues.
- A principle-based approach to trauma-informed care is effective because it promotes healing by reducing re-traumatization, decreasing suffering, enhancing coping, and promoting autonomy.
- Safety was identified as a priority, and encompasses physical, social, and psychological aspects. These include the location of the health facility, the atmosphere of the healthcare clinic, staff attitudes, ensuring that healthcare professionals are kept emotionally safe, and avoiding re-traumatization.
- We were made aware that people who have been intentionally harmed by others do not easily trust. Therefore, trust must be earned through compassionate connection, protecting a person's privacy, and being cautious with physical touch.
- Transparency involves openness in providing information about the care that is provided and ensuring that there are no hidden agendas. It is best achieved by promise-keeping, clearly explaining all expectations, and honouring confidentiality.
- There are times when confidentiality needs to be breached. However, the client/patient must be reassured that their information will be protected and not revealed to outsiders, unless required by extenuating circumstances or the law.
- Peer support consists of the help and encouragement received from others who have lived through similar experiences. The reason why people often value peer support is because they feel a connection to others who have gone through similar trials, and this normalizes their experience.
- Collaboration and mutuality foster a shared environment where everyone is equally involved in decision-making. Advice giving or false assurances should be avoided.
- Empowerment, voice, and choice are helpful ways to tap into a person's strengths to help them overcome adversity, to give them an opportunity to be listened to, and to make their own decisions.
- Empowerment programs that are successful in helping youth encourage their participation in decision-making in an environment of equally shared power.

- We need to do our best to create a safe place for people to tell their stories. We were also made aware of the power of empathy and other-focused listening.
- The importance of addressing cultural, historical, and gender issues was emphasized, including being aware of the influence of historical trauma and how it contributes to mistrust and other problems.
- We were informed that poor health outcomes experienced by people of the LGBTQ2S community, are highly correlated with stigma. Nurses were identified as harbouring prejudicial attitudes toward members of this population, and educational efforts were strongly suggested to change these behaviours.
- Cultural humility was recommended as an effective way to counteract racism and power difficulties through empowerment, excellence in care, and an atmosphere of mutual respect.
- Self-awareness and self-reflection were suggested as strategies to enhance cultural humility in nursing practice.
- Two Narrative Case Studies were presented. The first emphasized the importance of safely conducting a client assessment. We were made aware that adopting a caring demeanor, demonstrating genuine compassion, and offering clear expectations help to create a safe environment. We were also informed of the benefits of a strength-based approach and offering unconditional positive regard.
- The second Narrative Case Study explored how peer support helped a bereaved child. We learned that peer support can sometimes be more helpful for a young grieving child than individual therapy. The reasons often have to do with the child feeling comfortable with other children because they have also experienced loss and understand what they are going through.
- Four Learning Activities were suggested (*e.g.*, Strategies that Enhance the Environmental Safety of a Healthcare Facility, When Breaching Confidentiality is Necessary; Situations that Promote or Impede Trust, and Actively Communicating Other-focused Listening).
- The Chapter ended with a recommended self-care strategy that encourages mindfulness as a way to enhance coping.

RECOMMENDED READINGS

Cohen, J. A., Mannarino, A. P., and Deblinger, E. (2017). Treating trauma and traumatic grief in children and adolescents. The Guildford Press.

Fisher, J. (2017). Healing the fragmented selves of trauma survivors: Overcoming internal self-alienation (1st edition). Routledge.

Levine, P. A., (1997). Waking the tiger: Healing trauma. North Atlantic Books.

Rosenberg, M. B. (2003). Nonviolent communication: A language of life (2nd edition). PuddleDancer Press.

REFERENCES

Bulanda, J & Byro Johnson, T (2016) A trauma-informed model for empowerment programs targeting vulnerable youth. *Child Adolesc Social Work J*, 33, 303-12.
[http://dx.doi.org/10.1007/s10560-015-0427-z]

Burkhardt, MA, Nathaniel, AK & Walton, NA (2015) *Ethics and issues in contemporary nursing* Nelson Education Limited.

Canadian Nurses Association (CNA) (2017) *CNA code of ethics for registered nurses*https: //cna. informz. ca/cna/dat a/image s/Cod e_of_Ethic s_201 7_Ed itio n_Se cure _In teracti ve.pdf

Canadian Nurses Protective Society (2022) *InfoLAW: Confidentiality of health information.* Available from : https://ieeexplore.ieee.org/document/6567202

Carabez, R, Pellegrini, M, Mankovitz, A, Eliason, M, Ciano, M & Scott, M (2015) "Never in all my years . . ." Nurses' education about LGBT health. *J Prof Nurs*, 31, 323-9.
[http://dx.doi.org/10.1016/j.profnurs.2015.01.003] [PMID: 26194964]

Cohen, JA, Mannarino, AP & Deblinger, E (2017) *Treating trauma and traumatic grief in children and adolescents.*The Guildford Press.

Collin-Vézina, D, Brend, D & Beeman, I (2020) When it counts the most: Trauma-informed care and the COVID-19 global pandemic. *Dev Child Welf*, 2, 172-9.
[http://dx.doi.org/10.1177/2516103220942530]

Doncliff, B (2022) Trauma-informed care – What is it? Why is it important. *Kai Tiaki Nursing*, 6, 30-1.

Dowdell, EB & Speck, PM (2022) Trauma-informed care in nursing practice. *Am J Nurs*, 122, 30-8.
[http://dx.doi.org/10.1097/01.NAJ.0000827328.25341.1f] [PMID: 35348516]

Ferow, A (2019) Available from: https://dx.doi
[http://dx.doi.org/10.19044/ejes.s.v6a1]

Fleishman, J, Kamsky, H & Sundborg, S (2019) Trauma-informed nursing practice. *Online J Issues Nurs*, 24
[http://dx.doi.org/10.3912/OJIN.Vol24No02Man03]

Foronda, C, Baptiste, DL, Reinholdt, MM & Ousman, K (2016) Cultural humility. *J Transcult Nurs*, 27, 210-7.
[http://dx.doi.org/10.1177/1043659615592677] [PMID: 26122618]

Foster, P (2017) Available from: https://hdl.handle.net/2429/62470

Gillard, S (2019) Peer support in mental health services: where is the research taking us, and do we want to go there? *J Ment Health*, 28, 341-4.
[http://dx.doi.org/10.1080/09638237.2019.1608935] [PMID: 31070066]

Goddard, A (2021) Adverse childhood experiences and trauma-informed care. *J Pediatr Health Care*, 35, 145-55.
[http://dx.doi.org/10.1016/j.pedhc.2020.09.001] [PMID: 33129624]

Gottlieb, H (2021) The case for a cultural humility framework in social work practice. *Journal of Ethnic & Cultural Diversity in Social Work*, 30, 463-81.
[http://dx.doi.org/10.1080/15313204.2020.1753615]

Institute on Trauma and Trauma-informed Care (ITTIC) (2022) *What is Trauma-informed care?.* Available from: https: //social work. buffalo. edu/ social-research /institutes- centers /institute -on-trauma -and -trauma -informed-care /what- is-trauma -informed -care. html

Isobel, S (2015) Because that's the way it's always been done: Reviewing the nurse – initiated rules in a mental health unit as a step toward trauma-informed care. *Issues Ment Health Nurs,* 36, 272-8. [http://dx.doi.org/10.3109/01612840.2014.982842] [PMID: 25988593]

Isobel, S & Edwards, C (2017) Using trauma informed care as a nursing model of care in an acute inpatient mental health unit: A practice development process. *Int J Ment Health Nurs,* 26, 88-94. [http://dx.doi.org/10.1111/inm.12236] [PMID: 27291292]

Knight, C (2015) Trauma-informed social work practice: Practice considerations and challenges. *Clin Soc Work J,* 43, 25-37. [http://dx.doi.org/10.1007/s10615-014-0481-6]

Knight, C (2019) Trauma-informed practice and care: Implications for field instruction. *Clin Soc Work J,* 47, 79-89. [http://dx.doi.org/10.1007/s10615-018-0661-x]

Kusmaul, N, Wolf, MR, Sahoo, S, Green, SA & Nochajski, TH (2019) Client experiences of trauma-informed care in social service agencies. *J Soc Serv Res,* 45, 589-99. [http://dx.doi.org/10.1080/01488376.2018.1481178]

Lanphier, E (2021) Trust, transparency, and trauma-informed care. *Am J Bioeth,* 21, 38-40. [http://dx.doi.org/10.1080/15265161.2021.1906992] [PMID: 33945422]

Levenson, J (2020) Translating trauma-informed principles into social work practice. *Soc Work,* 65, 288-98. [http://dx.doi.org/10.1093/sw/swaa020] [PMID: 32676655]

Lomas, T, Medina, JC, Ivtzan, I, Rupprecht, S & Eiroa-Orosa, FJ (2018) A systematic review of the impact of mindfulness on the well☐being of healthcare professionals. *J Clin Psychol,* 74, 319-55. [http://dx.doi.org/10.1002/jclp.22515] [PMID: 28752554]

McCormick, A, Scheyd, K & Terrazas, S (2018) Trauma-informed care and LGBTQ youth: Considerations for advancing practice with youth with trauma experiences. *Fam Soc,* 99, 160-9. [http://dx.doi.org/10.1177/1044389418768550]

Menschner, C & Maul, A (2016) *Issue Brief: Key ingredients for successful trauma-informed care implementation*   Available   from: https://www.samhsa.gov/sites/default/files/programs_campaigns/childrens_mental_health/atc-whitepaper-040 616.pdf

Metel, M & Barnes, J (2011) Peer-group support for bereaved children: A qualitative interview study. *Child Adolesc Ment Health,* 16, 201-7. [http://dx.doi.org/10.1111/j.1475-3588.2011.00601.x] [PMID: 32847193]

Meyer, I H (2013) Prejudice, social stress, and mental health in lesbian, gay, and bisexual populations. *Conceptual issues and research evidence Psychology of Sexual Orientation and Gender Diversity,* 1, 3-26. [http://dx.doi.org/10.1037/2329-0382.1.S.3]

Mottaghi, S, Poursheikhali, H & Shameli, L (2020) Empathy, compassion fatigue, guilt and secondary traumatic stress in nurses. *Nurs Ethics,* 27, 494-504. [http://dx.doi.org/10.1177/0969733019851548] [PMID: 31284826]

Pedneult, KS (2002) *What is emotional validation?.* Available from: https://www.verywellmind.com/what-i--emotional-validatioon-425336

Porter, E (2016) Gendered Narratives: Stories and silences in transitional justice. *Hum Rights Rev,* 17, 35-50. [http://dx.doi.org/10.1007/s12142-015-0389-8]

Purkey, E, Patel, R & Phillips, SP (2018) Trauma-informed care: Better care for everyone. *Can Fam Physician,* 64, 170-2.https://www.cfp.ca/content/cfp/64/3/170.full.pdf [PMID: 29540379]

Rakel, D (2018) *The compassionate connection: The healing power of empathy and mindful listening.*W. W. Norton & Company.

Rajaraman, A, Austin, JL, Gover, HC, Cammilleri, AP, Donnelly, DR & Hanley, GP (2022) Toward trauma-

informed applications of behavior analysis. *J Appl Behav Anal,* 55, 40-61.
[http://dx.doi.org/10.1002/jaba.881] [PMID: 34525220]

Ranjbar, N, Erb, M, Mohammad, O & Moreno, FA (2020) Trauma-informed care and cultural humility in the mental health care of people from minoritized communities. *Focus Am Psychiatr Publ,* 18, 8-15.
[http://dx.doi.org/10.1176/appi.focus.20190027] [PMID: 32047392]

Ray, MA (2018) *Transcultural caring dynamics in nursing and healthcare* F. A. Davis Company.

Rogers, C (1980) *A way of being.*Houghton Mifflin.

Shalaby, RAH & Agyapong, VIO (2020) Peer support in mental health: Literature review. *JMIR Ment Health,* 7, e15572.
[http://dx.doi.org/10.2196/15572] [PMID: 32357127]

Spinelli, C, Wisener, M & Khoury, B (2019) Mindfulness training for healthcare professionals and trainees: A meta-analysis of randomized controlled trials. *J Psychosom Res,* 120, 29-38.
[http://dx.doi.org/10.1016/j.jpsychores.2019.03.003] [PMID: 30929705]

Stephany, K (2020) *The ethic of care: A moral compass for Canadian Nursing practice* Bentham Science Publishers Pte. Ltd..

Stylianou, P & Zembylas, M (2018) Peer support for bereaved children: Setting eyes on children's views through an educational action research project. *Death Stud,* 42, 446-55.
[http://dx.doi.org/10.1080/07481187.2017.1369472] [PMID: 29300136]

Substance Abuse and Mental Health Services Administration (2014) Available from: https: //store. samhsa. gov/sites /default /files/d7/ priv/sma14 -4816. pdf

Szczygiel, P (2018) On the value and meaning of trauma-informed practice: Honoring safety, complexity, and relationship. *Smith Coll Stud Soc Work,* 88, 115-34.
[http://dx.doi.org/10.1080/00377317.2018.1438006]

van der Kolk, B (2014) *The body keeps score: Brain, mind, and body in the healing of trauma.*Viking Penguin.

Wilson, C, Pence, DM & Conradi, L (2013) *Trauma-informed Care Encyclopedia of Social Work.*National Association of Social Workers Press and Oxford University Press.

Wolf, MR, Green, SA, Nochajski, TH, Mendel, WE & Kusmaul, NS (2014) We're civil servants: The status of trauma-informed care in the community. *J Soc Serv Res,* 40, 111-20.
[http://dx.doi.org/10.1080/01488376.2013.845131]

Client-Centered, Person-Centered, and Resilience-Based Approaches to Trauma-Informed Care

Abstract: Chapter three explores client-centered, person-centered, and resilience-focussed approaches to trauma-informed care, and although they differ somewhat, all three are strength-based and share the common goal of helping people who have experienced adversity. Client-centered care places the person and their capacity for growth and change at the heart of all that occurs. This approach prioritizes respect for the self-worth of every human being and promotes the practice of unconditional positive regard. The quality of the therapeutic relationship between the nurse and client/patient is important, as is the nurse's ability to apply professional knowledge and competence to the care they provide. A unique aspect of person-centered care is that it provides services to people with acute and chronic health issues that are holistic, and recovery-orientated. Collaboration and effective communication skills are essential features of this approach. Positive ways to offer person-centered care to people from these populations are reviewed, the elderly, those with a disability, people with dementia, palliative care patients, and persons suffering from mental illness and substance use. Specific components of recovery-oriented care that are included in the discussion are a person's capacity for change and courage, their responsibility for their growth, and the importance of finding purpose in their lives. Resilience is identified as the is the ability to carry on and bounce back to original functioning after experiencing a trauma. We are made aware that a resilient person becomes stronger despite adversity because they utilize positive emotions, develop a sturdy mindset, a renewed commitment to life, and welcome challenges. The remainder of the discussion focuses on how to safely conduct screening for trauma for everyone including survivors of interpersonal violence (IPV). Two Narrative Case Studies are presented. The first one demonstrates that when a client/patient crosses a professional boundary, a problem is created for the nurse. The second Case Study explores how a survivor of interpersonal violence (IPV) may require advocacy to help them stay safe. The following four learning activities are recommended, how to practice unconditional positive regard; exploring helpful strategies to utilize when conducting trauma screening; dispelling myths associated with IPV; and how to implement survivor-centered approaches when caring for someone who has experienced IPV. At the end of the Chapter, a self-care strategy is recommended that challenges nurses to set aside time to focus more on being present.

Keywords: Boundary violation, Client-centered care, Caring, Communication, Cognitive behavioral therapy (CBT), Collaboration, Dignity, Dementia, Empathy, Human connection, Implicit bias, Myth, Professional boundaries, Positive emotions, Palliative care, Patient-centered care, Person-centered care, Rescuing, Recovery-orientated care, Resilience, Respect for self-worth, Stress-hardy, Survivor-centered approaches to intimate partner violence (IPV), Stranger rape, Sturdy mindset, Strength-based approaches, Trauma-informed care, Trauma-screening, Transference, Therapeutic relationship, Unconditional positive regard, Victim blaming.

LEARNING GUIDE

After completing this chapter, the reader should be able to:

- Explain the differences and similarities between client-centered, patient-centered, person-centered, and resilience-focused approaches to trauma-informed care.
- Identify the essential features of client-centered care and understand why respect for self-worth and unconditional positive regard are a part of this strategy.
- Adopt ways to incorporate unconditional positive regard into nursing practice.
- Recognize the value of human connection, therapeutic relationships, and knowledge competence.
- Explain the basic premises and unique aspects of person-centered care.
- Gain an awareness of how the needs of special populations are addressed by person-centered care.
- Define resilience.
- Articulate why resilience-focused strategies facilitate positive functioning following a traumatic experience.
- Learn about the risk associated with not being properly trained to conduct trauma screening.
- Understand how to safely conduct a screening that includes survivors of interpersonal violence (IPV).
- Become aware of how implicit bias and myths perpetrated by nurses cause harm to survivors of IPV and how to prevent it.
- Review two narrative case studies and ensuing thematic analysis. The first one demonstrates that when a client/patient crosses a professional boundary, a problem is created for the nurse. The second one reveals how a survivor of IPV may require advocacy to stay safe.

- Participate in these Learning Activities (*e.g.*, How to Practice Unconditional Positive Regard; Helpful Strategies to Utilize when Conducting a Trauma-assessment; Dispelling Myths Associated with IPV; and Survivor-Centered Approaches to utilize when caring for people who have suffered from IPV).
- Consider utilizing a self-care strategy that challenges nurses to set aside time to focus more on being than doing.

INTRODUCTION TO CHAPTER THREE

"A helping hand can be a ray of sunshine in a cloudy world." Author Unknown

Chapter Three offers a comprehensive analysis of specific components of client-centered, person-centered, and resilience-focused approaches to trauma-informed care. What all these strategies share is the common goal of helping people to heal from adversity (Fig. **3.1**). The subtle differences between each of these techniques are explained, and recommended ways to implement them into nursing practice are suggested. Instructing healthcare professionals how to safely conduct screening for trauma and caring for survivors of interpersonal violence (IPV), are also presented. The goal is to transform intrinsic biases that may exist and encourage the practice of compassionate and safe care.

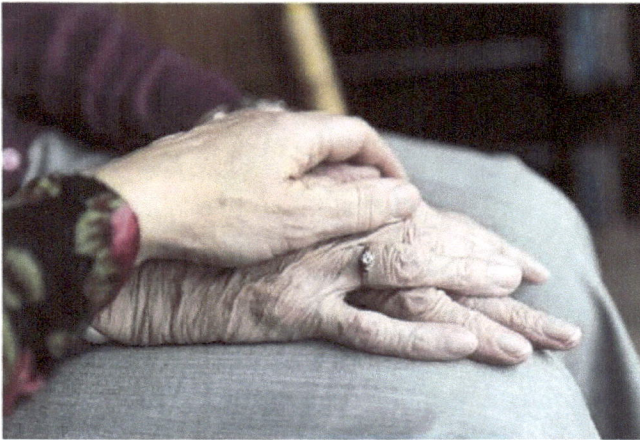

Fig. (3.1). Helping people to heal. Source: www.pixabay.com.

THE DIFFERENCES BETWEEN CLIENT-CENTERED, PATIENT-CENTERED, PERSON-CENTERED, & RESILIENCE-FOCUSED TRAUMA-INFORMED CARE

Client-centered, patient-centered, person-centered, and strength-based trauma-informed care share the common goal of alleviating suffering and helping people who have experienced trauma to heal. Many of the strategies associated with each of these approaches are also **strength-based** because they assist people who have experienced trauma to concentrate on the skills they have developed from surviving adversity (Brooke & Goldstein, 2003; Knight, 2015; Seligman, 2011). However, differences in their primary focus do exist and require clarification.

Client-centered care puts the person, their inherent capacity to grow and change, and their goals and hopes, at the heart of all that occurs (Gillen *et al.*, 2014; Stephany, 2020). **Patient-centered care** is derived from a biomedical model that primarily emphasizes diagnosing and treating disease. Traditionally it was based on the view that the ill patient who suffered from a sickness or injury, requires that a physician oversee and be in charge of that process (Zhao *et al.*, 2016). However, over the course of time, patient-centered care has expanded its focus to be more inclusive and holistic in its approach (Kwame & Petrucka 2021).

Person-centered care, although somewhat like patient-centered care, differs in that it places more emphasis on the individual at the center of decision-making, with a particular emphasis on respect for autonomous self-determination. It also considers biological, psychological, emotional, and social influences (Zhao *et al.*, 2017). A unique feature of person-centered care is its emphasis on assisting underrepresented groups, and a focus on recovery (Bassuk *et al.*, 2017; Quaile & Benyounes-Ulrich, 2021). Person-centered trauma-informed care specifically provides services to people with acute and chronic health issues, that include those who suffer from disabilities, mental illness, and substance use (Bassuk *et al.*, 2017). **Resilience** is the ability to bounce-back and re-build one's life after adversity. It is a crucially important attribute to possess, because people who have experienced trauma need to be aware they are more than what happened to them, and being resilient is about having the strength, hardiness, will, and determination to carry on (Collier, 2016; Levenson, 2020).

CLIENT-CENTERED CARE

Client-centered care can be applied to everyone including persons who have experienced trauma because it recognizes a person's autonomy, their capacity to play a central role in their own care and assists them in learning how to utilize their innate abilities to recover and heal (Knight, 2015). **Client-centered care** prioritizes the needs and desires of the client/patient in an environment that is safe, non-judgmental, and respectful through establishing trust, collaboration, compassion, respect, and shared power (Gillen *et al.*, 2014; Levenson, 2020; Stephany, 2020). The discussion that follows emphasizes these key trauma-focused components of client-centered care, respect for self-worth, unconditional positive regard, being kind on purpose, and the importance of the therapeutic relationship.

The Reality of Status and How Some People are Treated and Judged

Everyone deserves to be treated with dignity regardless of their social standing, but unfortunately, that is not always the case. What traditionally occurs is that people who occupy a higher socio-economic position, who work in positions of power or prestige, or who have achieved outstanding professional or personal achievement, are often viewed more favourably than others (Barclay, 2016). Similarly, people who occupy a lower socio-economic status, are labelled as underachievers, occupy blue-collar jobs, or are from marginalized populations, are often viewed less positively by others (Barkley, 2016). Additionally, those who suffer from a mental illness or substance use, or have made less than favorable life choices, are also judged negatively.

People Who have been Traumatized Also Feel Judged by Healthcare Professionals

People who have experienced trauma often have a distorted view of themselves, may have a long-standing history of being betrayed by people close to them, and may feel unworthy of being liked or loved (Dowdell & Speck, 2022). What can make matters worse for them is being subjected to judgment by healthcare professionals who are supposed to be there to help. In fact, one of the reasons some people who have a history of trauma do not reach out for help is because they want to avoid being stigmatized by health professionals. Yet, the hallmark of trauma-informed care is that it embraces diversity, and is inclusive and welcoming to everyone no matter the presenting situation of those accessing services (Dowdell & Speck, 2022). That is why a problem exists when this is not what is practiced.

SOMETHING TO REFLECT UPON

Think of a time when you were present when someone talked badly about a client/patient and what they said was discriminatory in nature. If you did not respond in anyway, why not? Were you afraid of being attacked too? What would you need in terms of support to respectfully challenge their views?

The Importance of Respect for Self-Worth & Unconditional Positive Regard

"Every life deserves a certain amount of dignity, no matter how poor or damaged the shell that carries it." Rick Bragg, American Journalist & Writer.

Respect for self-worth views each human being as deserving of honour and dignity, no matter what their circumstances, and is closely aligned with the notion of **unconditional positive regard,** which involves the act of caring for someone without conditions (Rogers, 1980; Stephany, 2020). It does not matter if someone has made less than favourable choices in life, they are human beings who are still worthy and serving dignity, respect, and compassion (Stephany, 2020). Although unconditional positive regard was briefly introduced in Chapter Two, a Learning Activity on how to practice it is included here (Box **3.1**).

Box 3.1. Learning activity: how to practice unconditional positive regard (as cited in Stephany, 2022, p. 30 and as adapted from Stephany, 2017).

This activity can be done on your own or as an in-class exercise. For each of the following four strategies, give examples of how you will demonstrate them in your personal and professional life.
1-Make unconditional positive regard a conscious choice.
It is not helpful to judge others. Therefore, you need to make a conscious choice not to judge.
2-Imagine that your client is someone in your life that you care about.
If you imagine that they are someone you love, you are less inclined to judge them.
3-Remind yourself that your client is human just like you.
This strategy was developed by Chopra (2005). Just like you your client has people in their life that love them. Just like you they have experienced joy and sorrow. Just like you, they will someday die. They deserve your respect.
4-Take time to listen to their story.
We are quick to judge when we do not understand what has happened to someone. Many people have experienced trauma. That is why listening to their story helps us to relate to them on a more compassionate level.

Actions that Undermine a Person's Self-Worth

Victim Blaming & Other Hurtful Behaviors

Victim blaming holds a person responsible for their set of circumstances without considering other contributing factors like life circumstances or social injustices. It also places the sole responsibility on the person for getting themselves out of their predicament (Stephany, 2020). Victim blaming is one of the biggest impediments to honouring a person's sense of self-worth because you will not treat someone well if you do not value them. Victim blaming has no place in nursing, especially when nurses are working with people who have survived adversity. The International Council of Nurses (ICN) (2021) mandates that all nurses act with respect, care, compassion, and empathy which includes honoring the dignity of everyone. (p. 9). Similarly, the Canadian Nurses Association (CNA) Code of Ethics (2017) mandates that nurses must "recognize the intrinsic worth of each person" and do whatever it takes to "support persons receiving care in maintaining their dignity and integrity" (p. 12). That means that no one should ever be treated with malice or a lack of compassion.

Victim blaming is only one example of disrespectful behavior. There are other ways that a person can feel denigrated in a healthcare setting (Barclay, 2016). Some examples include not being addressed personally by a healthcare professional, or being talked about by a couple of practitioners who are still in the room, as though they were not even present. Being watched by a whole bunch of students while a specialist conducts a physical examination, without obtaining consent, tops the list of insults. Being spoken to in a condescending manner, and not having their concerns addressed are two other blatant examples that are disparaging (Barclay, 2016). It also does not matter if the behaviour is intentional or unconscious, the negative effect on the client/patient is still apparent. What is therefore recommended is that all healthcare professionals, including nurses, regularly partake in self-reflective practice to increase their self-awareness with the goal of changing any insensitive behaviours (Stephany, 2020).

Strategies that Honour a Person's Self-worth

"You are worthy now. Not when you get that job, not when you lose twenty pounds, not when people know who you are now, simply because you exist" Nina Parker, American Journalist.

According to Perlman (1983), we can and should help people to understand that they are worthy of being loved, and she explained that someone who society has considered to be a failure can be shown their worth through a counter-narrative. The message that we need to help them adopt is that they do belong, that they are someone of value, and that they are so much more than their past or life choices. However, for someone with a poor self-concept to accept their own value may require actions by others that treat them as though they do matter (Perlman).

There are several ways for a healthcare professional to convey respect for someone. You can listen to their story and not judge them. Ensuring that you obtain informed consent before conducting any assessment or intervention is important. You can involve them in planning and decision-making. You can be cognizant of their fears and do what you can to alleviate them. Proceeding cautiously when asking them direct questions about trauma is advised so you do not re-traumatize them. Obtaining consent before including students in an examination for teaching purposes should be a common courtesy, as is asking them what they need or want (Cooper *et al.*, 2019; Haskins, 2019).

The Importance of Human Connection in Trauma-informed Care

The bonds that people develop with other people that they value and esteem are the hallmarks of **human connection** (Fig. **3.2**). In fact, being connected to other humans is also a basic social need in life, because without belonging, we feel alone in our experience (Ferrucci, 2006). Bonding with other people also matters because it helps people deal more effectively with life's problems and enhances their mental health (Harley *et al*., 2020). When someone is either emotionally or physically unwell, they often feel alone in their experience. They may have family or friends who care about them, or there may be no one who is there for them, and worse yet, they may be in a violent, and abusive relationship. Their need to feel a connection with someone like a nurse who is assessing or treating them, can be real and palpable, but first, their willingness to trust you must be earned.

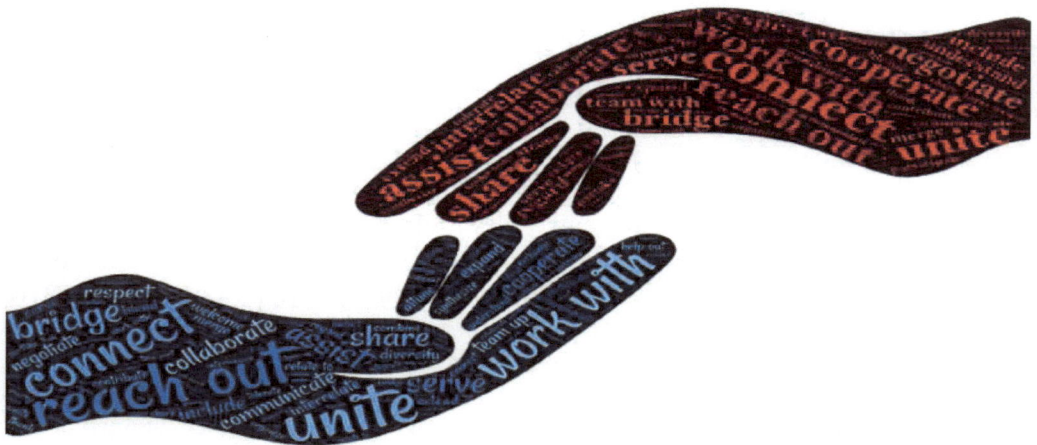

Fig. (3.2). Human connection matters. Source: www.pixabay.com.

Establishing Connection through Effective Communication

According to Jiwa (2018), the most valuable component associated with good patient outcomes is the quality of the person's connection with their caregiver. For example, the bond between a physician and client/patient is associated with decreased emotional distress in a person even if their present problem cannot be solved (Jiwa). Rakel (2018) further explains that the degree of confidence that someone has in their doctor is dependent on the physician's ability to effectively communicate genuine empathy and to listen with an intent to understand.

A trusting relationship between a nurse and client/patient is also correlated with positive mental health outcomes, and the nurse's capacity to demonstrate compassion has been ranked highest on the list of patient-identified essential components that facilitate healing (Hartley *et al*., 2020). Furthermore, an extensive review of healthcare literature by Sinclair *et al*., (2016) revealed three attributes of nurses' compassion that were declared by patients as essential. The first is the positive impact that compassion has on the person. People feel cared for when a nurse identifies with their suffering. The second consists of effective communication techniques that indicate that the nurse genuinely cares about what is going on for them and is willing to actively listen. The third is described as the nurse giving of their time and presence, with the intent of wanting to get to know the patient as a person (Sinclair *et al*.,).

The Value of the Therapeutic Relationship

"Let no one ever come to you without leaving better and happier." Mother Teresa, Catholic Nun & the Founder of The Missionaries of Charity.

Every encounter with another human being is an opportunity for caring to occur (Stephany, 2020). That is why a therapeutic relationship between the nurse and their client/patient is so vitally important. According to Duffy (2018), the word therapeutic is associated with help and healing, and the term we refer to as relationship implies a bond or alliance between two people. Therefore, a **therapeutic relationship** in nursing consists of the capacity of the nurse to know and understand their client/patient in such a way, as to be able to connect with them in a humane and meaningful manner (Mirhaghi *et al*., 2017). A relationship is deemed to be truly therapeutic when both the one who is being cared for and the one offering care each receive something positive from the interaction (Duffy).

We know that the quality of the therapeutic relationship between a healthcare professional and their client/patient is important, and studies have revealed this connection facilitates emotional healing, regardless of the specific strategies that are employed (Duffy, 2018; Levenson, 2020; Stephany, 2022). Yet, therapeutic relationships have not consistently been valued in healthcare in general (Duffy, 2018; Mirhaghi *et al*., 2017). Some evidence also indicates that although they are associated with positive health outcomes in people accessing mental health services, nurses are sometimes found to be lacking the necessary communication skills or deem caring relationships as not as important as other more task-orientated aspects of their practice (Duffy, 2018; Harley *et al*., 2020).

Caring Relationships & Knowledge Competence

Caring is an integral aspect of the therapeutic relationship and consists of actions and motivation directed toward a person, for their protection, their overall welfare, and their enhancement of well-being in the physical, emotional, psychological, and spiritual realms (Duffy, 2018: Noddings, 2013; Ray, 2018). When working with people who have experienced trauma a component of caring that I view as important but not always recognized is knowledge competence. **Knowledge competence** is the ability to apply what one knows to the situations at hand. For nurses it is about clinical competency and practicing within our scope, ensuring that our actions are evidence-based, that they align with best practices, and that we improve health outcomes by enhancing our expertise through on-going educational pursuits (Duffy, 2018; Schmidt, 2002; Stephany, 2020). Consequently, when caring for persons who have experienced trauma, caring and knowledge competency is best achieved by purposefully acquiring the necessary training and expertise to better serve this complex population.

PERSON-CENTERED CARE

Like client-centered care, **person-centered care** can be universally practiced in most nursing care settings, prioritizes the care that people receive, and emphasizes a collaborative relationship between healthcare professionals and recipients. It not only focuses on illness and services that hospitals and long-term care facilities provide but goes beyond that. It individualizes care that is catered to the person, no matter the setting, and is especially focused on those with unique needs. That is why attributes of person-centered care that have traditionally made it valuable consist of a holistic approach that is personalized, strength-based, empowering, and respectful (Zhao *et al.*, 2016). It treats everyone as you would want to be treated, especially those who have traditionally been ignored such as people suffering from acute and chronic illnesses, disabilities, mental illness, and substance use (Bassuk *et al.*, 2017; Stokes *et al.*, 2017). Key components of trauma-informed person-centered care that will be discussed here include the collaborative relationship between the care provider and the one accessing services; utilizing effective communication skills to facilitate change; and the needs expressed by special populations which include recovery-orientated strategies.

Collaboration

A collaborative relationship in person-centered trauma-informed care must be designed in a manner that views the person who needs help as the expert, and an active participant in the process (Hanga *et al.*, 2017). Therefore, **collaboration** must consist of a coordinated effort to include the individual in all aspects of the planning and implementation of care. It should involve establishing goals and a process that is safe and respectful, and that considers personal and cultural preferences (Knight, 2019; Isobel & Delgado, 2017). Shared power is also important because clients/patients do not want to be ignored, coerced into treatment, or treated in a condescending manner.

What may be required to ensure collaboration is that every person working in the setting be educated on how to deliver quality care in a cooperative and consultative manner. Administrators and staff should be trained in the necessary skills to make that a reality because as Miller *et al.*, (2017) point out, an attitude shift is sometimes needed in everyone who works in the setting and may need to begin with those in charge. They ideally should be educated with evidence-based data to understand that people can and do recover from the physical and psychological ramifications associated with trauma, that they have the capacity to improve their lives, and that they have the desire to be consulted in plans that involve them (Miller *et al.*,).

To create a safe space where a client/patient is made an equal partner in the process may require that a practitioner, that is used to being the sole decision-maker, take a step back in terms of what they think should occur. Instead, what may be required is that they do their best to honor the person's right to choose for themselves, even if some of those decisions may appear at face value to be less than desirable. There are valid reasons for this. Five clear goal setting strategies that encourage a person's participation in the collaborative process and that facilitate good outcomes were identified by Miller and Barnie (2016). They consist of identifying the purpose of every goal; ensuring that outcomes are personalized to the client/patient's needs; and that the person who is most affected by any decision be the center of decision-making. The plan also needs to be action focused with clearly stated steps toward achieving every goal (Miller & Barnie).

Utilizing Effective Person-Centered Communications Skills

Person-centered communication is a form of engagement that honors the person and their family's point of view, values their input, and seeks their active involvement in decisions. Effective communication skills are essential for person-centered trauma-informed care for the following valid reasons. Successful communication enhances the therapeutic alliance by validating the person's experiences, listening empathetically to their story and respecting their point of view (Kwame & Petrucka, 2021; Levenson, 2020). Best practices in communication are made possible when there is a clear two-way channel of discussion between the healthcare professional and client/patient, with both parties listening to understand, without interruptions, and where opinions are allowed to be shared even if they differ. This process includes seeking clarification to better understand (Kwame & Petrucka, 2021; Rosenberg, 2003).

Barriers to Person-Centered Communication

Unfortunately, research has revealed that there are obstacles to effective person-centered communication. Some consist of superficial interactions or lack of clarity (Isobel & Delgado, 2017). Other impediments are institutional and due to less-than-ideal circumstances like staffing shortages or increased workloads, which lead to nursing burnout. Some are environmentally induced, such as noisy surroundings, too many people in the unit, and a lack of privacy. Treating people as objects, being too task-orientated, harboring negative attitudes, and lacking in empathy also create tension. Miscommunication is another identified problem, which includes language barriers, disrespectful non-verbal gestures, and not taking the person's concerns seriously (Kwame & Petrucka, 2021).

OFFERING PERSON-CENTERED CARE TO PEOPLE FROM SPECIAL POPULATIONS

Let's briefly explore effective ways to offer person-centered care to people from these special populations: the elderly, those with a disability, people with dementia, palliative care patients, and persons suffering from mental illness and substance use.

The Elderly

According to Wanko Keutchafo *et al.*, (2022), non-verbal forms of positive, caring communication instigated by nurses have been identified as extremely important in offsetting the loneliness experienced by the elderly. For example, the evidence indicates that when nurses willingly communicate with compassion and care, many elderly patients get better faster and hospital stays are shortened. The opposite is also true. Attitudes by nurses that stem from ageism, that view older people in non-flattering ways, or that communicate overall disdain for members of this group have a negative effect on patient outcomes. The authors highly recommend that nurses who care for the elderly make it a priority to increase their self-awareness of any negative attitudes and non-verbal communication techniques with the intention of changing them (Wanko Keutchafo *et al.*,).

People With Disabilities

Scherer (2014) explains that in the later part of the 20th century, services designed for people with disabilities viewed these clients/patients as abnormal and in need of treatment to function in a world that was not designed with their needs in mind.

Fortunately, that focus has evolved over time toward efforts to customize treatment with an emphasis on the individual, but it is still less than ideal, as will be made apparent. For example, comprehensive research was conducted by Hanga *et al.*, (2017) involving people who suffer from disabilities that explored their critical views of what they disliked about existing person-centered programs, followed by recommendations for change. They identified the following as particularly problematic: issues accessing services, poor relationships with healthcare personnel and staff due to power struggles, and not having their needs met. They suggested that all future services be designed with their needs in mind. Additionally, they would prefer to be fully informed of what to expect before receiving care, that power differentials be properly addressed and eradicated, and that strategies that empower them to live their best lives be prioritized (Hanga *et al.*, 2017).

Persons Suffering from Dementia

In 2017, it was noted that dementia impacted at least 46.8 million people globally (Kim & Park, 2017). That number is likely higher today. Although there are various forms, **dementia** is generally used to describe a person's impaired capacity to function in everyday life due to memory loss, impaired language skills, or being incapable of thinking clear enough to solve the problem (Alzheimer's Association, n.d.). Research by Jim and Park (2017) has revealed that teaching staff to apply specific person-centered skills when caring for people with dementia results in enhanced overall well-being and quality of life when compared with the usual unspecified care. For example, in this extensive study, healthcare personnel were taught to apply all the elements of a **VIPS** scale for person-centered care. They consisted of "**V**, as the value of human life; **I**, for an evaluation of individuality; **P**, for an understanding of patient perspectives; and **S**, for positive social psychology to improve relative well-being" (Kim & Park, 2017, p. 382). Key positive results of this staff-instigated educational endeavor included a significant decrease in symptoms of depression and agitation and a reduction in other debilitating neuropsychiatric symptoms (Kim & Park).

People and Families Requiring Palliative Care

A key component of patient-centered strategies is **palliative care** with the goal of improving the quality of life of patients of all ages and their family members while they are dealing with problems associated with a life-threatening illness (World Health Organization (WHO), 2020). Dignity is a central component of palliative care, and there are no exceptions to this rule. **Dignity** in practice consists of the recognition that everyone possesses intrinsic worth and value and should be treated with respect, regardless of their situation or circumstances (I,

2017). Due to their health state and possible decreased life expectancy, people receiving palliative care have unique needs when it comes to preserving their dignity because they are often incapacitated and experience a deterioration in their ability to function and care for themselves, which can negatively affect their sense of self-esteem (Kuhl, 2002). What they need in these situations is to be treated as though they still matter, even if they are deemed to be weaker than their former selves. However, unfortunately they do not always receive the care that they deserve. For instance, a comprehensive review of the literature by Pringle at al. (2015) has shown that large numbers of recipients of palliative care in a hospital setting during the time leading up to and including their death, had a sense that they were not treated in a dignified manner. The authors of this study concluded that those working in all palliative care settings should be trained to manage their client/patient's symptoms more holistically. They recommended prioritizing more than pain management, and also prioritizing helping with emotional distress (Pringle *et al*.,).

Wisdom for Caring for People Who are Dying

"Only people with a terminal illness know what it is like to live with such an illness. They are the people who hold the knowledge. They are our best teachers."
Dr. David Kuhl, Author of the book called, *What Dying People Want*

Nurses working with palliative care experience emotional distress when caring for those who are going to die and attribute their difficulty to their early encounters with death as a new nurse, that was never properly dealt with. This, in turn, results in the emotional detachment of the nurse, which leads to diminished work satisfaction for them, and a decrease in the quality of care provided to their patients (Anderson *et al*., 2015). However, facing death and the fear and distress that is associated with it is a part of the experience of life, and more frequently than not, it is also part of doing the job as a nurse or doctor. Besides, people who are being cared for near the end of their lives often look to healthcare professionals for emotional comfort and solace in dealing with their fears. They are afraid of what will happen to those whom they will leave behind. They are anxious about the absoluteness of death and even question whether any part of them will exist after they are no longer alive (Kuhl, 2002). Nurses and doctors are not expected to act as clergy, counselors or advisors, so what can they do to help? They can choose to interact with these people in the following ways. Whenever possible, sit down and be with the person who is dealing with this particularly distressing situation. If it is okay with them, and with permission, you can reach out and hold their hand for a while because human touch matters a great deal.

Encourage them to talk if they want to, but also let them know that it is okay to remain silent if that is what they prefer. Sometimes, just being present can be enough. If they feel like speaking, do your best to listen with undivided attention. Look into their eyes. If they cry or get angry, let them know that it is okay for them to show emotion and to be scared. Let them know that you are there to listen to them if they want to talk about their life. Ask them what they need from you because you want to help them, as long as it is within your professional capacity to do so. Afterward, when the person dies, give yourself permission to grieve. In time, the emotional labor of nursing can take a toll on your well-being, so search for ways to keep yourself from being too negatively affected by the loss. Sometimes, that process involves reaching out for support from others in your close circle of family or friends, but it also may include getting professional help from a Counsellor. Connecting with the goodness of life in some way will ground you and keep you focused in the here and now. It also helps to be grateful to be alive.

People Suffering from Mental Illness and Substance Use

It is estimated that mental health and substance use affect 50% of people during their lifetime, resulting in poor health outcomes and a 25-year decrease in life span (Bassuk *et al.*, 2017). Being exposed to adverse childhood experiences predisposes people to develop mental illness or substance use in adult life (Goodman, 2017). Furthermore, general exposure to traumatic life experiences at any age is a contributing factor to many mental health illnesses, such as post-traumatic stress disorder (PTSD), depression, anxiety, and substance use (Nieforth & Craig, 2021). Substances are often used to self-medicate to offset the adverse psychological symptoms that people experience due to trauma and contribute to their decreased capacity to self-regulate their emotions (Levin *et al.*, (2021). Public stigmatization and negative stereotypes add to shame and poor self-worth and internalizing the public social stigma attributed to them, which creates a barrier to accessing services (Matthews *et al.*, 2017).

Person-centered trauma-informed care is recommended for those with mental health or substance use issues, and one specific strategy that is known to help is the words that we choose to refer to them (Bassuk *et al.*, 2017; Fadus, 2020). For example, they are often subjected to unfair and unkind labelling. Terms like *"crazy," "lunatic," "drug addict," "drug abuser,"* or *"junkie"* are insulting and degrading and should be completely avoided (Matthews *et al.*, 2017). Even the term *"addiction"* is no longer considered appropriate. What is more acceptable is to refer to the person as suffering from a mental illness or substance use. Consumers of mental health services have also made some specific recommendations that align well with person-centered care to improve the care that they receive (Bassuk *et al.*, 2017; Isobel *et al.*, 2021). A key request is to avoid causing harm by properly educating healthcare professionals on the prevalence of trauma in society, its negative impacts, and the key pillars of trauma-informed care. Those in professional helping roles should be taught to prioritize establishing trust relationships and safety, and actively including those accessing services in the planning of care and intervention. Compassion, empathy, and being responsive to their needs are categorized as necessary skills (Bassuk *et al.*,; Isobel *et al.*,).

THE VALUE OF RECOVERY-ORIENTED CARE

Healing relationships as an essential component of addressing the needs of people with all chronic conditions, and it is best achieved through efforts that support recovery-orientated care. **Recovery-orientated care** fosters wellness by respecting all people, honoring their unique strengths and qualities, valuing them as equal partners in their care, and being purposefully responsive to their needs. It is used in many settings but has been largely associated with the treatment of persons suffering from substance use (Bassuk *et al.*, 2017). There are tremendous benefits of recovery-orientated approaches. For instance, they cultivate change in a variety of situations, prioritize empathy and compassion, and combat stigma through acceptance, tolerance, and inclusion (Sowers, 2022). The following crucial components associated with recovery will now be explored: change and courage, responsibility for growth, how to deal with resistance, and the importance of meaning-making and hope.

Change & Courage

Most people who are referred for recovery services will be asked to alter some of the behaviours that have been detrimental to their overall physical to mental health. However, altering behaviour is not that easy, especially if what they have been accustomed to has served a purpose, such as self-medicating with substances to alleviate anxiety or traumatic memories. It, therefore, takes courage to change because altering habitual behaviours involves work, distress, and pain. The person must have the determination and perseverance to stay the course even with setbacks (Sowers, 2022). In fact, with most recovery processes, the teaching that needs to occur is that relapsing to old ways of being is often a part of the journey, especially when stressful events occur. Therefore, one must refuse to adopt an all-or-nothing approach to healing and exchange this view for one that acknowledges that recovery is a process and that setbacks do occur. It is beneficial to remind then that valuable insight can be drawn from what did not work but that they may require additional support to re-embark on their recovery journey when they have relapsed.

Responsibility for Growth

For any alteration in behaviour to occur, the person must take responsibility for making it happen. No one can do it for them. They must be willing to give up beliefs that no longer serve them (Sowers, 2022). They have to recognize specific behaviours that need changing and be assisted in developing a plan of action that is achievable in steps. This process is, therefore, collaborative, with the person needing help being guided by those offering care. In this fashion, the healthcare professional acts in the role of coach (Sowers, 2022).

How to Deal with Resistance to Change

Resisting change is quite common for most people at some point in their lives, and individuals who are in the process of recovery are no exception. There are many ways that resistance may manifest. Denial and not believing that they have a problem is common, as is convincing themselves that they have the situation handled and do not need any help. Some may get defensive and express anger (Perlman, 1979). Even after consenting to alter their behaviour, hesitancy and uncertainty may still be evident because there is a degree of comfort in sticking to what you know. Therefore, it helps to explain that for most people, any major change can be scary, and it is normal to vacillate. Assurances that they will be supported in the process and not judged if they are hesitant is also helpful. Encouraging them to make a list of all the pros and cons of staying with what no longer serves them *versus* moving forward can help them to visualize real benefits associated with changing their behaviour (Levenson, 2020).

THE POWER OF RESILIENCE

"Life doesn't get easier or more forgiving; we get stronger and more resilient," Dr. Steve Maraboli, Behavioral Scientist.

People who have experienced trauma need to be aware they are more than what happened to them, and that they do have the skills and fortitude to move forward and live their lives more fully (Levenson, 2020). **Resilience** is the ability to bounce-back and carry on despite experiencing a trauma. It consists of constructive attributes of endurance, strength, and the will and motivation to move forward, despite what has occurred (Collier, 2016) (Fig. **3.3**).

In fact, people who have experienced trauma and are **resilient**, are able to eventually return to their former degree of functioning. Initially, they may feel sad, upset, defeated, or hopeless, but they do not want to remain there. They possess a willingness and capacity to move forward with their lives that makes them more sturdy and able to weather future life challenges when and if they occur (Seligman, 2011). People who are resilient often possess healthy skills of adaptation along with support from family, friends, or community (Brooks & Goldstein, 2003). There are attributes that contribute to a person's capacity for resilience, and the ensuing discussion will emphasize some of them such as the role of positive emotions, the importance of adopting a sturdy mindset, and how to effectively deal with mistakes.

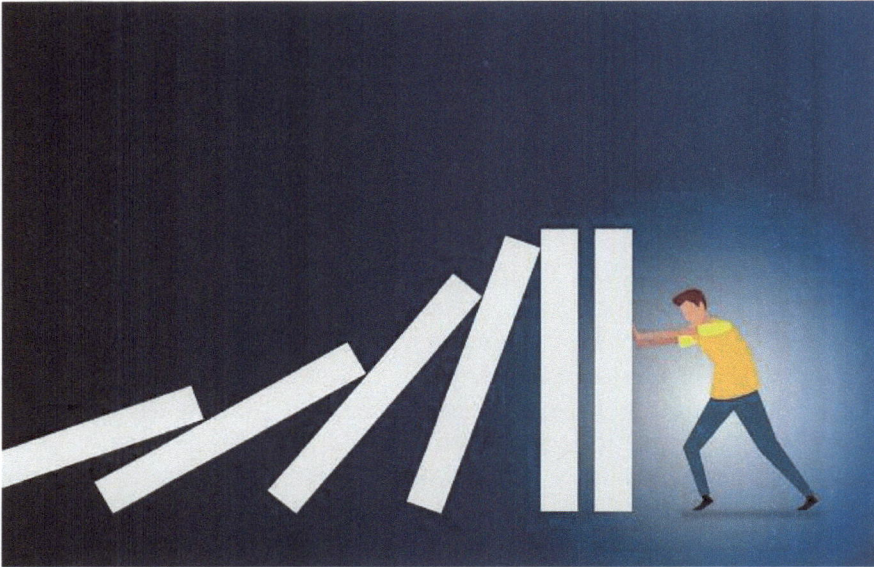

Fig. (3.3). Resilience. Source: www.pixabay.com.

Attributes of Resilience

There are attributes that contribute to a person's capacity for resilience. The ensuing discussion will emphasize some of them, such as the role of positive emotions, the importance of adopting a sturdy mindset, and how to effectively deal with mistakes.

The Role of Positive Emotions

Resilient people usually possess positive attitudes and beliefs about themselves that influence their behaviors and their ability to handle stress after adversity (Brooks & Goldstein, 2003). For instance, there is evidence that the ability to move forward optimistically following trauma is facilitated by **positive emotions** like happiness, joy, gratitude, and appreciation, which in turn enhances the overall experience of life (Poseck *et al.*, 2006; Seligman, 2011).

Seligman (2011) explains how positive emotions improve life after trauma. Willingly adopting an optimistic outlook leads to enthusiasm, an openness to change, and being more fully engaged with everyday activities. Resilient people tend to cope with their adverse experiences by utilizing creativity, positive thinking, and humour. Furthermore, positive emotions act in a protective capacity by helping to somewhat shield a person from developing anxiety and depression (Fredrickson, 2003; Poseck *et al.*, 2006).

Adopting a Sturdy Mindset: The Importance of a Commitment to Life & Challenge

Unfortunately, stress is an inevitable aspect of life, and none of us can escape it completely. However, chronic stress is somewhat problematic and can contribute to an array of physical and psychological issues, such as heart disease, stomach problems, diabetes, depression, and anxiety. Additionally, too much stress can also decrease the overall quality of life (Brooks and Goldstein, 2003). There are some simple ways to increase one's capacity to deal with stress by altering lifestyle choices that enhance wellness, which may include getting enough exercise, eating a proper diet, avoiding substance use, and getting enough hours of sleep. Nevertheless, it is not always the amount of stress that causes the biggest problems; it is the inability to cope with stress (Brooke & Goldstein, 2003).

Conversely, people who effectively deal with life's pressures possess personality traits that make them **stress-hardy,** which enables them to respond to demanding situations in an adaptive manner. So, what is the difference between a sturdy mindset *versus* one that is not? Much of what we now know about stress-hardiness comes from studying professional athletes (Sheard, 2013). Let's use analogy drawn from sprinting competitions. Imagine two athletes with a similar build, physical stamina, training, and coaching competing in an event like short-distance running. One of them wins the race by a big margin, while the other loses badly. What may have separated their chances of succeeding? The one who won the race most likely possessed an attitude of *"I can do this,"* whereas the other did not (Sheard, 2013). The good news is that a person can learn to develop a stress-hardy mindset by adopting certain ways of behaving in their everyday life.

The first component of a **sturdy mindset** is a commitment to being fully engaged with life. It is about having a reason to get up in the morning and looking forward to the challenges of the day with a sense of excitement. It is not that different from meaning-making (Stephany, 2012). Sometimes a good place to start when helping someone to develop a more optimistic outlook, is to ask them questions they may not have considered. *"What gives you purpose? What makes you feel fully alive, and what sort of activities help you feel more engaged? Would you consider doing* *some of those things?"* (Brooke & Goldstein, 2003, p. 53). Another action that helps to connect people with the goodness in life is being compassionate and serving others (Stephany, 2022). When someone identifies with the suffering of another it helps them to move away from their own predicament. When they help someone in a small way they realize that they are capable of making a difference and that they do matter (Brooks & Goldstein, 2003; Stephany, 2022).

The challenge is another aspect of a strong mindset because people who are stress-resilient usually view trying situations as opportunities in disguise (Brooke & Goldstein, 2003). When someone is seeking guidance because they are afraid of change, a good place to begin is to gently nudge them out of their comfort zone by suggesting that they try something new. It doesn't have to be anything huge. They can have coffee in a different location, take a walk in a park, visit a library, paint or color a picture, volunteer, or try a new recipe. Challenging themselves to be a little bit more adventurous can be inspirational and build confidence. Success with each new adventure usually leads to a sense of satisfaction and achievement. The result is that the person is more inclined to become fully engaged with life one small step at a time. When they succeed, they are also more inclined to repeat that behavior and to feel positive and hopeful (Stephany, 2012).

Learning How to Deal with Mistakes

The way that we respond to errors that we make reveals a great deal about us. People who are resilient tend to see mistakes as an opportunity to learn from what transpired, and as opportunities rather than obstacles (Brook & Goldstein, 2003; Stephany, 2012). Those who view errors as a direct reflection of their intrinsic flawed character support an internal narrative that they are the problem and, therefore incapable of change. However, thinking you are a failure and incapable of success is just an idea that you believe to be true. Simply put, if you think you can, you will. If you think you can't, you won't.

Subsequently, to deal more effectively with failure, the person needs to change their thinking. As a starting point they can be taught to understand that how they feel about their situation is not necessarily due to facts but due to their beliefs about their situation (Seligman, 2011). The next step is to challenge their preconceived notions with the following types of questions. *"Did you fail due to your own stupidity or bad choices? Were there other mitigating factors that contributed to the problem that had nothing to do with you? Identify those additional circumstances that contributed to an unfavorable outcome. Can you see that everything that occurred was not only due to you?"* As a therapist, I ask them to show me the verification that what happened was completely their fault, and most often, they have no proof, because when closely examined, the evidence demonstrates factors that are unrelated to them. Next, I have them review all the facts. When they are confronted with the truth, they start questioning some of their unsubstantiated ideas about the specific incident (Stephany, 2012).

Professional assistance is sometimes required. However, as previously mentioned, facilitating change in beliefs that have been longstanding often requires personal effort and assistance from others. That is why professional help in the form of **cognitive behavioral therapy (CBT)** may still be required to change strongly imbedded negative self-scripts. CBT assists people to become aware of their negative beliefs and how they influence their actions. The goal of CBT is to teach the person to identify their negative and unsubstantiated beliefs, to challenge those ideas with the truth, and to think of themselves in a more optimistic way (McLeod, 2023). Change in their thinking happens when CBT therapy is offered long enough for the person to acquire new habits of thinking, speaking, and acting, which results in a more hopeful and positive outlook toward the world and themselves.

Individualism versus Community Well-being

Waters *et al.*, (2022) point out that there is a caveat worth addressing, and that is the fact that not every culture prioritizes individualism. Some, in fact, assert that the wellbeing and honor of family and community take precedence over the needs of the person. For example, the individual's right to make autonomous choices may be considered less significant than the needs of a larger community to which they belong (Waters *et al.*, 2022). Therefore, one must be careful not to promote ideas like the pursuit of self-actualization without first ensuring that this perspective does not conflict with cultural norms because to do so may inadvertently cause them harm (Waters *et al.*,).

CONDUCTING TRAUMA-SCREENING IN A SAFE MANNER

The current discussion diverts our attention to the topic of safely screening people for trauma. Although there may be some slight overlap in the content presented in the two previous Chapters, the current dialogue offers additional beneficial information. Furthermore, while reading through what will be advised, consider what was just learned about offering client-centered, person-centered, and resilience-focussed trauma-informed care and how these approaches may be helpful when assessing people for trauma.

Why Training in Trauma-Screening is Needed

Healthcare professionals need to be adequately trained to safely conduct trauma assessments because although trauma is quite prevalent in society, the rate of trauma-screening that occurs in healthcare settings is still quite low in comparison to other forms of assessment (Cooper *et al.*, 2019). Furthermore, all health professionals should know how to properly screen for trauma in anyone who presents for care, so that no one who has experienced adversity is missed in the process (Haskins, 2019). This is extremely important since many people who have been traumatized are not forthcoming in disclosing their history due to memory suppression or the fear of being judged. Additionally, becoming aware of a person's history of trauma may facilitate a more comprehensive plan of care, such as treatment for medical or behavioral issues and referral to needed community resources (Knight, 2015; Jones *et al.*, 2021).

Risks Associated with a Lack of Training in Trauma-Screening

There are risks associated with a lack of training in trauma-screening. For example, if unchecked, a healthcare professional's implicit biases and stereotypes may surface and be acted upon, causing harm. An additional problem occurs when an unskilled healthcare professional conducts a quick upfront screening before rapport building is established. They may unknowingly violate the person's sense of autonomy by undermining their experience, excluding them in the assessment and planning process, or unfairly judging them. These actions hinder trust and often result in the person either leaving early, refusing to return for further treatment, or both (Menschner & Maul, 2016).

Being Aware of Someone's Trauma History is Helpful

There are benefits associated with a healthcare professional becoming aware of a person's history of trauma if they compassionately approach this sensitive subject. For instance, gaining an understanding of someone's trauma history may facilitate a connection between the caregiver and client/patient that builds rapport and trust through empathy. This, in turn, may improve the likelihood of their participation, enhance their adherence to a treatment plan, and result in better health outcomes (Brewerton & Alexander, 2019; Menschner & Maul, 2016).

Take Measures to Avoid Re-Traumatization

Gaining an understanding of someone's trauma history is quite different from asking them to tell their whole story. You, therefore, are required to do whatever you can to prevent re-traumatization. Best practices advise that you respectfully inform the person not to disclose specific aspects of their trauma because it is not necessary and may cause them harm. If they still insist on disclosing trauma-related details, a polite interruption may award you an opportunity to educate them. What also works best is for you to remind them that you are there to help them, that they are safe, and that you will not judge them (Kusmaul & Anderson, 2018).

An Unskilled Practitioner Must Not Set Out to Uncover Repressed Memories

Sometimes, the memory of a traumatic event is unconsciously suppressed as a way of coping and surviving. Dr. Bessel van Der Kolk (2014) points out that memory loss can occur after any trauma, but most often, it is associated with war, serious disasters, being abducted, living in a concentration camp, and being physically or sexually abused. When memory suppression happens after a traumatic event or set of circumstances, it can be somewhat adaptive (Mary *et al.*, 2020). The opposite experience is that of post-traumatic stress disorder (PTSD), where someone is tortured by mental flashbacks that they cannot control.

Neuroscience research has revealed that when a suppressed memory is carefully retrieved and uncovered under controlled circumstances by a professional expert, the act of telling the story can sometimes facilitate meaning-making for the person and may even contribute to their capacity to become resilient (Mary *et al.*, 2020; van Der Kolk, 2014). However, memory recovery after the suppression of a previous trauma is a very sensitive process and, if not conducted properly, can cause additional psychological harm to the trauma survivor. It must only be undertaken by a trained and skilled professional, such as a Social Worker, Psychiatrist, or Psychologist. The responsibility for such an undertaking must never reside in someone who is a novice and is well beyond the scope of most nurses.

Up-Front *Versus* Later Trauma-Screening

Before proceeding to suggest strategies for conducting trauma-screening, it must be pointed out that any proposed approach is not intended to be used to diagnose, nor are they suitable in every situation. Rather, they are meant to be considered as possible adjuncts to other important aspects of thorough history taking and other health assessments.

Although screening for trauma is viewed as a key component of trauma-informed care, there are still differences in opinion on when this screening should ideally occur (Menschner & Maul, 2016). Some recommend up-front screening that is universal and investigates everyone for trauma as soon as possible. Advocates for this approach argue that universal screening decreases the likelihood of cultural stereotypical biases, may enable the healthcare professional to obtain a more comprehensive assessment of the person's trauma history, be better informed when planning treatment options, and can contribute to data collection (Menschner & Maul, 2016).

Those who are opposed to upfront screening and prefer later screening allege that time is needed to build a trust relationship between the person conducting the assessment and the client/patient before posing questions about their trauma history. They also assert that asking too many questions before the person is ready may hinder progress or lead to re-traumatization (Menschner & Maul. 2016). Even though opinions may differ as to when to conduct trauma screening, the following general components are viewed as ideal by both sides (Box **3.2**).

Box 3.2. General components of trauma-screening (as adapted from Menschner & Maul, 2016).

-The Treatment Setting Should Guide How Quickly the Screening Occurs. For instance, up-front screening may be more appropriate in a primary clinic where someone may be presenting for the first time, and later screening is more suitable for a mental health setting where the person is known.
-The Focus of Screening Should Benefit the Client/Patient. If any healthcare concerns are identified during the screening process, appropriate treatment options must be offered, or they should be referred elsewhere for follow-up care.
-Re-Screening Must be Avoided. Re-screening usually includes asking the person to repeat their story about the trauma and can lead to re-traumatization. To minimize this potential risk, information sharing between medical treatment centers accessed by the client/patient is suggested, but only if protection of privacy is guaranteed.
-All Professional and Non-Professional Staff Need to Be Trained in Trauma Screening. Everyone working in a setting that conducts trauma assessments needs to be trained in how to conduct the initial and subsequent screenings, with particular attention given to cultural or ethnic variables.

How to Begin an Assessment for Trauma

When proceeding to conduct an assessment for past or present trauma, ProQuest (2020 highly recommends that the healthcare professional make a positive connection with the person. What does that consist of? The first step should be to establish a trust relationship based on wanting to get to know the client/patient in the form of a friendly, non-threatening conversation, with you doing the listening and them doing most of the talking. Once you get the sense that there is a degree of comfort in them, you may proceed to gently inquire about other things. However, you are still advised to start by asking what is generally going on for them, like what makes them feel sad, stressed out, or unable to cope. If their comfort will allow for it, you may ask more directly about any history of trauma (ProQuest, 2020). The most crucial areas to explore during trauma-screening are listed in Box (**3.3**). A Learning Activity is suggested in Box (**3.4**) to explore ways that may prove helpful during assessment.

Box 3.3. Crucial areas to cover for trauma-screening (as adapted from Corbett in ProQuest, 2020; Quaile & Benyounes-Ulrich, 2020; Stephany, 2022).

- Ask the client/patient to tell you about symptoms they are experiencing that they think are related to trauma.
- Inquire about symptoms of depression (*e.g.*, lack of interest in things pleasurable, negative self-reference, and negative world reference).
- Are they experiencing any sleep disturbances (*e.g.*, too little or too much sleep)?
- Have they ever been diagnosed with a mental-disorder, and if yes, are they being treated for one?
- Can they tell you what type of trauma they may have experienced without giving any details?
- Is substance use an issue?
- Do they have adequate social supports or access to other helpful resources?
- Have they experienced episodes of self-harm or suicide attempts or violence toward others?
- Are there any health issues that they are suffering from?

For Specific Tools to Assess for Trauma Visit

Substance Abuse and Mental Health Services Administration (SAMHSA) (2014). Trauma-Informed Care in Behavioral Health Services. Treatment Improvement Protocol (TIP) Series 57. HHS Publication No. (SMA) 13-4801. Rockville, MD: Substance Abuse and Mental Health Services Administration. https: //store. samhsa.gov /sites/ default/files/ d7/priv/ sma14-4816.pdf

Box 3.4. Learning activity: explore ways that may be helpful in trauma-screening (as adapted from Knight, 2015).

Background Data Prior to Discussion: The following is a list identified by trauma survivors that they perceive to **NOT** be helpful when they are being assessed and screened for trauma.
1-The clinician avoids talking about trauma all together or minimizes the negative effects of trauma when it is disclosed.
2-They give the impression that what has happened to a person does not matter.
3-Being asked too much detail about the trauma is re-traumatizing.
4-Trying to get the person to talk about their feelings before they are ready impedes trust.
Learning Activity: In a general class discussion or in small groups, talk about specific strategies that may be used by a nurse that may be helpful when screening someone for trauma.

Healing Often Begins with Acknowledging that Trauma has Occurred

"Trauma is personal. It does not disappear if it is not validated. When it is ignored or invalidated, the silent screams continue internally, heard only by the one held captive. When someone enters the pain and hears the screams, healing

can begin". Danielle Bernock, Clinical Psychologist, Author, and Trauma-informed Coach

Healing often begins when someone is able to admit that the trauma occurred, and minimizing or pretending that it did not happen is harmful and may impede recovery. For example, a client came to see me for counselling after she had a less than favourable experience with a Volunteer Counsellor in the Community. She explained what occurred in her session with this person. When the client disclosed that she had been violently assaulted and was having difficulty sleeping and coping, the Counsellor advised that she forget that it happened and just move on. This client left the session and said that she wanted them to understand that if it were that easy, she would have done that. Danielle Bernock (2014) who is a Clinical Psychologist, recommends that a person's trauma be recognized because keeping it hidden as though it never occurred does not make it go way and may obstruct or prolong their journey toward healing (Bernock, 2014). Likewise, staff who are not trained and proficient in trauma-informed care should not proceed to give advice because their lack of knowledge can do more harm than good.

The Role of Validation

Although having a person relive the details of past trauma can be harmful, acknowledging that trauma has occurred, followed by intentionally validating and normalizing a person's emotional response to adversity, can be helpful (Knight, 2015). **Validation** in trauma-informed care recognizes and accepts that what a person has experienced did happen, and what they are feeling is justifiable (Knight, 2015). However, a word of caution is advised. Before proceeding with this strategy, ensure that you have established rapport and trust with the person and that you have reminded them that they are safe (O'Hara, 2019).

There are many benefits to validation. The person feels heard by someone who genuinely does care and wants to understand what they have been going through. Acknowledging a person's experience of trauma without exploring any specific aspects can be beneficial in that it allows them to admit that something terrible did happen, legitimizes their experience without prejudice, and can set the stage for healing to begin. It can also have a profound emotional effect on them, especially if they have been prone to feeling guilt and shame (Knight, 2015; Naparstek, 2014).

THE IMPORTANCE OF SETTING PROFESSIONAL BOUNDARIES

It is vitally important that healthcare professionals sensitively but firmly communicate and set professional boundaries when assessing or caring for someone who has experienced trauma. A **professional boundary** in nursing is a limit that dictates how far a relationship can go and when it is unacceptable to continue (Stephany, 2020). It is about knowing what is right or wrong when caring for clients/patients (Fig. **3.4**). Nurses are advised to ensure that their relationships are solely for the benefit of the person(s) they are caring for. They must not take advantage of their affiliation with clients/patients for personal or financial gain or enter into any liaison that is romantic or sexual in nature (CNA, 2017).

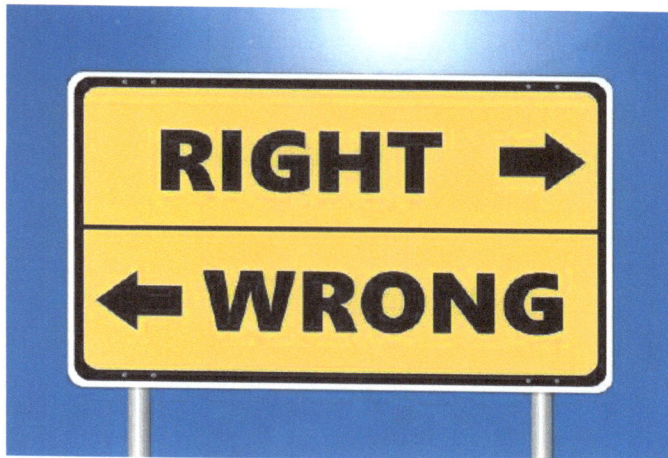

Fig. (3.4). Boundaries are about Knowing What is Right or Wrong Action. Source: www.pixabay.com.

Avoiding Boundary Violations

A **boundary violation** happens when the actions between two people go against well-accepted social expectations. A professional boundary violation may be instigated by either the client/patient or by the healthcare professional. It may occur when a client/patient acts toward their caregiver in a socially unacceptable way or when the help that a healthcare professional offers them is too personal in nature (Knight, 2015). An example of a client/patient crossing a boundary can be in the form of giving gifts, wanting to socialize with their caregiver outside of the clinical setting, or acting toward them in an overly caring or romantic manner. A healthcare professional may also overstep their professional role by offering their client/patient gifts, acting too much like a friend, or providing shelter in their home. All these actions are unprofessional and prohibited.

Rescuing is Unacceptable

"People don't need to be saved or rescued, people need knowledge of their own power and how to access it." Tammy Plunkett, Certified Life Coach and Author.

Nurses must do everything in their power to avoid situations that violate professional boundaries, which include resisting the temptation to assume the role of rescuer. **Rescuing** is a form of helping in a professional capacity that is not beneficial for the recipient. It consists of doing things for a person rather than helping them become more self-sufficient or empowered (Psych Central, 2018). Clients/patients who have experienced trauma do not need to be rescued because it places them in the victim role and can also create unhealthy dependence. What they do require is to become more aware of their strengths and abilities. Healthcare professionals need to be reminded that there is a power differential between them and the person they are caring for, with the client/patient occupying a subservient position. Furthermore, people who have experienced trauma may be used to others making decisions for them, so if a caregiver replicates an authoritarian role, they may perpetuate a harmful reliance (Valente, 2017). What is more beneficial is to assist them to explore how they can achieve their goals, one small task at a time, which builds their self-esteem and encourages self-reliance.

Clear Communication is Needed when Establishing Professional Boundaries

You can be empathetic and not cross a boundary when you thoughtfully set limits that clearly communicate the specific aspect of your role as a professional helper (Valente, 2017). Make it clear from the onset that you are their professional caregiver, and even though you have their best interests at heart, and you cannot get over involved in personal aspects of their lives. You may further explain that overstepping this position could jeopardize your job and even compromise your care. You may also have to address any situation that arises when it occurs if it has the potential to violate a professional boundary. For instance, if they inquire about your personal life, politely remind them that it is not appropriate for you to talk about your private affairs. If they ask for you to have coffee with them, respectfully decline. If they want to be your friend or offer you gifts, politely remind them that as their nurse this is not appropriate. The following case study illustrates how a violation of a professional boundary creates difficulties for a nurse. Refer to Box (**3.5**).

Box 3.5. Narrative case study one: when crossing a professional boundary becomes a problem.

Larissa is a new nurse who just started working in a Community Health Center that caters to troubled youth. She works alongside a team of other health professionals, such as other nurses, social workers, counselors, and physicians. The type of services offered at this Center include physical and mental health assessments, assistance with accessing housing, and referral to other Community Services as needed. Larissa likes this new role. She feels like she does a fairly good job of establishing trusting relationships with most of the

(Box 3.5) cont.....

young people who attend the clinic; she believes that she has something in common with many of the youth because she is not a whole lot older than most of them. Over the course of the past two weeks, one specific 15-year-old client named Rosemary has been coming to the Health Center for support and has taken a special liking to Larissa. In fact, Rosemary insists that Larissa is the only person she is willing to see, regardless of her presenting issue. Larissa was initially somewhat flattered by Rosemary's attachment to her, but she was also beginning to feel uncomfortable with this situation. One of the social workers pointed out to Larissa that Rosemary's recent behavior may be the beginning of an unhealthy dependence and that she needs to set some professional boundaries between herself and Rosemary. Larissa was aware that Rosemary suffers from generalized anxiety and does not trust very many people. She also believes that Rosemary would really benefit from being seen by one of the Counsellors at the clinic and was planning to make a referral for her. On this particular visit Larissa was surprised to hear from Rosemary that she had been abused by a family member as a child, and that was why she ran away from home. Larissa did what she could to validate Rosemary's experience and avoided asking about details of what exactly happened to her. Larissa explained to Rosemary that what occurred was not her fault, and that she was safe here at the clinic and would not be judged. Without warning, Rosemary hugged Larissa and uttered her appreciation.

"Thank-you, thank-you for being my friend. You are so wonderful to me. I don't know what I would have done without you. You are like a mother to me. I think I love you and I don't want anyone else to look after me, only you. I love you."

In shock, Larissa gently pulled away from Rosemary. For a moment, Larissa felt kind of flattered by what her client had just stated and then quickly realized that a serious professional boundary had just been crossed. Larissa knew that if she did not appropriately address this situation, she would be perpetrating an unhealthy dependence, but she also feared that if she rejected Rosemary, she could jeopardize the connection that developed between them. Larissa didn't know what to do next.

NARRATIVE CASE STUDY ONE: IDENTIFICATION OF THEMES & ANALYSIS

Two key themes were identified from this story.

Theme # 1: In this situation, transference occurred when Rosemary hugged her nurse, told her she viewed her as a friend, that she was wonderful, loved her, and likened her to a mother substitute.

Theme # 1 Analysis: Transference most often occurs between a client and therapist but may happen in any relationship (Positive Psychology, n.d.). In counselling or healthcare settings, it happens when a person projects strong feelings that they may have had for someone else in their life, usually in childhood, toward the healthcare professional who is treating them. The client/patient does not see their professional helper as they are, and their automatic behaviors associated with past relationships, whether beneficial or harmful, are transposed into this current one (Perlman, 1983).

Theme # 2: Rosemary's behavior toward Larissa resulted in a boundary violation. However, Larissa felt that she lacked the ability to properly navigate through the situation.

Theme # 2 Analysis: When caring for persons who have experienced trauma, offering empathy and validating the person's feelings in the moment can decrease their sense of isolation. However, the caring that is communicated must not be too intimate in nature. When a transference issue arose for Larissa, the best way for her to manage it was to refuse to play the role designated by the process. She could politely remind her client that her relationship is solely professional and also solicit direct peer support and advice from a more experienced professional colleague, on how best to proceed (Positive Psychology, n.d.). For example, after Rosemary hugged Larissa and uttered words of affection toward her, Larissa could have stated something to Rosemary like, *"I am glad that I have been able to help you, but I cannot act as your friend or take the place of your mother because I am your nurse. My role has to remain professional."* There is, of course, the reality that addressing the boundary violation may result in the rapport between Larissa and Rosemary being severed, even just temporality. However, not addressing what occurred would be unprofessional and may impede the person's progress (Valente, 2017).

QUESTION FOR FURTHER REFLECTION

1-Pretend that you are Larissa. What would you do next and why?

TRANSFORMING IMPLICIT BIAS & MYTHS AIMED AT SURVIVORS OF INTIMATE PARTNER VIOLENCE & STRANGER RAPE

Intimate Partner Violence (IPV) & Stranger Rape

Survivors of sexual violence do not just include women but can be experienced by persons of all gender identities, and these acts include intimate partner violence and stranger rape. **Intimate partner violence (IPV)** consists of violent sexual or physical acts inflicted by a person who has a relationship with the survivor, either currently or in the past. Violence may also include stalking or purposefully inflicting psychological harm (Sullivan & Goodman, 2019). In **stranger rape,** the perpetrator of the sexual assault and the victim do not know one another. However, it needs to be pointed out that intimate partner violence is much more common than stranger rape (Welfare-Wilson, 2022).

Implicit Bias & Unsubstantiated Myths Cause Harm

The subject of implicit bias was briefly presented in Chapter One of this Textbook. In this current discussion, it is re-introduced along with the notion of myths to specifically address stigma toward survivors of intimate partner violence (IPV). **Implicit bias** consists of prejudicial attitudes and beliefs aimed at a specific group of people, and **myths** are assumptions of the cause of something that may or may not be based on fact but is presumed to be true. Perceptions that blame the trauma survivor are hurtful, impede trust and may cause them to refrain from seeking medical attention (Welfare-Wilson, 2022). In order for trauma-informed, client-centered care to help those who have survived sexual violence, all encounters with others, especially those in healthcare, must be free of stigma and implicit bias.

One of the negative effects of being a trauma survivor is being subjected to the stigma exhibited by healthcare professionals (Dowdell & Speck, 2022). Unfortunately, the evidence indicates that some nurses have been known to blame or harshly judge sexual assault survivors (Pemberton & Loeb, 2020; Taccini & Mannarini, 2023). Yet, this fact is problematic because, given the prevalence of sexual violence, nurses, especially those working in a mental health setting, are more likely than most, to be caring for survivors of intimate partner violence or stranger rape (Welfare-Wilson, 2022).

Challenging the Myths

One way to challenge nurses' and other healthcare professionals judgmental attitudes toward survivors of IPV is by openly challenging some of the myths that exist (Taccini & Mannarini, 2023). What bias exists concerning sexual assault? Many, if not all of them, blame and shame the victim in some way. For example, the belief that you would not have been a victim of such an event if you were more careful, like not walking alone, having too much to drink, or wearing the wrong clothing, or not wearing enough clothes. You are not believed because there was a delay in reporting the event to the police, or because you were in a relationship with the perpetrator (Welfare-Wilson, 2022). Many other myths exist. What nurses need to understand is that not being believed is a second form of trauma for the survivor and feeds into the sequela of self-blame and shame (Welfare-Wilson, 2022; Pemberton & Loeb, 2020).

The Reality of the IPV Survivor's Experience of Being Judged

"Judging others makes us blind, whereas love is illuminating. By judging others, we blind ourselves to our own evil and to the grace which others are just as entitled to as we are", Dietrich Bonhoeffer, German Philosopher, Pastor, and WW II Anti-Nazi Activist.

It is crucially important for nurses and other healthcare professionals to dispel the myths associated with IPV, by becoming educated by the evidence, by not participating in the blame game, and by replacing judgment with an empathetic understanding of the person's experience. A good place to start this process is to become informed of what it is like to be someone who has experienced sexual violence. For example, after a sexual assault, the survivor suffers from a whole range of responses that are long-term and affect them in many areas of personal functioning (Taccini & Mannarini, 2023; Welfare-Wilson, 2022). They no longer feel safe; they may be perplexed by anxiety, and the fear of being alone or leaving home. Everyday tasks like going to work or caring for a home or family may be interrupted. Remaining close relationships with those they do still trust may be eroded, due to fear and avoidance. Self-injurious behaviours or suicide attempts are also not uncommon, especially if the person is made to feel responsible in some way for what occurred, either by the abusive perpetrator, family members, or even healthcare personnel (Taccini & Mannarini; Welfare-Wilson). Furthermore, due to the risk of retaliation from their perpetrator, especially if they remain in a relationship with them, a survivor may feel intense fear and anxiety related to disclosing the trauma to anyone, including a clinician or nurse (Pemberton & Loeb, 2020). For a Learning Activity that explores additional myths concerning survivors of IPV and how to change them, refer to Box **(3.6)**.

Box 3.6. Learning activity: dispelling the myths associated with IPV.

Review the evidence to identify other myths that exist concerning survivors of IPV. Then brainstorm and come up with strategies that you can adopt to challenge and change these views amongst colleagues and the general public.

Adopt a Survivor-Centered Approach

Healthcare professionals, including nurses, need to adopt a **survivor-centered approach** to IPV that works co-operatively with survivors, prioritizes safety, honours their choices and needs, and strengths their ability to cope (Goodman *et al.*, 2016; Kulkarni *et al.*, 2015). Refer to Box **(3.7)** for specific aspects of survivor-centered approaches to use when caring for persons who have lived through IPV. A Learning Activity is included to help you consider ideas that may help you to implement these approaches into your practice.

Box 3.7. Survivor-centered approaches to caring for persons who experienced intimate partner violence (as adapted from goodman *et al.*, 2016; Kulkarni *et al.*, 2015).

Learning Activity: In small groups, discuss each of the following survivor-centered approaches and identify specific actions to actualize each of them in real life.
1-A survivor of IPV indicates that they want to have their safety prioritized, which must include a plan. What would that plan include?
2-They would also like guidance and support with the implementation of a plan for safety. How would you offer them that support?
3-They require assurance that their plan for safety is comprehensive enough to not negatively impact other areas in their lives. What do you think that may consist of?

(Box 3.7) cont.....

4-They would like assistance in making good choices. What would that help look like?
5-They prefer that their relationships with Service Providers and healthcare professionals be cooperative and collaborative, especially regarding decision-making. What measures need to be implemented to include them?
6-Any action plan that is developed should validate their experiences and support them to maximize their strengths. If you are unfamiliar with a strength-based approach to caring for people who have survived IPV, what will you need to do to ensure that they get the assistance that they need?
7-Any obstacles that limit their opportunities for success should also be addressed (*e.g.*, issues related to the legal system or social services).

Advocacy & Survivors of Intimate Partner Violence (IPV)

Few would argue against programs prioritizing the safety of survivors of IPV. However, Sullivan & Goodman (2019) point out that in addition to ensuring immediate safety needs, other forms of assistance are also important, such as external support in the form of referrals for resources, housing, income assistance, or safe guarding the person's rights within the legal justice system. Therefore, a form of advocacy is sometimes needed. At the personal level, **advocacy** involves being the voice for a client/patient to address their needs, especially if they feel disempowered or too afraid to act on their own. (Stephany, 2020, p. 50). If survivors of IPV could advise those whose job it is to assist them, they would likely point out that regardless of the support offered, what needs to occur first is to establish a strong, trusting relationship with them and to follow their lead when deciding to make plans (Sullivan & Goodman). What often needs to also occur is for someone to advocate for what they may additionally need to keep them safe, not just in their present situation but beyond that. The following Narrative Case Study demonstrates how crucially important advocacy may be. Refer to Box (**3.8**).

Box 3.8. Narrative case study two: when a survivor of intimate partner violence requires advocacy.

Angela is a Psychiatric Nurse who, for the past five years, worked in an Emergency Room in the role of a Psychiatric Liaison. In that job, Angela was quite accustomed to assessing people and referring them for adjunct services when and if they were needed. However, Angela just started a new position in an Outpatient Community Resource Referral Center for persons who have experienced domestic violence. Although Angela was new at this clinic, she knew some of the other professionals who worked there because she had worked with them in the past. Today was Angela's first day in this new role. Her dealings with the first two clients seemed quite routine in that they were both stable and had returned to the clinic for a follow-up Group Therapy session. However, a problem arose when Angela was required to do an intake assessment of a 20-year-old woman named Shannon, who had been living with her boyfriend, who was abusing her on a regular basis. Shannon had been referred to this Resource Center by a women's shelter where she had spent the weekend. She had just been released from the hospital, where she was treated for

(Box 3.8) cont.....

facial trauma and a concussion, injuries she had sustained at the hands of her partner. When Angela walked into the examination room, she couldn't help but notice that Shannon had two black eyes and, multiple facial bruising and sutured facial lacerations. Feeling slightly overwhelmed, Angela took a deep breath to get grounded, then proceeded to introduce herself to her client with the goal of making Shannon feel safe.

"Hello, my name is Angela, and I will be your nurse today. I will be asking some routine questions so I can get a better understanding of why you are here, and how we can best help you. I want you to know that this is a safe place. You will not be judged by me. Anything you share here will stay here and only be disclosed to other members of the team on an as needed basis. However, I will have to breach confidentiality if you admit to me that you intend on hurting yourself or anyone else. Does that make sense to you?"

Shannon was looking down at her shoes and did not attempt to make eye contact. She seemed so tired and a bit distracted. Angela paused to observe her client's demeanor, and after a few minutes, she spoke again.

"Is there anything you would like to ask me about the process, what my role is, or how I can help you?"

Jane shook her head from side to side, indicating a "No" as her non-verbal response. Angela waited before questioning her client again. To her surprise, Shannon looked up, appeared somewhat angry, then began to speak.

"You are just like the rest of them. This isn't my first time at a place like this. I have been beaten by my boyfriend many times before. I get taken by the police to the hospital. They tend to my injuries, then the police try and push me to lay charges against my partner. They say that a restraining order will help, but they are wrong. When I refuse to lay charges, they drop me off at a women's shelter. Then I get sent to a place like this where you try and teach me to be more assertive and to be stronger, or to attend groups where other women who have been beaten talk about how they cope, but none of that ever works out for me, none of it."

Shannon was now visibly crying. Huge tears were streaming down her injured face. She appeared so vulnerable, and her sense of hopelessness was paramount. Feeling somewhat uncomfortable, Angela proceeded to speak again but carefully chose her words so not to cause any more injury to an already tentative situation.

"I hear your pain and frustration. I am so sorry that we have let you down in the past. I am not sure what you want or need. What about if you tell me what you need so I can see what we can do to help you this time."

Shannon made eye contact with Angela for the first time. She wiped some of the tears away from her face with a Kleenex and responded to Angela's comments but in a much more subdued manner.

"Yes, I think that might be okay."

Angela proceeded to do her best to encourage Shannon to tell her what she needed, but Angela feared that Shannon would not trust her enough, after all, the system had clearly failed her in the past, and on more than one occasion.

"Shannon, I want to do my best to help you. Would you please tell me what you need for us to do."

Shannon spoke quietly but truthfully.

"You see, what I really need is to get away from my partner. A restraining order never works because he never obeys it. It just makes him more angry and more violent towards me. I must get away from him for good. The beatings have been getting more frequent and worse. He says that if I leave him, he will kill me, and I believe he will. I can't go back to my Mom because he will come to her house and take me away to beat me. That has happened before. Can you please help me this time? Please help me. I have to get away from him before he kills me."

(Box 3.8) cont.....

Angela could hear the fear, desperation, and urgency in her client's voice, and she wanted to help her. She then took a moment to choose her words carefully and then promised to seek the assistance of someone she knew would actually advocate for her client.

Shannon, I will tell you what I can do. I am going to go and speak with our Social Worker, someone who has the role of helping you to be able to go somewhere where you will feel safe and not be found by your attacker. I know her, I worked with her in the hospital, and she has experience helping people just like you. I have seen firsthand how she is able to get what needs to be done. If I were in a situation like you are in, she would be the person I would want to have fighting for me. I will go and speak with her right now and then bring her in to see you as soon as she is available. I need to warn you though, that what she has done before is to involve the police so they can arrest your boyfriend, charge him, and place him in a cell. That gives her time to make the necessary arrangements to keep you safe, which will involve you being somewhere he cannot easily find you, both in the short term, and in the long term. I promise you that she is discreet and is known as someone who is the voice for people like you who have survived terrible situations. Social Services will also be part of the plan to arrange for safe lodging, food, and other necessities. Are you willing to see our Social Worker to talk more about how she can help you? Her name is Susan."

Shannon looked up and made eye contact with Angela.

"Yes, I would like to see her, but can you tell her to please include me in the plans before making any big decisions, okay? I need to know what to expect."

Angela reassured Shannon that she would be consulted with the planning and implementation process before actions were taken. She then left the room to go and get the Social Worker.

NARRATIVE CASE STUDY TWO: IDENTIFICATION OF THEMES & ANALYSIS

Three key themes were identified from this story.

Theme # 1: Shannon was courageous enough to communicate to her nurse that the help she had received from Community Services in the past had not been enough to keep her physically safe from her partner's abuse. In fact, the violence had recently escalated, and she now feared for her life.

Theme # 1 Analysis: IPV negatively impacts the lives of those who are afflicted, and the violence often gets worse with time. Unfortunately, sometimes only short-term solutions are offered, even though what is needed is something much more. What is needed is a long-term strategy to keep the person safe from their perpetrator (Pemberton & Loeb, 2020).

Theme # 2: Angela was willing to advocate for Shannon by consulting with a Social Worker who would be the best person to implement a plan of action that would help to keep her safe.

Theme # 2 Analysis: Although immediate safety is a priority when assisting survivors of IPV, advocacy may also be needed for adequate safety to be implemented and sustained over time. Offering the person a more permanent and safe refuge from their abuser, temporary housing, financial support, legal aid, and other forms of assistance may be required (Sullivan & Goodman, 2019).

Theme # 3: Shannon clearly indicated that she wanted to be included in any plans that were developed on her behalf.

Theme # 3 Analysis: Any advocacy effort to keep a survivor of IPV safe from future harm must include them collaboratively in the planning process before actions are taken. It is about working with the survivor to honor voice and choice, and to address their individual and unique needs. This process enhances trust, empowers them to have a sense of control over their lives, and makes it more likely that they will go along with the specified plan of care (Cattaneo *et al.*, 2021).

QUESTIONS FOR FURTHER DISCUSSION

1-In your opinion, what did Angela do well? What, if anything, could she have done better?

2-Advocacy was mentioned as an intervention that is sometimes not a crucial part of the services offered to this population. If you were working at this Community Center, what would you like to see changed to make it more helpful to other survivors of IPV?

SELF-CARE STRATEGY: LEARNING HOW TO FOCUS MORE ON BEING THAN DOING

"The present moment is the only one that matters, and what you are doing right now is as delightful as anything else." Victor Shamas, Psychologist, Lecturer, and Author.

In our busy lives, we need to take the time to be present (Fig. **3.5**). The reality of our present-day world is that social media bombards us with ongoing distractions that beckon our constant attention. In current-day nursing practice, the pressure to do so is also paramount. So many tasks need attending to, so there is little or no time for being present. In fact, nurses have become used to excessive workloads and balancing high-acuity patients' needs with less time and scarce resources. They are led to believe that this is the new norm. Duffy (2018) points out that these types of excessive job-related pressures contribute to decreased work satisfaction, disrupt a sense of internal calmness, and, more importantly, can cause physical or emotional illness in the nurse. However, when a nurse is permitted to spend some time purposefully being present, they can slow down just long enough to reflect on their practice and to be aware of how their work may be negatively impacting them. Reflection may lead to increased awareness of how being confronted with human pain and suffering on an ongoing basis without the time or means to address it, is negatively affecting their emotional well-being (Duffy, 2018). Conversely, learning how to be more mindful and present assists in de-stressing and relaxation, and enhances a nurse's ability to cope.

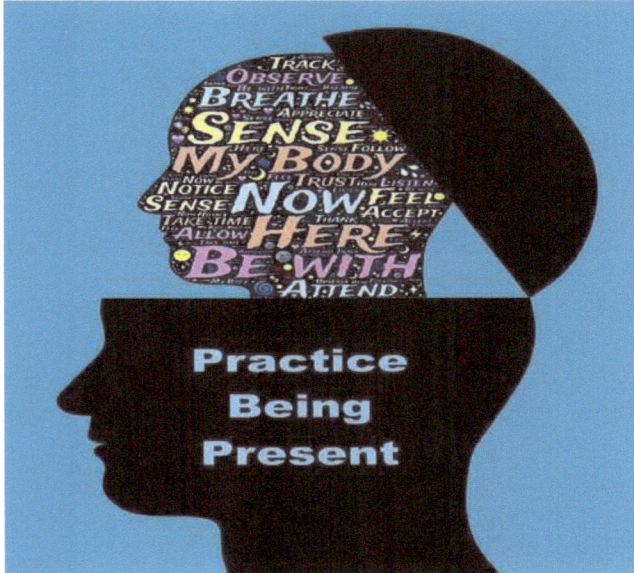

Fig. (3.5). Practice Being Present. Source: www.pixabay.com.

Therefore, to change the roller-coaster of *"doing," "being"* needs to be incorporated into a nurse's daily round. Duffy (2018) recommends setting aside 15 minutes a day for this crucially important undertaking. You can pick whatever time of day you feel is best for you. Your time for *"being"* can begin with some solitude in silence. Closing your eyes and becoming aware of your breathing is calming and is a great place to start. For others, you may want to participate in a creative activity that is awareness-raising, such as participating in art, music, writing, praying, or gardening. Some of you may even choose to join a yoga or meditation group (Duffy).

The Self-Care Challenge: Making Time to Focus More on Being than Doing

1-Every day, choose the time that suits you best and commit 15 minutes to being fully present and mindful. If inclined, reflect and write about your experiences in a journal. Hopefully, you will feel some benefit from this endeavor.

Note: Any suggested strategies are not intended to be a substitute for medical or psychological advice from a trained professional. The reader is, therefore, encouraged to seek medical or other professional help in any matters related to their physical or emotional health.

CONCLUSION

- Chapter Three explored crucial components of client-centered, person-centered, and resilience-focused approaches to trauma-informed care.
- We learned that although they differ in some ways, what each of these approaches has in common is the goal of helping people who have experienced trauma to heal.
- Essential features of client-centered care were identified. They include placing the person and their capacity for growth and change at the heart of all that occurs, prioritizing respect for the self-worth of every human being; and promoting strategies that foster unconditional positive regard.
- We learned that respect for self-worth is a hallmark of client-centered care because it embraces diversity, is inclusive, and welcomes everyone regardless of their situation.
- Unconditional positive regard consists of caring for someone without any conditions. Even if someone has made less favourable choices in life, they are still worthy of respect and compassionate care.
- These four ways to practice unconditional positive regard were recommended. Make this way of being a choice. Imagine that your client is someone in your life that you care for. Recognize that they are human, just like you. Take the time to listen to their story.
- In the client-centered care, the quality of the therapeutic relationship between the nurse and client/patient was deemed important for healing, as was the nurse's ability to apply professional knowledge competence to the care they provide.
- Not unlike client-centered care, person-centered care is built on the premise of putting the individual first. However, what is unique about person-centered care is its emphasis on assisting underrepresented groups like people with acute and chronic health issues and its focus on recovery.
- Collaboration and effective communication skills were declared essential features of a person-centered approach.
- Unique and beneficial ways to care for people from these populations were reviewed: the elderly, those with a disability, people with dementia, palliative care patients, and persons suffering from mental illness and substance use.
- Specific components of recovery-oriented person-centered care that were included in the discussion were a person's capacity for change and courage, their

responsibility for their own growth, and how to help them deal with resistance to change.

- Resilience is the ability to carry on and bounce back to original functioning after experiencing a trauma. We learned that a resilient person becomes stronger despite adversity because they develop a sturdy mindset a renewed commitment to life, utilize positive emotions, and learn from their mistakes.

- The discussion then moved to the importance of safely conducting trauma screening.

- It was pointed out that interpersonal partner violence (IPV) consists of violent acts sexual or physical in nature, by a person in a relationship with a survivor. Stranger rape differs somewhat in that the perpetrator of the sexual assault and the victim do not know one another. However, it needs to be pointed out that IPV is much more common than stranger rape.

- How to conduct screening safely and respectfully for survivors of IPV was presented, with the goal of challenging and transforming implicit biases and myths that exist in healthcare.

- Two Narrative Case Studies were reviewed. The first one demonstrated that when a client/patient crosses a professional boundary, a problem is created for the nurse. In this case, transference was identified as the reason for what happened. Nurses are advised to do their best to professionally address the boundary violation as soon as it occurs so that it will not progress any further.

- The second Narrative Case Study revealed that sometimes more than assessment is required when caring for a person who has experienced IPV. What may be needed is for the nurse to advocate for the individual to receive extra assistance when required to keep them safe from the risk of life-threatening harm.

- These four learning activities were recommended (*e.g.*, How to Practice Unconditional Positive Regard; Helpful Strategies to Utilize when Conducting a Trauma-assessment; Dispelling Myths Associated with IPV; and Survivor-Centered Approaches to utilize when caring for people who have suffered from IPV).

- At the closing of the Chapter, a self-care strategy was recommended that challenged nurses to set aside time to focus more on *being* than *doing*.

RECOMMENDED READINGS

Duffy, J. R. (2018). Quality caring in nursing and health systems. Springer Publishing Company.

Frankl, V. (2006). Man's search for meaning. Beakon Press.

Kuhl, D. (2002). What dying people want: Practical wisdom for the end of life. Anchor Canada.

Perlman, H. H. (1983). Relationship: The heart of helping people. The University of Chicago Press.

Rakel. D. (2018). The compassionate connection: The healing power of empathy and mindful listening. W. W. Norton and Company.

REFERENCES

Alzheimer's Association *What is Dementia?*. n.d. Available from: https://www.alz.org

Anderson, NE, Kent, B & Owens, RG (2015) Experiencing patient death in clinical practice: Nurses' recollections of their earliest memorable patient death. *Int J Nurs Stud,* 52, 695-704.
[http://dx.doi.org/10.1016/j.ijnurstu.2014.12.005] [PMID: 25577307]

Barclay, L (2016) In sickness and in dignity: A philosophical account of the meaning of dignity in health care. *Int J Nurs Stud,* 61, 136-41.
[http://dx.doi.org/10.1016/j.ijnurstu.2016.06.010] [PMID: 27351830]

Bassuk, EL, Latta, RE, Sember, R, Raja, S & Richard, M (2017) Universal design for underserved populations: Person-centered, recovery-oriented, and trauma-informed. *J Health Care Poor Underserved,* 28, 896-914.
[http://dx.doi.org/10.1353/hpu.2017.0087] [PMID: 28804068]

Bernock, D (2014) Emerging wings: A true story of lies, pain, and the love that heals. *4F Media.*

Brewerton, TD, Alexander, J & Schaefer, J (2019) Trauma-informed care and practice for eating disorders: personal and professional perspectives of lived experiences. *Eat Weight Disord,* 24, 329-38.
[http://dx.doi.org/10.1007/s40519-018-0628-5] [PMID: 30565188]

Brooks, R & Goldstein, S (2003) *The power of resilience: Achieving balance, confidence, and personal strength in your life.*McGraw Hill.

Canadian Nurses Association (CNA) (2017) *CNA code of ethics for registered nurses* Available from: https://cna.informz.ca/cna/data/images/Code_of_Ethics_2017_Edition_Secure_Interactive.pdf

Chopra, D (2005) *Peace is the way.*Three Rivers Press.

Collier, L (2016) Growth after trauma: Why some people are more resilient than others, and can it be taught. *J Trauma Stress,* 9, 455-71.
[http://dx.doi.org/10.1007/BF02103658]

Cooper, C, Coleman, J, Irvin, N, Lee, A & Antoine, D (2020) Personal trauma among healthcare providers: Implications for screening practices. *Women Health,* 60, 570-84.
[http://dx.doi.org/10.1080/03630242.2019.1683122] [PMID: 31665985]

Dowdell, EB & Speck, PM (2022) CE: Trauma-informed care in nursing. *Am J Nurs,* 122, 30-8.
[http://dx.doi.org/10.1097/01.NAJ.0000827328.25341.1f] [PMID: 35348516]

Duffy, JR (2018) *Quality caring in nursing and health systems.* Springer Publishing Company.
[http://dx.doi.org/10.1891/9780826181251]

Fadus, MC (2020) Rethinking the language of substance abuse. *Curr Psychiatr,* 19.
[http://dx.doi.org/10.12788/cp.0019]

Ferrucci, P (2006) *The power of kindness: The unexpected benefits of leading a compassionate life.* Penguin Group Inc.

Frankl, V (2006) *Man's search for meaning.* Beakon Press.

Fredrickson, B (2003) The value of positive emotions: The emerging science of positive psychology is coming to understand why it's good to feel good. *Am Sci,* 91, 330-5. https://www.jstor.org/stable/27858244
[http://dx.doi.org/10.1511/2003.26.330]

Goodman, LA, Cattaneo, LB, Thomas, K, Woulfe, J, Chong, SK & Smyth, KF (2015) Advancing domestic violence program evaluation: Development and validation of the Measure of Victim Empowerment Related to Safety (MOVERS). *Psychol Violence,* 5, 355-66.
[http://dx.doi.org/10.1037/a0038318]

Goodman, R (2017) Contemporary trauma theory and trauma-informed care in substance use disorders: A conceptual model for integrating coping and resilience. *Adv Soc Work,* 18, 186-201.
[http://dx.doi.org/10.18060/21312]

Haas, M (2015) *Bouncing forward: Transforming bad breaks into breakthroughs.* Atria & Enliven.

Hanga, K, DiNitto, DM, Wilken, JP & Leppik, L (2017) A person-centered approach in initial rehabilitation needs assessment: Experiences of persons with disabilities. *Alter,* 11, 251-66.
[http://dx.doi.org/10.1016/j.alter.2017.06.002]

Hartley, S, Raphael, J, Lovell, K & Berry, K (2020) Effective nurse–patient relationships in mental health care: A systematic review of interventions to improve the therapeutic alliance. *Int J Nurs Stud,* 102, 103490.
[http://dx.doi.org/10.1016/j.ijnurstu.2019.103490] [PMID: 31862531]

Haskins, J (2019) *What if we treated every patient as though they had lived through trauma?.* Available from: https://www.aamc.org/news-insights/what-if-we-treated-every-patient-though-they-had-lived-through-trauma

International Council of Nurses (ICN) (2021) *The ICN Code of Ethics for Nurses* Available from: https://www.icn.ch/system/files/2021-10/ICN_Code-of-Ethics_EN_Web_0.pdf

Isobel, S & Delgado, C (2018) Safe and collaborative skills: A step towards mental health nurses implementing trauma-informed care. *Arch Psychiatr Nurs,* 32, 291-6.
[http://dx.doi.org/10.1016/j.apnu.2017.11.017] [PMID: 29579526]

Isobel, S, Wilson, A, Gill, K & Howe, D (2021) 'What would a trauma-informed mental health service look like?' Perspectives of people who access services. *Int J Ment Health Nurs,* 30, 495-505.
[http://dx.doi.org/10.1111/inm.12813] [PMID: 33219725]

Jiwa, M (2018) The value of human connection in health care. *J Healthc Des,* 3, 139-40.
[http://dx.doi.org/10.21853/JHD.2018.68]

Kelly, JD, IV (2022) Your best life: In the lowest moments, an opportunity for post-traumatic growth. *Clin Orthop Relat Res,* 480, 33-5.
[http://dx.doi.org/10.1097/CORR.0000000000002070] [PMID: 34812794]

Jones, LM, Nolte, K, O'Brien, AJ, Trumbell, JM & Mitchell, KJ (2021) Factors related to providers screening children for behavioral health risks in primary care settings. *J Pediatr Nurs,* 59, 37-44.
[http://dx.doi.org/10.1016/j.pedn.2020.12.014] [PMID: 33460878]

Kelly, JD, IV (2022) Your best life: In the lowest moments, an opportunity for post-traumatic growth. *Clin Orthop Relat Res,* 480, 33-5.
[http://dx.doi.org/10.1097/CORR.0000000000002070] [PMID: 34812794]

Kim, SK & Park, M (2017) Effectiveness of person-centered care on people with dementia: a systematic review and meta-analysis. *Clin Interv Aging,* 12, 381-97.
[http://dx.doi.org/10.2147/CIA.S117637] [PMID: 28255234]

Knight, C (2015) Trauma-informed social work practice: Practice considerations and challenges. *Clin Soc Work J,* 43, 25-37.
[http://dx.doi.org/10.1007/s10615-014-0481-6]

Knight, C (2019) Trauma-informed practice and care: Implications for field instruction. *Clin Soc Work J,* 47, 79-89.
[http://dx.doi.org/10.1007/s10615-018-0661-x]

Kuhl, D (2002) *What dying people want: Practical wisdom for the end of life.* Anchor Canada.

Kulkarni, S J, Herman-Smith, R & Ross, T C (2015) Measuring intimate partner violence (IPV) service

providers' attitudes: The development of the survivor-defined advocacy scale (SDAS). *Journal of Family Violence,* 30, 911-21.
[http://dx.doi.org/10.1007/s10896-015-9719-5]

Kusmaul, N & Anderson, K (2018) Applying a trauma-informed perspective to loss and change in the lives of older adults. *Soc Work Health Care,* 57, 355-75.
[http://dx.doi.org/10.1080/00981389.2018.1447531] [PMID: 29522384]

Kwame, A & Petrucka, PM (2021) A literature-based study of patient-centered care and communication in nurse-patient interactions: barriers, facilitators, and the way forward. *BMC Nurs,* 20, 158.
[http://dx.doi.org/10.1186/s12912-021-00684-2] [PMID: 34479560]

Lantz, J (1992) Franklian psychotherapy with adults molested as children. *Journal of Religion and Health,,* 31, 297-37.

Levenson, J (2020) Translating trauma-informed principles into social work practice. *Soc Work,* 65, 288-98.
[http://dx.doi.org/10.1093/sw/swaa020] [PMID: 32676655]

Levin, Y, Lev Bar-Or, R, Forer, R, Vaserman, M, Kor, A & Lev-Ran, S (2021) The association between type of trauma, level of exposure and addiction. *Addict Behav,* 118, 106889.
[http://dx.doi.org/10.1016/j.addbeh.2021.106889] [PMID: 33735776]

Mary, A, Dayan, J, Leone, G, Postel, C, Fraisse, F, Malle, C, Vallée, T, Klein-Peschanski, C, Viader, F, de la Sayette, V, Peschanski, D, Eustache, F & Gagnepain, P (2020) Resilience after trauma: The role of memory suppression. *Science,* 367, eaay8477.
[http://dx.doi.org/10.1126/science.aay8477] [PMID: 32054733]

Matthews, S, Dwyer, R & Snoek, A (2017) Stigma and self-stigma in addiction. *J Bioeth Inq,* 14, 275-86.
[http://dx.doi.org/10.1007/s11673-017-9784-y] [PMID: 28470503]

McCormick, A, Scheyd, K & Terrazas, S (2018) Trauma-informed care and LGBTQ youth: Considerations for advancing practice with youth with trauma experiences. *Fam Soc,* 99, 160-9.
[http://dx.doi.org/10.1177/1044389418768550]

McLeod, S (2023) Available from: https://www.simplyPsychology.org/cognitive-therapy.html

Menschner, C & Maul, A (2016) *Issue Brief: Key ingredients for successful trauma-informed care implementation.* Available from: https://www.samhsa.gov/sites/default/files/programs_campaigns/childrens_mental_health/atc-whitepaper-040616.pdf

Miller, E & Barnie, K (2016) *Personal Outcomes: Learning from the meaningful and measurable project: Strengthening links between identity, action, and decision-making Summary Version.* Healthcare Improvement Scotland.

Miller, E, Stanhope, V, Restrepo-Toro, M & Tondora, J (2017) Person-centered planning in mental health: A transatlantic collaboration to tackle implementation barriers. *Am J Psychiatr Rehabil,* 20, 251-67.
[http://dx.doi.org/10.1080/15487768.2017.1338045] [PMID: 31632212]

Miller, WR & Moyers, TB (2015) The forest and the trees: Relational and specific factors in addiction treatment. *Addiction,* 110, 401-13.
[http://dx.doi.org/10.1111/add.12693] [PMID: 25066309]

Mirhaghi, A, Sharafi, S, Bazzi, A & Hasanzadeh, F (2017) Therapeutic relationship: Is it still heart of nursing? *Nurs Rep,* 7
[http://dx.doi.org/10.4081/nursrep.2017.6129]

Naparstek, B (2014) *Invisible heroes: Survivors of trauma and how they heal.* Bantam.

Nieforth, LO & Craig, EA (2021) Patient-centered communication (PCC) in equine assisted mental health. *Health Commun,* 36, 1656-65.
[http://dx.doi.org/10.1080/10410236.2020.1785376] [PMID: 32586134]

Noddings, N (2013) *Caring: A relational approach to ethics and moral education.* University of California Press.

O'Hara, C (2019) From therapy to therapeutic: The continuum of trauma-informed care. *Children Australia: Special Conference Issue – The Neuroscience of Trauma and Development in Everyday,* 44, 73-80.

Pemberton, JV & Loeb, TB (2020) Impact on women: Trauma-informed practice and feminist theory. *J Fem Fam Ther,* 32, 115-31.
[http://dx.doi.org/10.1080/08952833.2020.1793564]

Perlman, HH (1983) *Relationship: The heart of helping people.* The University of Chicago Press.

Poseck, BV, Baquero, BC & Jimenez, MLV (2006) The traumatic experience from positive psychology: Resiliency and post-traumatic growth. *Pap Psicol,* 27, 40-9.http://www.cop.es/papeles

Positive Psychology n.d. Available from: https://postivepsychology.com

Pringle, J, Johnston, B & Buchanan, D (2015) Dignity and patient-centred care for people with palliative care needs in the acute hospital setting: A systematic review. *Palliat Med,* 29, 675-94.
[http://dx.doi.org/10.1177/0269216315575681] [PMID: 25802322]

ProQuest (2020) Available from: https:// www.proquest.com /trade-journals/ pps-alert- long- term- care-2020- index.do

Psych Central (2018) *Rescuing, resenting, and regretting: A codependent pattern.* Available from: https://www.psychcentral.com/blog/imperfect/2018/06/rescuing-resenting-andregrettin--a-codependent-pattern#what-is-rescuing

Purkey, E, Patel, R & Phillips, SP (2018) Trauma-informed care: Better care for everyone. *Can Fam Physician,* 64, 170-2.
[PMID: 29540379]

Quaile, H C & Benyounes-Ulrich, J (2021) Trauma-informed are part I: The road to its operationalization. *A Clinical Journal for NPs and Women's Healthcare,* 9, 1-7.

Rakel, D (2018) *The compassionate connection: The healing power of empathy and mindful listening.*W. W. Norton & Company.

Ray, MA (2018) *Transcultural caring dynamics in nursing and health care* F. A. Davis Company.

Rogers, C (1980) *A way of being.*Houghton Mifflin.

Rosenberg, MB (2003) *Nonviolent communication: A language of life.*Puddle Dancer Press.

Scherer, MJ (2014) From people-centered to person-centered services, and back again. *Disabil Rehabil Assist Technol,* 9, 1-2.
[http://dx.doi.org/10.3109/17483107.2013.870239] [PMID: 24304239]

Seligman, M (2011) *Flourish: A new understanding of happiness and well-being – and how to achieve them.*Nicholas Brealey Publishing.

Sheard, M (2013) *Mental toughness: The mindset behind sporting achievement.* Routledge Taylor & Francis Group.

Sinclair, S, Norris, JM, McConnell, SJ, Chochinov, HM, Hack, TF, Hagen, NA, McClement, S & Bouchal, SR (2016) Compassion: A scoping review of the healthcare literature. *BMC Palliat Care,* 15, 6.
[http://dx.doi.org/10.1186/s12904-016-0080-0] [PMID: 26786417]

Sowers, WE (2022) Recovery and person-centered care: Empowerment, collaboration, and integration. In: Sowers, W.E., McQuistion, H.L., Ranz, J.M., Feldman, J.M., Runnels, P.S., (Eds.), *Textbook of Community Psychiatry* Springer 21-32.
[http://dx.doi.org/10.1007/978-3-031-10239-4_3]

Stephany, K (2012) Each day is a new creation: Guidelines on living a life on purpose. *Balboa Press: A Division of Hay House.*

Stephany, K (2017) *How to help the suicidal person to choose life: The ethic of care & empathy as an indispensable tool for intervention.*Bentham Science Publishers Pte. Ltd.

Stephany, K (2020) *The ethic of care: A moral compass for Canadian nursing practice.* Bentham Science Publishers Pte. Ltd.

Stephany, K (2022) *Cultivating empathy: Inspiring health Professionals to communicate more effectively* Bentham Science Publishers Pte. Ltd.
[http://dx.doi.org/10.2174/97898150364801220101]

Stokes, Y, Jacob, JD, Gifford, W, Squires, J & Vandyk, A (2017) Exploring nurses' knowledge and experiences related to trauma-informed care. *Glob Qual Nurs Res,* 4.
[http://dx.doi.org/10.1177/2333393617734510] [PMID: 29085862]

Substance Abuse and Mental Health Services Administration (SAMHSA) (2014) *Trauma-Informed Care in Behavioral Health Services* Available from: https://store.samhsa.gov/sites/default/files/d7/priv/sma14-4816.pdf

Sullivan, CM & Goodman, LA (2019) Advocacy with survivors of intimate partner violence: What it is, what it isn't, and why it's critically important. *Violence Against Women,* 25, 2007-23.
[http://dx.doi.org/10.1177/1077801219875826] [PMID: 31718528]

Taccini, F & Mannarini, S (2023) An attempt to conceptualize the phenomenon of stigma toward intimate partner violence survivors: A systematic review. *Behav Sci (Basel),* 13, 194.
[http://dx.doi.org/10.3390/bs13030194] [PMID: 36975219]

Valente, SM (2017) Managing professional and nurse-patient relationship boundaries in mental health. *J Psychosoc Nurs Ment Health Serv,* 55, 45-51. https://di.org/10.3928/02793695-20170119-09
[http://dx.doi.org/10.3928/02793695-20170119-09] [PMID: 28135391]

van der Kolk, B (2014) *The body keeps score: Brain, mind, and body in the healing of trauma.* Viking Penguin.

Wanko Keutchafo, EL, Kerr, J & Baloyi, OB (2022) A model for effective non-verbal communication between nurses and older patients: A grounded theory of inquiry. *Healthcare,* 10, 2119.
[http://dx.doi.org/10.3390/healthcare10112119] [PMID: 36360461]

Waters, L, Algoe, SB, Dutton, J, Emmons, R, Fredrickson, BL, Heaphy, E, Moskowitz, JT, Neff, K, Niemiec, R, Pury, C & Steger, M (2022) Positive psychology in a pandemic: Buffering, bolstering, and building mental health. *J Posit Psychol,* 17, 303-23.
[http://dx.doi.org/10.1080/17439760.2021.1871945]

Welfare-Wilson, A & J, B (2023) "Were you wearing underwear?" Stigma and fears around sexual violence: A narrative of stranger rape and considerations for mental health nurses when working with survivors. *J Psychiatr Ment Health Nurs,* 30, 141-7.
[http://dx.doi.org/10.1111/jpm.12864] [PMID: 35962647]

World Health Organization (WHO) (2020) *Palliative care defined* Available from: https://www.who.int/teams/integrated-health-services/clinical-services-and-systems/palliative-care

Zhao, J, Gao, S, Wang, J, Liu, X & Hao, Y (2016) Differentiation between two healthcare concepts: Person-centered and patient-centered care. *Int J Nurs Sci,* 3, 398-402.
[http://dx.doi.org/10.1016/j.ijnss.2016.08.009]

Trauma Recovery from a Positive Psychology and Post-Traumatic Growth Perspective

Abstract: The aim of **Chapter Four** is to demonstrate that living a better life after adversity is possible when adequate support is offered. Therefore, positive psychology and post-traumatic growth are two recovery-focused trauma-informed approaches that are highly recommended to help people who have experienced adversity. Positive psychology studies human well-being and optimal functioning. Post-traumatic growth refers to positive changes in someone's coping that occur from sorting through their experience of trauma. Three different responses to traumatic stress are explained. For instance, certain people bounce right back after an adverse event, others develop maladaptive functioning, and a third reaction results in post-traumatic growth. The particular response that a person experiences is somewhat context-dependent. After trauma occurs, positive changes in brain function are made possible through neuroplasticity. Positive Psychology and trauma-informed care share the common goal of helping people to live better lives, but they also differ. For instance, positive psychology strategies are designed to be used by everyone and are therefore not limited to those who have experienced trauma. The five key elements of well-being theory called PERMA are presented, such as positive emotions, engagement, relationships, meaning, and accomplishment. Positive emotions are deemed essential for life satisfaction. Work-related well-being was later developed and called PERMA+4 and is associated with physical health, mindset, work environment, and economic security. Flourishing is a central component of well-being theory and consists of the capacity to be satisfied with one's life achievements and being involved in something that is meaningful. The following strategies are known to facilitate well-being, being grateful, a positive attitude, random acts of kindness, and positive psychotherapy. Positive psychotherapy is an effective method to treat trauma because it focuses on a person's strengths and weaknesses but also uses a person's character signature strengths to help them move forward. Appreciation for life, new possibilities, relating to others, personal strength, and spiritual change are the five domains of post-traumatic growth. Meaning-making, instillation of hope, and self-compassion are identified as additional life-enhancing responses to adversity. Two Narrative Case Studies are presented. The first one identifies how a student nurse felt unprepared to discuss spiritual issues with her patient. The second case study demonstrates how nurturing mindful self-compassion helps a teen to heal from childhood trauma. The following three learning activities are suggested, debating the value of positive emotions, understanding the 24 signature strengths of positive psychotherapy, and lessons learned from those who have experienced post-traumatic growth. The chapter ends by recommending specific gratitude-enhancing self-care strategies.

Kathleen Stephany

Keywords: Accomplishment, Character Strengths, Coherence, Creative Visualization, Economic Security, Emotional Intelligence, Engagement, Existential Reevaluation, Flourish, Flow, Gratitude, Gratitude Journal, Gratitude Visit, Guilt, Hope, Humanistic Psychology, Interpretive Reality, Kindness, Logotherapy, Meaning, Meaning-Making, Meditation, Mindful Self-Compassion, Mindfulness, Mindset, Neuroplasticity, Ontology, Perception Of Reality, Perma, Perma+4, Physical Health, Positive Emotions, Positive Psychology, Positive Psychotherapy, Positive Psychotherapy Sessions, Post-Traumatic Growth, Psychological Preparedness, Purpose, Relationships, Religion, Self-Compassion, Shame, Signature Strengths, Significance, Social Intelligence, Spirituality, Strengths Due To Suffering, Subjective Well-Being, Trauma-Informed Care, Traumatic Stress Response, Well-Being Theory, What-Went Well Exercise, Will To Meaning, Work Environment, 24 Signature Strengths.

LEARNING GUIDE

After completing this chapter, the reader should be able to:

- Explain the three different outcomes to a traumatic stress response.
- Gain an awareness of how neuroplasticity enables the human brain to change.
- Describe positive psychology, what it shares with trauma-informed care and how they differ.
- Gain an understanding of the five key elements of well-being theory, the framework for work-related well-being, and the core components of flourishing.
- Learn about positive psychology strategies that foster well-being.
- Recognize the value of positive psychotherapy and how it is implemented.
- Describe post-traumatic growth, explain how it differs from resilience, and the role that struggling plays in recovery.
- Describe the three models, two interpretive stages, and the five domains of post-traumatic growth.
- Understand the similarities and differences between religion and spirituality, and when participation in these practices may be inappropriate in relation to trauma-informed care.
- Identify three additional life-enhancing responses to adversity that facilitate positive outcomes.
- Review two Narrative Case Studies and ensuing Thematic Analysis. The first one identifies how a student nurse felt unprepared to discuss spiritual issues with her patient. The second one demonstrates how nurturing mindful self-compassion helps a teen to heal from childhood trauma.

- Participate in these learning activities (*e.g.*, Debating the Value of Positive Emotions; Understanding the 24 Signature Character Strengths of Positive Psychotherapy; and Lessons Learned from Those who Experienced Post-Traumatic Growth following Adversity).
- Consider adopting at least one of three suggested gratitude enhancing self-care strategies.

INTRODUCTION TO CHAPTER FOUR

"Success is not final; failure is not fatal. It is the courage to continue that counts" Winston Churchill, Former Prime Minister of the United Kingdom.

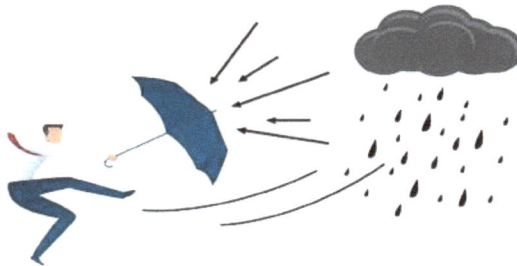

Fig. (4.1). Post-traumatic Growth and Perseverance. Source: www.pixabay.com.

Trauma-informed care sets out to help people who have experienced trauma and focuses on prevention, intervention, and treatments that are evidence-based and cater to the needs of those who have experienced adversity (Menschner & Maul, 2016). Subsequently, chapter four presents a variety of ways to facilitate trauma-informed recovery from a positive psychology and post-traumatic growth perspective. **Positive Psychology** is the scientific study of human well-being, optimal functioning, and flourishing (Seligman, 2011). Positive Psychology and trauma-informed care share the common goal of helping people to live better lives. However, positive psychology strategies are designed to be used by everyone, including those who have not experienced adversity (Ginwright, 2018). **Post-traumatic growth** consists of positive changes in a person's life following trauma that develops as a direct result of their struggle to work through and persevere in spite of what happened to them (Fig. **4.1**). What will become apparent in the ensuring discussion is that living a more fulfilling life is possible for those who have survived adversity, especially if they receive adequate support. The chapter begins by pointing out that the responses to traumatic stress are not always negative.

THE TRAUMATIC STRESS RESPONSE

Three Different Responses

A **traumatic stress response** usually consists of a specific but normal neuropsychological reaction to an abnormal event. It may include a sequela of emotional responses that usually subside with time. However, what needs to be emphasized, is that the outcome of all psychological stress does not always result in negative repercussions. These three different outcomes of a traumatic stress response may occur. The first is a normal reaction and consists of an immediate emotional reaction followed by a quick return to normal functioning. The second response can result in the development of maladaptive functioning, and a third reaction may stimulate post-traumatic growth (Christopher, 2004).

The Context-Dependent Individual Response to Stress

The particular response to stress that a person experiences is somewhat context-dependent, and is somewhat due to the absence or presence of support. An unhealthy response is more likely when chronic stress occurs in the absence of personal or social support. This may result in alterations in brain function that lead to a decreased ability to function normally, and an array of short-term or long-term physical and emotional abnormalities, such as physical diseases, mental disorders, substance use, and an overall decreased life span (Christopher, 2004; Oral *et al.*, 2016).

Conversely, the opposite is also true. If a child or adult who has experienced an adverse event, exists in a loving and empathetic environment, the stress they experience may be more tolerable, can result in less negative repercussions, and does not necessarily interfere with coping (Oral *et al.*, 2016). Furthermore, someone who can positively work through and adapt to the effect of adversity and become stronger because of it, experiences post-traumatic growth (Kelly, 2022). These people usually possess strong self-esteem, view life's challenges with resilience, and are involved in healthy relationships with significant others (Christophe, 2004).

NEUROPLASTICITY

"An influx of new research explores how our brains do continue to change and how our very thoughts impact those changes. This natural tendency of our brains to rewire is neuroplasticity, which can be influenced by external and internal factors." Tina Hallis, Scientist & Author.

The Human Brain's Capacity for Change

There is a need to move beyond a focus on the negative repercussions of adversity and to pay attention to factors that can improve the lives of those who have survived trauma (Leitch, 2017). What is exciting to report is that a person's ability to adapt and learn healthy ways of coping after experiencing adversity is supported by the research conducted into neuroplasticity (van de Kolk, 2014) (Fig. **4.2**).

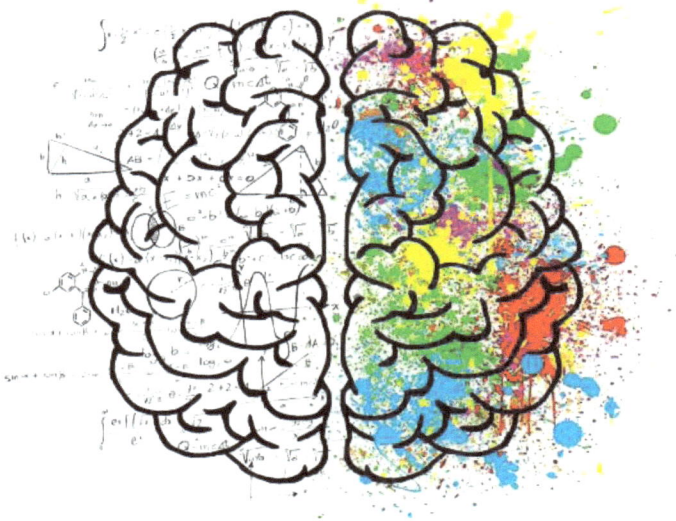

Fig. (4.2). The Human Brain. Source: www.pixabay.com.

Neuroplasticity refers to the brain's intrinsic ability to change and its ongoing capacity to do so, by developing new neural connections that are experience-based (Costandi, 2016; Pal & Elbers, 2018). The good news is that evidence from research supports the hypothesis that the brain can positively adapt to strategies that redirect its functioning through beneficial behaviours. For example, a study into brain neuroplasticity conducted by Shaffer (2016) on older individuals demonstrated that lifestyle interventions like increased exercise, a healthier diet, and improved sleep, not only improved their overall physical health, but also enhanced brain function (Shaffer, 2016). Additional research into brain plasticity by McEwen (2016) and the effect of nonpharmacological health-enhancing strategies also revealed promising results. They found that brain functioning improved through regular physical activity, mindfulness meditation, increased social support, and finding purpose in life. The results also revealed an increase in cognitive ability, enhanced emotional regulation, and increased resilience, all following the introduction of healthy lifestyle interventions (McEwen).

POSITIVE PSYCHOLOGY

"The aim of Positive Psychology is to catalyze a change in psychology from a preoccupation only with repairing the worst things in life to also building the best qualities in life." Martin Seligman, American Psychologist, Educator, and Author

Positive Psychology involves the empirical study of what is good about humans, and their capacity for strength, growth, and endurance (Macfarlane & Carson, 2019) (Fig **4.3**). Its optimistic effects are apparent on both the personal and collective level. On an individual level, Positive Psychology places the emphasis on subjective experiences as lived by the person, and their capacity to develop traits that contribute to their overall well-being, happiness, courage, hope, wisdom, and optimism. On a more collective level, Positive Psychology is concerned with a sense of civic duty, responsibility for others, tolerance, inclusivity, and a noble work ethic (Csikszentmihalyi & Seligman, 2014). Positive Psychology and trauma-informed care share the common goal of helping people to live better lives. However, Positive Psychology strategies are designed to be used by everyone, including those who have not experienced adversity. The discussion about Positive Psychology that ensues will focus on some historical background; the five key elements of well-being; its positive effects on physical health; interventions that promote wellness in nursing practice; and strategies that can be applied in everyday life.

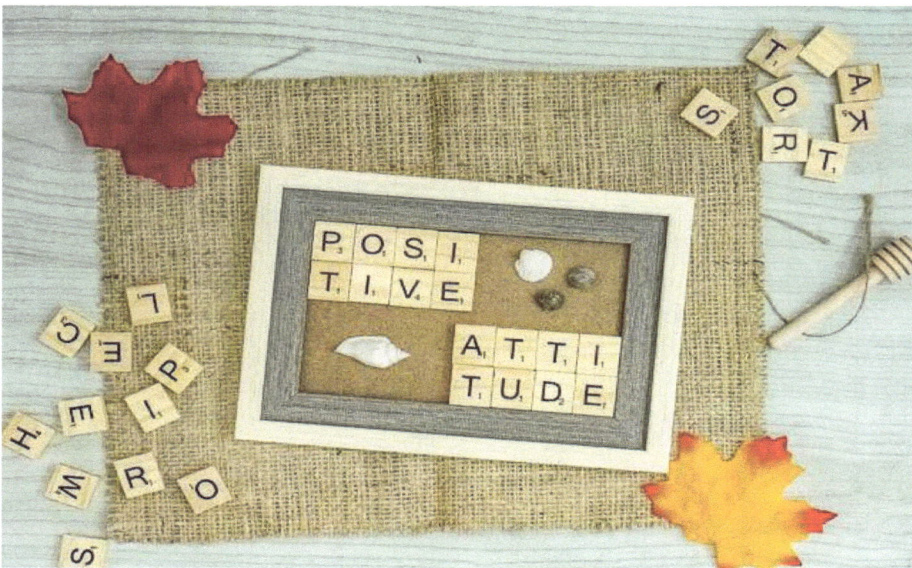

Fig. (4.3). Positive Attitude & Positive Psychology. Source: www.pixabay.com.

Historical Underpinnings of Positive Psychology: From A Focus on Pathology to Higher Functioning

Although Positive Psychology became more widely noticed near the end of the 20th Century, its roots are thought to run deep and can be traced as far back as the early 1900s and the work of William James on human consciousness and emotions (Froh, 2004). Yet, despite early interest in the notion of positive psychological functioning, Psychology in general remained primarily focused on pathology for the first half of the 20th Century. This emphasis was based on the assumption that humans do not necessarily possess the right character traits to be empowered to overcome obstacles and setbacks (Csikszentmihalyi & Seligman, 2014). Nevertheless, in the 1950s Psychologists in the Humanistic Psychology movement became disillusioned with the disease-obsessed approach to human functioning and replaced it with something hopeful and optimistic (Froh, 2004). For example, **Humanistic Psychology** proposed a view of human beings as uniquely bestowed with a capacity for growth and change, and a desire for well-being and happiness (Maslow, 1954). These notions are not unlike those later proposed by proponents of Positive Psychology. However, one key difference between the Humanistic movement and Positive Psychology did exist. Although Humanistic study explored what it meant to be human, it was more qualitative and experienced based on its approach to studying human behaviour. Whereas, from the onset, Positive Psychology insisted that there be a strong emphasis on ensuring that any findings and conclusions concerning the study of human functioning, be substantiated by rigorous and quantifiable empirical research (Cabrera & Donaldson, 2023; Froh, 2004).

Positive Psychology Gets Its Historical Debut

Historical accounts of Positive Psychology associate its public recognition with a Presidential address given to the American Psychological Association in 1998 by Dr. Martin Seligman (Linley *et al.*, 2007). In his speech, Dr. Seligman admitted publicly that the discipline of Psychology had concentrated for far too long on a disease-orientated mental deficit focus, and that a different, more positive, and empirically supported new approach to Psychology was needed (Cabrera & Donaldson, 2023). Prior to and following that notorious address Dr. Seligman was instrumental in attracting and sustaining substantial and on-going funding to conduct research into this new area (Seligman, 2011). He was also able to attract prominent scientists, and other major academics and professionals, into being involved in this scientific inquiry. Soon the influence was expanded beyond psychology to include other disciplines like economics, sociology, and anthropology (Linley *et al.*,). Presently the discipline of Positive Psychology exists as a credible therapeutic service and evidence-based psychological movement, with an expanding research base, and continued world-renowned interest (Cabrera & Donaldson).

Seligman (2011) also coined the term **flourishing** to describe how Positive Psychology can positively impact a person's life by increasing happiness, improving relationships, enhancing purpose, and providing people with the confidence to pursue their dreams. The subsequent discussion presents an overview of key elements of Positive Psychology's well-being theory, followed by the core components of flourishing.

PERMA: The Five Key Elements of Well-being Theory

Dr. Seligman (2011) believed that people not only pursue happiness for their own sake, but what they specifically focus on, varies and is quite individual in nature. He concluded that well-being is the key subject of Positive Psychology and not authentic happiness, which was his earlier choice. Seligman's reasons for replacing a theory of happiness had to do with his conclusion that happiness is too focused on cheerfulness, good mood, and other positive emotions, and did not adequately reflect what people intentionally choose to make them happy. Subsequently, Seligman developed a **well-being theory** that consists of elements that are measurable and are comprised of what people are willing to choose as contributing factors to their life satisfaction (Seligman). Seligman and colleagues subsequently came up with five key elements of **well-being theory** represented by the acronym **PERMA**, which stands for positive emotion, engagement, relationships, meaning, and accomplishment (Seligman) (Fig. **4.4**).

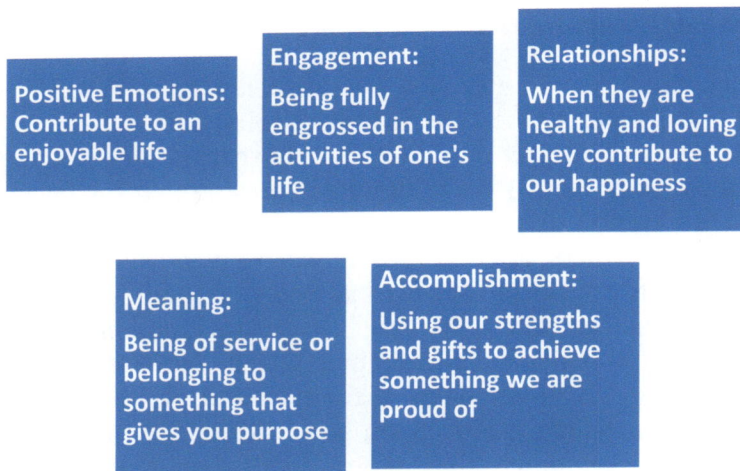

Positive Emotions: Contribute to an enjoyable life

Engagement: Being fully engrossed in the activities of one's life

Relationships: When they are healthy and loving they contribute to our happiness

Meaning: Being of service or belonging to something that gives you purpose

Accomplishment: Using our strengths and gifts to achieve something we are proud of

Fig. (4.4). PERMA: The five key elements of well-being (as adapted from Donaldson *et al.*, 2022; Seligman, 2011).

Positive Emotions

The ongoing investigation of what makes life worth living was the impetus for recognizing specific positive emotions and their importance (Donaldson, 2022: Fredrickson, 2003). Therefore, it is not surprising to learn that the first component of well-being theory is **positive emotions** because they contribute to life satisfaction and happiness. The following positive emotions have been specifically identified as significant, the capacity to feel happy, and the experiences of joy, love, and gratitude (Donaldson; Seligman, 2011). Why are positive emotions so important? The experience of positive emotions leads to feeling pleasure, comfort, and pleasantness in life which contributes to an enjoyable and significant experience of living (Seligman). For instance, psychological research revealed that when people experience positive emotions they think more expansively and creatively, and it benefits them in other ways (Fredrickson). They appear to enjoy what they are doing at the moment and are more fully engaged with life. A habitual focus on positive emotions instead of negative ones is also correlated with improved overall health, an increase in longevity, enhanced social bonds with others, and other life-enhancing effects (Csikszentmihalyi & Seligman, 2014; Fredrickson).

Engagement

The art of **engagement** in well-being theory is the ability to be fully engrossed in the activities of one's life. When someone is fully engaged in something of interest, they become totally captivated by what they are doing (Donaldson *et al.*, 2022). Another way to describe this experience is being in the flow. **Flow** is a term in Positive Psychology that was coined by Mihaly Csikszentmihalyi. To be in the flow is to be so fully absorbed in an activity that you love that nothing else matters, and it is as if time stands still. For example, when you are in the flow you are mindfully present, while wholeheartedly participating in an activity that challenges you and makes you feel productive and happy (Nakamura & Csikszentmihalyi, 2014). Flow may happen when you are creating something new, listening to music, or doing something else that you totally enjoy, but it also occurs when you are doing work that you really love (Nakamura & Csikszentmihalyi; Seligman, 2011). However, to experience this phenomenon, you must be able to identify what your unique gifts and abilities are and pursue them (Seligman). For me, being in the flow happens in one of these ways, when I am gardening, researching, or writing.

Relationships

In the well-being theory, ideal **relationships** are healthy and loving and contribute to our happiness (Donaldson *et al.*, 2022). The late Helen Perlman (1979) wrote an amazing book called, *Relationship: The Heart of Helping People.* I can remember reading this book in one sitting and feeling forever changed by what I learned. In her writings, Perlman said a great deal about relationships. What really stood out for me was her comparison of what it is like to be alone when experiencing stress and adversity, *versus* being deeply cared for by another person. She explained that our feeling of loneliness in an hour of extreme difficulty with no one to turn to can make that experience unbearable. Conversely, Perlman pointed out how the opposite is also true. When we feel defeated, there is nothing more comforting, than to experience a genuine sense of being understood and accepted unconditionally by another human being who cares about us, and our situation. In her own words, "(t)hat is what a helping relationship is all about" (Perlman, 1979, p. 11).

In well-being theory relationships are important for similar reasons because people are naturally social creatures, and meaningful connections with others are an integral part of the human experience (Khaw & Kern, 2014). Healthy relationships with others are also known to decrease one's risk for depression and other mental illnesses, contribute to increase physical health, can prolong one's lifespan, and decrease suicidal risk (Khaw & Kern; Tay *et al.*, 2013). Being able to maintain, sustain, and nourish healthy, loving, and beneficial relationships with others, also contributes positively to our overall wellness and happiness (Donaldson *et al.*, 2022). Some aspects of a relationship that make it good consist of the ability to give and receive appreciation, demonstrate mutual respect, and be trustworthy (Walker, 2010). Not judging is another essential component, especially in situations where someone has experienced trauma and feels shame (Ashley, 2020; Stephany, 2020).

Meaning

The well-being theoretical notion of **meaning** involves being of service to a cause or belonging to something that gives you purpose (Donaldson *et al.*, 2022). Meaning is not solely based on subjective experience but must meet three clear criteria. It must add to one's overall well-being. It is usually sought after for its own sake, and the meaning that is experienced exists without the prerequisite of positive emotion (Seligman, 2011).

Martela and Steger (2016) have identified three ways that meaning is experienced in life that are similar yet different in certain ways. They consist of coherence, purpose, and significance. **Coherence** refers to making sense of one's life and the direction it has taken. For example, your life is considered to be coherent when you can make plans, successfully carry them out, and feel comfort in the predictability of the outcome. The opposite of coherence is a feeling of uncertainty. **Purpose** consists of a person's reason for getting up in the morning and knowing where they are headed. It entails having clear goals and pursuing and achieving them. However, in comparison, a life without purpose consists of a loss of direction and feeling stuck. **Significance** is the belief that somehow one's life is worthwhile, means something, and that you have something to look forward to. Alternatively, a life without significance may be experienced as aimless (Martela & Steger).

Accomplishment

In well-being theory, **accomplishment** is the ability to use our strengths and gifts to achieve something that gives us deep satisfaction (Rashid & Seligman, 2018). What gives a person a sense of accomplishment can be a part of their job or career, or it can be something outside of work. However, the key is that it makes the individual feel productive and happy, and they pursue this activity for its own sake, even if there is no positive reward for engaging in it (Seligman, 2011). It is the act of participation that makes them feel good when they are fully engaged in that particular activity. Accomplishment is also not about merely winning for winning sake, nor does it entail having excessive possessions. It is about living an achieving lifestyle where you pursue goals that challenge and interest you (Donaldson *et al.*, 2022).

PERMA+4: A Framework for Work-Related Well-being

Seligman (2011) never intended for well-being theory to be restricted to only a few elements of a person's life but argued that this theory was rather fluid in nature, and dependent on what free people would choose to identify with. Therefore, it is not surprising that four additional components of well-being were developed that are associated with work or employment added to the original five PERMA. They were identified as **PERMA+4** which consists of a framework for work-related well-being and these four elements, physical health, mindset, work environment, and economic security (Donaldson *et al.*, 2022) (Fig. **4.5**). These specific elements were chosen because they were empirically validated as contributing to a person's work-related well-being, enhanced and sustainable work achievement, and overall success (Donaldson *et al.*, 2022).

| Physical Health: An essential ingredient to buffer someone from mental illness | Healthy Mindset: Is about work success | Work Environment: When it is positive it leads to increased work satisfaction | Economic Security: Is crucially important to people |

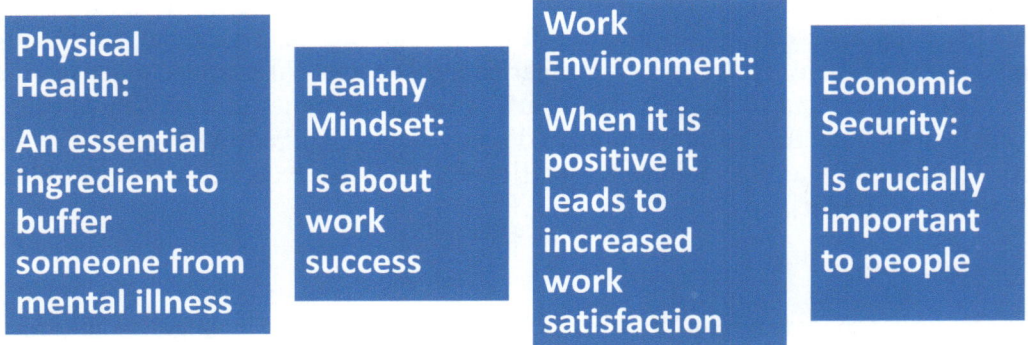

Fig. (4.5). PERMA+4: A Framework for Work-Related Well-being (as adapted from Donaldson *et al.*, 2022).

Physical Health

In the PERMA+4 work-related framework, physical health was declared as an essential and necessary ingredient to buffer a person from developing mental stress or illness. The following aspects of physical wellness were identified as important, physical fitness, healthy diet, overall general health, absence of disease, the ability to execute work-related duties, and one's overall psychological functioning. For instance, a person who excels in their work, in terms of performance, achievement, and personal satisfaction, usually scores high in all areas of health functionality (Cabrera & Donaldson, 2023: Donaldson *et al.*, 2022).

Mindset

A healthy mindset was chosen as an additional element of work-related success. That is because in addition to their work ethic and innate skills, a positive mindset results in employment success due to a person's intrinsic belief that they can and will succeed. For example, people with a healthy frame of mind welcome challenges and learn from their mistakes. Conversely, those who hold a fixed closed mindset believe that they are incapable of change. They avoid challenges, view mistakes as directly due to their intrinsic flaws, and are less prone to succeed in work (Donaldson *et al.*, 2022).

Work Environment

It has been verified that a work environment can have a considerable impact on a person's physical and emotional well-being, especially since most people spend roughly a third of their life time in some form of employment. Positive workplace atmospheres that are aesthetically appealing, comfortable to work in, with good ventilation, free of noisy distractions, and where employees feel valued, contribute to work satisfaction. Furthermore, work environments that support close connections and good relationships with others have a direct and significant impact on workplace satisfaction and overall employee performance (Donaldson *et al*.,).

Economic Security

According to Donaldson *et al*., (2022), a person's income, their ability to save for the future, and to feel a sense of economic security and stability have been the most compelling predictors of work-related well-being. The reasons attributed to this empirically verifiable finding have to do with the fact that if someone cannot meet their basic physiological needs, like housing, adequate food, and paying bills, they develop increased stress, and may develop mental illness in the form of anxiety and depression. Those who find themselves in extreme financial debt with little ability to rectify their predicament also experience a higher risk of suicide. Alternatively, when someone feels a sense of security about their overall current and future financial situation, they are more likely to engage with life and make plans for their future. That is why research evidence indicates that strategies that teach people how to better manage their financial situation are effective in positively affecting their overall health and happiness (Donaldson *et al*., 2022; Lowe *et al*., 2018).

Flourishing: Pursuing What Really Makes Us Happy

Flourishing in Positive Psychology has been identified as the central component of well-being theory and consists of the capacity to feel a sense of satisfaction and contentment with our lives and accomplishments. It is about being involved in something that is meaningful, gives us a sense of purpose, and fosters close social connections with others (Seligman, 2011).

The Core Components of Flourishing

Positive emotions, optimal functioning, optimistic thoughts, and healthy supportive relationships, have all been identified as key components to flourishing. According to Seligman (2011), to flourish, a person must possess all of these three core features, positive emotions, engagement/interest, and meaning/purpose. They must also display three of these six additional features, self-esteem, optimism, resilience, vitality, self-determination, and positive relationships. Fredrickson (200) identified positive emotions as the foundation for all the other elements because evidence indicates that they contribute to the increased quality of life, life success, and longevity. Increased life span is thought to be due to a positive outlook that in turn enhances coping, adaptability, resilience, perseverance, and hope. A Learning Activity is suggested in Box (**4.1**) that encourages debate over the value of positive emotions.

Box 4.1. Learning activity: debating the value of positive emotions.

You have just read about Positive Psychology, well-being theory and flourishing. In small groups spend time reviewing additional empirical evidence that supports why positive emotions are beneficial and then come to together as a whole class to share your findings.

POSITIVE PSYCHOLOGY STRATEGIES THAT FOSTER WELL-BEING

Positive Psychology strategies are evidence-based activities that are known to foster well-being, especially if they are practised on a regular basis. They can improve a person's mood and even enhance their overall physical and emotional health if practiced on a regular basis (Macfarlane & Carson, 2019). The following specific recommended approaches are presented along with the rationale for their usefulness, being grateful, possessing a positive attitude, random acts of kindness, and positive psychotherapy. The first three strategies can be easily incorporated into a person's daily life without additional professional assistance. However, positive psychotherapy components are therapeutic modalities that are usually implemented by a trained professional like a Psychiatrist, Psychologist, Social Worker, or Counsellor.

Being Grateful

"Gratitude unlocks the fullness of life. It turns what we have into enough, and more. It turns denial into acceptance, chaos to order, confusion to clarity. It can turn a meal into a feast, a house into a home, a stranger into a friend. Gratitude makes sense of our past, brings peace for today, and creates a vision for tomorrow." Melody Beattie, Author

Gratitude involves being thankful for the people, situations, or things in your life. In Positive Psychology, being grateful is used to enhance well-being because it makes life happier and more fulfilling (Seligman, 2011). Being thankful despite life's circumstances acts as a beneficial psychological measure that increases a person's capacity to appreciate aspects of living that they may have overlooked (Emmons & McCullough, 2003). Gratitude reduces stress-related sickness and when appreciation is conveyed toward other people, our relationships with them are strengthened (Armenta *et al.*, 2017). Another important result is worth-mentioning. Being grateful is known to function as a catalyst for habitual positive attitudes and behaviors that consistently endure over time (Xiang *et al.*, 2018).

Gratitude Related Approaches

Three specific gratitude-related strategies that have been known to be life-enhancing consist of *The Gratitude Journal, The Gratitude Visit,* & *The What-Went-Well Exercise.* I can personally attest to the benefit of *The Gratitude Journal.* Many years ago, I began a habitual routine where every night before going to sleep, I chose to write down five things for which I was thankful. Somedays it was not as easy as others to identify things to be grateful for, but forcing myself to examine the good in my day helped me to change what I focused on. Even when something went wrong, I looked for the lesson. Over the course of time this one strategy improved my life. For instance, I consistently felt less pessimistic, and more optimistic, hopeful, and appreciative of many of the little things that I would normally have overlooked.

Seligman (2011) has developed two additional gratitude related strategies that are positive and impactful. The first one is called *The Gratitude Visit.* It consists of writing a letter of gratitude to a person whom you never formally thanked, who did something special for you in the past. The exercise consists of writing a letter to this person to tell them in explicit and heartfelt detail how much you appreciate what they have done for you. Then you arrange to meet with them. At some point during your visit, you open the letter and read it to them aloud. What usually transpires is that a person feels very appreciated, and you feel a sense of accomplishment in having done the right thing. This experience has been known to strengthen your relationships with others who you may have previously taken for granted. It is also known to decrease depressive symptoms (Seligman, 2011).

Another approach by Seligman (2011) is *The What-Went-Well Exercise* which is also referred to as *The Three Blessings.* The goal of this strategy is similar to *The Gratitude Journal* but a bit more specific in its focus. The objective is to help you focus on what is going well instead of what is not. In this assignment, you are asked to spend 10 minutes every night to write down three things in your journal that went well that day, and then spend time assessing and writing about why they went well. Seligman (2011) advises that you do this exercise for at least a week, and then evaluate how it is working out, and if needed, you can continue doing it for a longer time or even indefinitely.

A Cheerful Outlook is Beneficial

Positive attitudes lead to successful outcomes. However, a **positive attitude** is not just about spouting off optimistic cliches. It entails responding to life's challenges with a hopeful viewpoint, and the perseverance and vision to continue toward your goals despite setbacks (Donnelly, 2017). Besides, making it your daily practice to do your absolute best to be positive is beneficial to your overall well-being. A review of research conducted by Diener and Chan (2011) revealed that happy people tend to live longer, more fulfilling, and satisfying lives than those who are prone to negativity. The results of their study demonstrated that subjective well-being, life satisfaction, optimism, and positive emotions, in conjunction with an absence of negative emotions, are what specifically contribute to enhanced health outcomes and longevity (Diener & Chan, 2011, p. 1). In this same study, people with a positive outlook experienced increased subjective well-being. **Subjective well-being** refers to a personal and individualized measure of a person's feelings and moods, including sorrow or joy. Furthermore, a positive emotional demeanor is known to reduce the incidence of stress-related physical and mental illnesses (Armenta *et al.*, 2017).

Practice Kindness on Purpose

"When we choose to intervene in someone's life by doing good, we make a difference in someone's life, no matter how small." Margot Silk Forrest, Author, and Motivational Speaker.

Unfortunately, no one can force us to be kind. You can mandate it, but any genuine act of benevolence must be performed freely otherwise it is counterfeit (Forrest, 2003). What I advise is that we make it our conscious intention to practice being kind to others. To be **kind on purpose** consists of actions that are thoughtful, caring, genuine, warm, respectful, and benevolent (Ferrucci, 2006). We can practice skills of being thoughtful and considerate of family and friends, especially those who are not that easy to love, and even though you may not be able to change a person's inherent behaviour, some people will respond positively to your loving attention.

I also believe strongly in forming good life habits and attest to the motto that whatever we focus on grows. Therefore, intentionally acting with kindness will undoubtedly help us to incorporate benevolence into our way of being. Saying hello to a person who seems alone, smiling back at someone who smiles at you, taking an interest in wanting to get to know an individual who is being ignored by others, are a few small examples of being kind. Regina Brett (2012) wrote an amazing book called, *Be the Miracle: 50 Lessons for Making the Impossible Possible.* In those lessons she shares compelling stories of how lives were positively changed by people who were not afraid of doing something caring and kind. She calls these acts miracles, but the actions she refers to are not something supernatural, they are within reach of anyone willing to follow where their heart leads. This is how Regina describes it.

Miracles aren't what other people do. They're what happens when ordinary people take extraordinary action. To be a miracle doesn't mean you have to tackle problems across the globe. It means making a difference in your own living room, cubicle, neighborhood, community (Brett, 2012, p. 2).

> ## SOMETHING TO REFLECT UPON
>
> **Think of a time when something out of the oridinary happened when you or someone else did something that made a positive difference in another person's life. What stood out for you? Was it a feeling of joy in knowing that someone's life was made better? What would it take for you to consider doing more of these sort of helping actions?**

Research into The Benefits of Kindness

"No kind action ever stops with itself. One kind action leads to another. Good example is followed. A single act of kindness throws out roots in all directions, and the roots spring up and make new trees. The greatest work that kindness does to others is that it makes them kind themselves" Amelia Earhart, American Aviation Pioneer, and Writer.

Research has demonstrated that offering random acts of kindness boosts life satisfaction. For example, Buchanan and Bardi (2010) conducted a study into the effects of kind acts. The participants were in the age range of 18 – 60 years old and took part voluntarily. They were randomly assigned to one of three groups. Group one was asked to perform acts of kindness. Group two were asked to participate in novel acts, and Group three were advised not to participate in any acts. Life satisfaction was measured before and after the interventions. The results demonstrated that acts of kindness and those that were novel increased overall life satisfaction, whereas no acts resulted in no change. Another more recent study by Rowland and Curry (2019) set out to investigate the effects of seven days of different acts of kindness to ascertain if there were any changes in subjective happiness. The results confirmed that performing acts of happiness for a week increased happiness, and there was a positive correlation between the number of kind acts and an enhanced level of self-reported joy. An unexpected finding was that the person performing the act of kindness and the one observing it measured equally on the degree of happiness that was experienced. The conclusion derived from this finding was that kindness benefits the giver and the receiver (Rowland & Curry).

Offer Kindness While Doing the Work of Nursing

We can still offer kindness when doing the work of a nurse even when we are under pressure to get the tasks done and when the chores that need attending to take up almost all our time. I have heard nursing students tell me that they do not have enough time to listen to their client's stories, or to establish a relationship of trust with them. The guidance that I give them, is that it costs no extra time to be kind. When time is a scarce commodity, thoughtfulness can be the element that happens in the process of doing the tasks, and still be felt by the client/patient. For example, greeting them with a smile and a hello at the beginning of your shift while introducing yourself to them, sets up at atmosphere of trust. You can do a check-in when giving them medications, changing a dressing, hanging a new IV bag, or ambulating them. Once you have given them a sense that you care about them, they will be more inclined to share their fears and concerns, which helps you to do a more comprehensive job of planning their care in a client-centered way. Getting to know them better may also provide you with valuable information to advocate for them when they need it. Furthermore, it will increase your overall job satisfaction because you will know that you have helped them in someway.

POSITIVE PSYCHOTHERAPY: A BALANCED APPROACH TO TREATMENT

Positive psychotherapy is a therapeutic approach derived from Positive Psychology and Chris Peterson's (2006) work on character strengths. It is based on the premise of creating balance in therapy by focusing on a person's strengths and weaknesses and focusses on a person's strengths as means to well-being. This approach differs from traditional psychotherapy that concentrates on changing or fixing personal deficits (Rashid, 2015; Seligman, 2011). In contrast, positive psychotherapy pays equal attention to a person's positive and negative symptoms. However, as a strategic intervention it concentrates more intensely on positive emotions, relationships, and resources, in conjunction with self-motivation. Opponents of this approach criticized it for an over-emphasis on strengths, and not enough attention paid to personal problems (Rashid, 2015). Although, some of the criticism has been labelled as unwarranted because positive psychotherapy still pays equal attention to both negative and positive emotions. However, even though negative emotions are acknowledged, strengths are used as the means to address them. Nevertheless, the effectiveness of positive psychotherapy has been empirically supported in pilot studies and further research is welcomed (Rashid, 2015).

The Three Assumptions of Positive Psychotherapy

According to Rashid (2015) there are three key assumptions of positive psychotherapy that are associated with "the nature, cause, course, and treatment of behavioral patterns" (p. 26). The first supposition is that pathology in the form of mental unwellness is a direct result of psychological and sociocultural influences. These effects impede a person's ability to grow, be fulfilled, and stay well. The second assumption identifies positive emotions and strengths as authentic, and just as important as symptomology of a mental disorder. The third postulation is that through discussing positive personal character traits and experiences, valuable and trusting relationships with therapists can be created. This professional trust relationship then serves the purpose of instilling hope and helping the person to own their inherent strengths (Rashid, 2015).

The Three Phases of Positive Psychotherapy

Rashid (2015) also identified three phases of implementing positive psychotherapy. In the first phase the client develops a stable narrative where they are required to explore their signature strengths from varying perspectives. They are then encouraged to actualize their signature strengths into the creation of meaningful goals, that are made to decrease psychological stress and improve functioning and well-being. The second stage is to foster positive emotions to deal with negative memories. The third and last phase consists of exercises that nurture positive relationships, and the importance of creating meaning and purpose in one's life (Rashid, 2015).

How Positive Psychotherapy is Implemented

Positive psychotherapy is based on operationalizing Seligman's (2011) scientifically measurable concepts of wellbeing known as PERMA into therapy (*e.g.*, positive emotion, engagement, relationships, meaning, and accomplishment) (Rashid, 2015). Positive psychotherapy utilizes specific positive exercises that emphasize a person's chosen signature character strengths, and incorporating them into treatment (Peterson & Seligman, 2004). **Signature strengths** in Positive Psychology consist of character strengths that are closely aligned with who we are, and what is vitally important to us. The ones that we choose have the following characteristics. We tend to take ownership of them and feel excited when we can show them (Peterson & Seligman). We want to make use of them, feel invigorated when the opportunity to apply them arises, and pursue projects that prioritize them. We also feel enthusiastic and joyful when utilizing them (Seligman, 2011).

There are twenty-four signature strengths in total and some of the main categories that they fall under consist of wisdom, courage, humanity, justice, temperance, and transcendence (Peterson & Seligman, 2004). Every one of us possesses all twenty-four but to varying degrees (Values in Action (VIA) Institute on Character, 2023). Emotional intelligence is one of the character strengths that warrants some explanation because it is crucially important for personal growth and change. **Emotional intelligence** refers to the ability to be aware of our feelings and those experienced by other people (Goleman, 2005). Self-awareness, the capacity to offer empathy, and adequate social skills are all necessary components of emotional intelligence (Goleman). **Social intelligence** is a part of emotional intelligence and consists of the capacity to feel and act in a socially acceptable manner (Stephany, 2022). A Learning Activity in Box (**4.2**) challenges you to gain a better understanding of each of the twenty-four signature strengths. In Box (**4.3**) how each of the Fourteen Character Strengths are explored in actual Positive Psychotherapy Sessions are clearly articulated.

Box 4.2. Learning activity: understanding the twenty-four signature strengths of positive psychotherapy (as adapted from *via* Institute on Character, 2023).

As a personal or class assignment spend time discussing how each of the following signature strengths are operationalized in real life. Ensure that you use examples when possible.
appreciation of beauty, bravery, creativity, curiosity, fairness, forgiveness, gratitude, honesty, hope, humility, humor, judgment, kindness, leadership, love, love of learning, perseverance, perspective, prudence, self-regulation, emotional/social intelligence, spirituality, teamwork, and zest.

Box 4.3. Character strengths positive psychotherapy (PPT) sessions (as adapted from Peterson and Seligman, 2004; Rashid, 2015, pp. 28-29; Stephany, 2022, pp. 115-116).

Session 1 Topic: Orientation to PPT & Lack of Positive Resources. Psychological distress is discussed including deficits in positive emotions such as PERMA. **Exercise:** Positive introduction to the therapy. The client is asked to write a one-page realistic story about their best attributes that ends positively. **Character Strength:** Emotional intelligence, Authenticity, Courage
Session 2 Topic: Character Strengths. Character strengths are introduced, and the topic of engagement and flow are discussed. **Exercise:** Client identifies their signature strengths during the session, and they complete an on-line self-report measure at home. Two other people (a family member and friend) are also asked to identify their five most significant signature strengths. **Character Strength:** Emotional Intelligence, Perspective
Session 3 Topic: Signature Strengths & Positive Emotions. Signature strengths are discussed. The client puts together their signature strengths profile with various perspectives included. **Exercise 1:** The client devises specific, measurable, and achievable goals that target specific problems, and the benefits of positive emotions is also discussed. **Character Strength:** Creativity, Hope, Optimism, Gratitude
Session 4 Topic: Good *versus* Bad Memories. The role of negative emotions and how they make psychological symptoms worse is discussed. The role of good memories is also emphasized. **Exercise:** The client writes about feelings of anger and bitterness and identifies how they instigate emotional distress. **Character Strength:** Gratitude, Appreciation of Beauty, and Excellence

(Box 4.3) cont.....

Session 5 Topic: Forgiveness. Forgiveness is promoted to transform anger and negative emotions into either neutral or positive feelings. **Exercise:** The client describes a wrongdoing, the emotional aftermath, and promises to forgive the perpetrator. A deliverable letter is not required. **Character Strength:** Forgiveness and Mercy, Kindness, Social Intelligence, Self-regulation
Session 6 Topic: Gratitude. Gratitude is discussed as an enduring trait. The role of both good and bad memories is re-visited with the focus on gratitude. **Exercise:** The client writes and then delivers in person a gratitude letter to someone that they never properly thanked. **Character Strength:** Gratitude, Love, Social and Emotional Intelligence, Authenticity
Session 7 Topic: Mid-therapy check. The forgiveness and gratitude assignments are re-visited. Experiences associated with the signature strengths and Blessing Journal activities are reviewed. The client and therapist identify obstacles and ways to overcome them. **Exercise:** The client completes the Forgiveness and Gratitude assignments. **Character Strength:** Perseverance, Perspective, Self-regulation
Session 8 Topic: Satisfying *versus* maximizing. Concepts like satisfying (meaning good enough) and maximizing are reviewed. **Exercise:** The client develops ways to increase satisfying. **Character Strength:** Self-regulation, Gratitude
Session 9 Topic: Hope and optimism. Hope and optimism are discussed in depth. The client is asked to reflect on occasions when things were grim but also recall good opportunities that presented themselves. **Exercise:** The client is asked to think of three doors that closed and identify what doors opened afterwards. **Character Strength:** Hope & Optimism
Session 10 Topic: Positive communication. A technique of positive communication called active-constructive is the goal. **Exercise:** The client looks for opportunities to communicate actively and constructively. **Character Strength:** Love, Kindness, Curiosity, Social Intelligence
Session 11 Topic: Signature strengths of others. The goal is to appreciate the character strengths of family members. **Exercise:** Family Strengths Tree: The client is required to ask family members to complete a signature strength measure. A family tree of strengths is created and then discussed at a family meeting. **Character Strength:** Love, Social Intelligence
Session 12 Topic: Savoring. Savoring is the focus in conjunction with an awareness of safeguarding against adaptation. **Exercise:** The client plans a savoring activity using specific strategies. **Character Strength:** Appreciation of Beauty, Excellence, Gratitude
Session 13 Topic: Positive Legacy & Gift of Time. The client is asked to imagine a positive legacy and the therapeutic benefits of being helpful to others. **Exercise:** Positive Legacy: The client is asked to write out how they would like to be remembered. **Gift of Time:** The Client makes plans to give a gift of time utilizing their signature strengths. **Character Strength:** Teamwork, Kindness
Session 14 Topic: The Full Life. Full life is identified as the amalgamation of pleasure, engagement, and meaning. Therapeutic gains and experiences are reviewed and ways to help sustain the positive changes that have been achieved. **Character Strength:** Perspective

THE ROLE OF POST-TRAUMATIC GROWTH IN RECOVERY

Post-traumatic Growth & How It Differs from Resilience

People are capable of enduring emotional struggle following adversity and still able to move forward (Collier, 2016). This process is referred to as post-traumatic growth, which is a strategy closely affiliated with Positive Psychology. **Post-traumatic growth** growth consists of positive changes in a person's life following trauma, that develops as a direct result of their struggle to work through what happened to them (Kelly, 2022; Poseck *et al.*, 2006). However, post-traumatic growth is different than resilience. **Resilience** is a personal attribute that involves the capacity to bounce back to normal functioning after experiencing trauma and does not involve a struggle. A resilient person is not that disturbed by what happened, and their belief system is not necessarily challenged by the adverse event. In contrast, **post-traumatic growth** occurs due to the psychological struggle associated with the trauma, and the effort required to recover from it (Collier, 2016). Nevertheless, the process of post-traumatic growth is not inferior to resilience, it is just different, and the resultant learning can be quite profound (Collier, 2016; Tedeschi *et al.*, 2015). For instance, the person realizes that because they were able to endure and cope with what happened, they now have increased confidence in their ability to deal with future travesty when it occurs. Working through the struggle forced them to survive, which in turn made them feel vulnerable, but also stronger (Calhoun & Tedeschi, 2000, Haas, 2015; Poseck *et al.*, 2006).

Stress & Psychological Growth

Although everyone is not able to move on after a traumatic experience and may develop distressing symptoms, research has revealed that a psychological growth is a key response to stress and trauma (Calhoun & Tedeschi, 2000; Christopher, 2003; Poseck *et al.*, 2006). Dr. Seligman (2011) explains that although a significant number of people may suffer from serious bouts of depression, anxiety and even PTSD following trauma, many of these same individuals develop enhanced strategies that lead to higher psychological functioning. For example, as illustrated in Fig. (4.6), despite less-than-ideal conditions a flower can grow in a crack in concrete. Similarly, perseverance and hope, and positive change can be cultivated in humans, even under less than favorable circumstances.

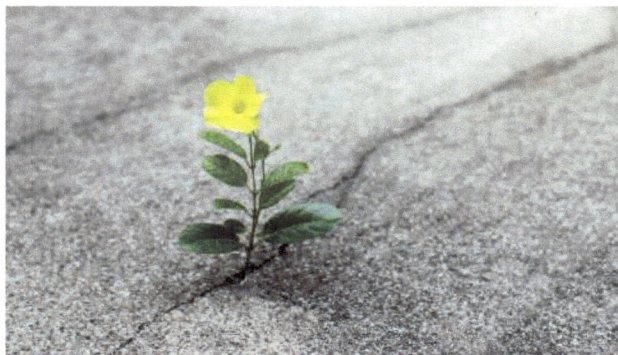

Fig. (4.6). Growth in less-than-ideal circumstances. Source: www.pixabay.com.

Learning from the Struggle

After someone has had their view of the world destroyed by travesty, many of their previous assumptions are no longer valid, like a belief that the world is a safe place. It is as if they awaken to the realization that some of their former plans and goals are no longer attainable, and this initially presents itself as a loss that must be grieved (Poseck *et al.*, 2006; Tedeschi *et al.*, 2015). Negative emotions are also often a part of that experience, and working through those feelings with the support of others is beneficial in warding off the risk of depression, and in fostering progress (Henson *et al.*, 2021). By sharing what they have gone through with other people who have endured similar adversity, their experiences are normalized, and they subsequently feel less alone. Conversely, people who suppress their memories of the trauma, hide what they are feeling, or try to return to normal functioning without getting any help, seldomly experience post-traumatic growth (Kashdan & Kane, 2011).

The Four Components of Post-Traumatic Growth

Post-traumatic growth is made possible after a person has grieved the loss of what was, and what could have been, and when they feel ready to move forward. According to Tedeschi *et al.*, (2015) there are four key components associated with the process of post-traumatic growth. The first element points out that post-traumatic growth happens most often after a major life crisis, and not following ordinary life stress. Secondly, it quite frequently coincides with a profound, and life transforming change. Thirdly, the person experiences it as a product of their experience and not just as enhanced coping, and fourthly, traumatic circumstances cause the person to question their basic assumptions of what is important in life. They actually feel motivated to derive meaning from what transpired (Tedeschi *et al.*, 2015). A Learning Activity is suggested in Box (**4.4**) that suggests exploring lessons learned from people who have experienced post-traumatic growth after adversity.

Box 4.4. Learning activity: lessons learned from those who experienced post-traumatic growth following adversity.

Have an open discussion to identify people in history who have experienced trauma and developed a new outlook on life, because of struggling to recover from what transpired. Share their story with the rest of the class. Then open the discussion to explore why you think the lessons they learned are important for all of us to hear about. To get you started you may want to consider exploring the life lessons learned by Nelson Mandela.

Things to Consider When Helping Someone on their Journey Toward Post-Traumatic Growth

There are a few things to consider when helping people move toward post-traumatic growth. We need to be cognizant of the fact that many of the tragic life crises endured by our clients/patients are catastrophic in nature (Tedeschi & Calhoun, 1996). They may have had their hopes and dreams shattered, are often in a very vulnerable and distressed state, and therefore they require a tender and gentle approach (Tedeschi *et al.*, 2015). According to Ashley (2020) paying attention to the power differential between you and them is important. They may view you as the expert which in turn makes them assume that they are somewhat inferior to you. Make it your goal to balance this power difference by being genuine and nonjudgmental, and reminding them of their strengths. When exploring the suffering that they have endured, make sure this happens in a safe environment, and that you display tolerance for some of their negative nuances. You must also be cautioned not to focus on the adverse event in your discussions (Ashley; Tedeschi *et al.*,).

POSITIVE CHANGE DUE TO POST-TRAUMATIC GROWTH

A review of the literature on post-traumatic growth reveals that many people who experience positive change after struggling with significant life circumstances, associate their life improvements as directly related to the loss (Calhoun & Tedeschi, 2000; Henson *et al.*, 2021; Poseck *et al.*, 2006; Tedeschi *et al.*, 2015). What is important to emphasize is that adverse events are not the source of positive change. Rather, it is the person's understanding of what happened to them, the meaning they have derived from it, and the new life they develop, that makes them stronger (Rendon, 2015). Furthermore, they also often embark on a journey of changing their story from one of victim to successful survivor (Tedeschi *et al.*,).

Three Explanatory Models of Post-Traumatic Growth

Janoff-Bulman (2004) designed three explanatory models of post-traumatic growth that happen after experiencing adversity. They are summarized as strengths due to suffering, psychological preparedness, and existential reevaluation. **Strengths due to suffering** occur in the form of self-reassessment and questioning one's belief system. **Psychological preparedness** concerns becoming better able to deal with adverse events when they happen in the future. **Existential reevaluation** is about inner work, pursuing meaning, and being awakened to the precious aspect of life (Janoff-Bulman,2014).

Two Interpretive Stages of Post-traumatic Growth

It has long been postulated that post-traumatic growth is also an interpretive process where the individual passes through two specific stages of coping with what transpired (Filipp,1999). Both stages act as an adaptive means to sort through what happened and psychologically adjust.

The first stage is about working through a **perception of reality** that consists of deceiving themselves by adopting an unrealistic optimism and hope about what happened. Apparently, this mechanism is a form of psychological denial that is used to sort through the magnitude of what transpired and acts as an emotional buffer. Following that stage there is an **interpretive reality**, where they begin to analyze and ruminate over what happened, and why, and draw their own subjective conclusions as another means to cope (Filipp, 1999).

THE FIVE DOMAINS OF POST-TRAUMATIC GROWTH

A Post-Traumatic Growth Inventory that consists of a self-report was originally developed by Tedeschi and Calhoun (1996) to evaluate how well someone was doing on their journey toward post-traumatic growth. Their work culminated in the identification of five domains as a means to assess progress. They consist of appreciation of life, new possibilities, relating to others, personal strength, and spiritual change. However, Tedeschi and Calhoun (2004) argue that not all five domains are needed for a person to experience post-traumatic growth. Nevertheless, due to their importance, all five domains from this inventory guide the discussion that ensues.

APPRECIATION OF LIFE

"Healing from trauma can also mean strength and joy. The goal of healing is not a papering over the changes in an effort to preserve or present things as normal. It is to acknowledge and wear your new life – warts, wisdom, and all – with courage." Catherine Woodiwiss, Author of *The Ten Things I've Learned About Trauma*

Post-traumatic growth and positive ways of coping following adversity is possible, because after loss, grief, and acceptance, gaining a new appreciation of life occurs (Henson *et al.*, 2021). In fact, the evidence points out that increased distress often acts as a springboard for post-traumatic adjustment (Kashdan & Kane, 2011). What changes is someone's priorities. Malhotra and Chebiyan, (2016) point out that the experience of certain serious traumas that actually posed a threat to someone's life, can often result in the most profound change in someone's outlook. For example, it can cause a reaction of sincere appreciation for still being alive, and a realization that new opportunities are still possible, like pursuing goals, and dreams. The little things that once seemed so important also matter less, and the people or situations that they often take for granted matter more. However, adopting a new way of thinking after loss often still involves a journey (Malhotra & Chebiyan, 2016).

NEW POSSIBILITIES

On the journey of post-traumatic growth, it is not the trauma in and of itself that causes the growth, but the new life story, and possibilities for the future that instigates the change. It is as though the person realizes that life is a gift and that it is meant to be lived fully (Kelly, 2022). Many people feel somewhat compelled to do the things they would have normally put off to sometime in the future, because time now is seen as what it really is, a limited commodity. Subsequently the person prioritizes what is really important, like family, friends, nature, serving others, and spirituality (Kelly, 2022; Janoff-Bulman, 2004). While working through post-traumatic growth some people feel compelled to give back to society and a renewed appreciation for all of life. They develop increased compassion, and a willingness to actively participate in helping others who suffer or who are in need. Service becomes an integral part of their healing process and becoming strong again (Malhotra & Chebiyan, 2016).

RELATING TO OTHERS

Relationships with others often change following trauma. Some report that their relationships with family and friends have improved, and they are more willing to get emotionally close to them. Some even feel receptive to the help offered to them by others when they formerly would have been reluctant to accept assistance due to pride. However, some relationships get worse following trauma. So, identifying who they can trust becomes important. For example, some people you thought would be there for you disappear. Yet others who you may not have noticed before, rise to the challenge, check in on you, just to see how you are doing, and if you require help (Macfarlane & Carson, 2019; Poseck *et al.*, 2006).

A Need for Social Connection

Healthy social connections with others accelerates post-traumatic recovery, and after experiencing a tragedy, the desire to form and sustain healthy and trustworthy relationships becomes a priority for many people (Macfarlane & Carson, 2019; Poseck *et al.*, 2006). This occurs because our need for connection is crucially important for our general well-being and happiness. For instance, as humans we are pre-programmed to bond with other people, not only to survive, but because we are social creatures who have an inherent desire to feel a sense of belonging (Seligman, 2011). Social connection is also beneficial because it enhances coping and is known to ward off serious mental illness (Macfarlane & Carson, 2019).

Sharing Experiences with Others

An additional encouraging effect on relationships following a trauma consists of a willingness to share personal experiences with others. However, cognitive processing of adverse events in this way is only helpful if the social environment is supportive. For instance, even sharing negative emotions with someone who is trusted is associated with post-traumatic growth (Calhoun & Tedeschi, 2013). Furthermore, the benefit of disclosure is heightened when the trauma survivor shares their story with someone who has experienced a similar adverse event. This is because disclosing to someone who truly understands what you have gone through legitimizes and normalizes your experience (Henson *et al.*, 2021).

Engaging in supportive interpersonal communication with others after a traumatic disaster has also been shown to be helpful. For instance, a study conducted by First *et al.*, (2018) specifically set out to explore the role of certain factors on post-traumatic growth after a tornado. They discovered that engaging in a discussion of the event with family members, friends, and fellow survivors resulted in increased post-traumatic growth, positive outcomes, and enhanced lasting interpersonal connections (First *et al.*, 2018).

PERSONAL STRENGTH

Surviving trauma can make a person feel stronger (Malhotra & Chebiyan, 2016). They often gain a new awareness of themselves, develop increased empathy, humility, enhanced creativity, and a desire to become more involved in humanitarian causes (Macfarlane & Carson, 2019; Tedeschi & Calhoun, 1996). Post-traumatic growth can also be a catalyst for enduring and optimistic changes in a person's personality traits, and although individual differences exist, character attributes associated with wisdom and enhanced self-confidence are known to be more common than others (Jayawickreme *et al.*, 2021). Apparently, the process of developing increased wisdom following adversity is more likely to happen once the person can distance themselves from the event. Conversely, if someone is stuck in negative emotional renumeration, their growth in wisdom character traits is impeded.

Changing One's Story: From Victim to Strong Survivor

Increased self-confidence is more likely to develop when the survivor revises their story following the tragic event from one of being defeated and victimized, into becoming a strong survivor with renewed hope. The meaning they derive from what transpired gives them a new vision of who they want to be in the future and the added confidence to pursue their goals (Jayawickreme *et al.*, 2021. Additionally, it is not uncommon for people who have survived trauma to gain new confidence and courage in their ability to deal with future adversity. Self-reliance, and the belief that you can handle troubles when they occur and seeing yourself as more capable and stronger than you first realized, are all due to the experience of surviving the trauma (Malhotra & Chebiyan, 2016; Poseck *et al.*, 2006).

SPIRITUAL CHANGE

As a part of their journey of post-traumatic growth following adversity, some individuals have an increased interest in religious or spiritual matters. However, before exploring this phenomenon and how it helps, the difference between religion and spirituality is presented. Reasons why participation in religious or spirituality may not be an appropriate treatment regime for some people is also explained.

The Similarities & Differences between Religion and Spirituality

Both religion and spirituality consist of universal experiences that are rooted in a quest for a greater meaning of human existence, and a relationship with either a higher deity or a spiritual essence (National Alliance on Mental Illness (NAMI), 2016). However, they also differ in several ways. **Religion** involves the worship of a being or greater power outside of human material existence. It may consist of following sacred texts, books, rules, formal prayers, or engaging in worship. It often includes community gatherings with those of a similar faith (NAMI, 2016; Stanford, 2010). Alternatively, **spirituality** emphasizes the energy that exists within the person and their connection with a universal source of power that is a part of all of life. It is broader in its focus and may involve practices of reaching alternative dimensions through specific rituals, meditation, or transcendence (Balboni *et al.*, 2014; NAMI, 2016; Ray, 2016).

When Participation in Religious or Spiritual Practices May Not Be Appropriate

Before proceeding to explore some of the general benefits of religious and spiritual practices as a strategy of post-traumatic growth, a word of caution is needed. For example, there are specific situations where trauma recovery should not include religion or spiritual involvement. The first condition involves those who have suffered physical or sexual abuse at the hands of people in positions of higher power in spiritual and religious settings (Cashwell & Swindle, 2018). The second situation involves people who have not been abused in a religious environment but may still have completely lost all faith and trust. They view their tragic circumstances as a form of spiritual abandonment or act of being punished by God for things they have done (Werdel *et al.*, 2014). For both groups of people their traumatic experiences are closely and negatively aligned with a religious affiliation. Therefore, religious or spiritual strategies of intervention may not be appropriate and may need to be avoided.

A Change in Religious or Spiritual Focus After Experiencing Trauma

"A way to understand spirit is that it's the part of you that is drawn to hope, that will not give in to despair. The part of you that has to believe in goodness; that has to believe in something more" Caroline Myss, American Author

People who have experienced an adverse event, especially those that are quite distressing or life threatening, often feel philosophically, religiously, or spiritually drawn to questions surrounding the meaning of life. They realize that their time on earth is limited, and they start to ponder a variety of questions about what is important about life (Malhotra & Chebiyan, 2016; Stephany, 2012). Even those with no previous belief in anything outside material existence prior to the adverse event, may turn to spiritual pursuits. Although those with previous experience with religion or spirituality are more likely to make sense of what happened through this avenue. Even those with no previous belief in anything outside material existence prior to the adverse event, may turn to spiritual pursuits (Malhota & Chebiyan). What specific spiritual activities are people drawn to participate in? Some report feeling drawn to praying, being grateful to God for help, and having a stronger affiliation with a formal religion or specific faith (Tedeschi *et al.*, 2015). Others admit being primarily preoccupied with trying to understand the greater meaning of life and helping others (Tedeschi & Calhoun, 2004).

Mental Health Benefits of Religion & Spirituality

For those who have not had bad prior experiences, being involved in religion or spirituality can improve their mental health. However, the specific advantages differ between the two theological approaches (NAMI, 2016). A key mental health benefit of religion comes from believing in something greater than yourself that you can rely on, especially in trying circumstances. Another value is derived from a sense of belonging by formal meetings with, and receiving support from, people of a similar faith (NAMI). Teachings that involve guidelines for living, and that foster gratitude, forgiveness, and compassion facilitate increased serenity. Research also suggests that involvement in religious activity can reduce rates of suicide and substance use (NAMI). Spirituality assists people to gain a better understanding of how they fit into the world and the meaning of life. It promotes stress reducing strategies that positively affect physical and mental well-being, like exercise, yoga, self-reflection, and meditation. Spirituality can also lead to living a more meaningful existence though an increased connection with other people, nature, and aesthetics (NAMI).

Additional Benefits of Religious & Spiritual Activities & Trauma Recovery

How much does engaging in religious or spiritual activities help in trauma recovery? Research by Hipolito *et al.*, (2014) into vulnerable trauma afflicted populations revealed that praying, reading holy scriptures, meditating, and participation in other spiritual practices positively influences a person's sense of empowerment. Empowerment in trauma-recovery is important because it enhances a person's willingness to reach out for help when they need it. Other benefits derived from increased participation in religious or spiritual activities post trauma include a decrease in depression, suicidal ideation, self-harm, and substance use. An increased experience of overall well-being, life satisfaction, and positive emotions are also readily experienced (Hipolito *et al.*,).

Knowledge Deficits in Nursing Education Concerning Spirituality

We have been made aware that practices associated with religion and spirituality can sometimes be helpful in trauma recovery, and nursing as a profession has been known to include spirituality as a part of holistic care (Watson, 2008). However, nurses admit that their formal training has not necessarily prepared them to implement spiritual care into their practice (Kuven & Giske, 2019). For example, a very comprehensive literature review was conducted at the University of Sunderland in the United Kingdom by Gulnar *et al.*, (2018) between the years of 1993 - 2017. The objective was to identify knowledge and practice deficiencies in nursing education. The results revealed four themes. The first demonstrated that a deficit in ontology was apparent in nursing content. **Ontology** explores the nature of what is and focuses on gaining a better understanding of the human capacity for being and becoming (Watson, 2008). Incorporating increased self-awareness, compassion, caring, and cultural and religious sensitivity into nursing education was recommended as a remedy for this problem (Gulnar *et al.*, 2018, p. 31). The second identified problem was a knowledge gap concerning phenomenology and the value of human experience. This issue was attributed to an over emphasis on the science of nursing, and less on the subjective and relational components of nursing practice. A third deficit was a lack of adequate content in nursing school curriculum on the general topic of spirituality. The fourth was faculty being inadequately trained in how to teach this subject to student nurses. The authors recommended that there be a shared discussion among nursing faculty and those working in the field on how best to develop, train, and mentor future nurses in spirituality. They also emphasized the value of spirituality becoming a recognized standard for future nursing school curriculum development (Gulnar *et al.*,). The following Case Study reveals a challenge that is not necessarily uncommon for student nurses, that of feeling somewhat unprepared to assist a client/patient in spiritual matters. Refer to Box (**4.5**).

Box 4.5. Narrative case study one: when a student nurse feels unprepared to talk to their client/patient about spiritual issues.

Zara is a fourth-year student nurse in her last Semester and Preceptorship in a Bachelor in Psychiatric Nursing Program. One of the people Zara was assigned to care for was Mrs. Colbert who was just admitted to hospital due to a major depression precipitated by the tragic death of her only daughter in a motor vehicle accident six months ago. Zara heard in report that Mrs. Colbert had requested to be visited by a Member of Clergy because she felt that she needed spiritual guidance in dealing with her grief, anger, and depression. Zara felt a bit worried that Mrs. Colbert would ask her questions about spirituality when caring for her because she was not affiliated with any form of religion and considered herself an atheist. When morning care was completed Mrs. Colbert asked Zara if they could have a talk sometime later that day about spiritual stuff. Zara reluctantly agreed but she was really concerned that her patient would ask her questions that she could not answer. On the advice given to her by a senior and supervising nurse, Zara decided to telephone her instructor during her lunch break for advice on how best to proceed. Zara was quite open when speaking with her instructor about her lack of faith, and her feeling of being inadequately prepared to talk about things of a spiritual or religious nature. Yet, she also expressed a genuine desire to do what she could to help her patient. The following consists of the conversation between Zara and her Instructor.
"Zara, I am glad that you called me. I want you to know that it is okay for you to feel somewhat unsettled about talking to your patient about spiritual issues. I think that we need to do a better job of preparing our future nurses to deal with these important topics when and if they arise. Do you have a specific question that you want to ask, or do you want me to share my thoughts based on my experience?"
Zara felt a little bit bewildered and asked for what she needed.
"I want to hear what you have to say and then maybe ask some questions about things that come up for me. Is that okay?"
Following Zara's lead, her instructor proceeded to share her wisdom.
"I am not sure if you remember some of the material you were taught in your first year in nursing school, but in Relational Practice we talked about the importance of holistic care and taking care of the body, mind, and spirit of our patients. The spiritual focus is often neglected not because we don't care about it, but due to our own unfamiliarity with the subject matter, and for fear of saying or doing the wrong thing. What I have always done when a patient brings up the subject matter is to tell them that I may not be able to answer their big questions, but that I am there to listen to them and will do what I can to help. I encouraged them to tell me what they are feeling and to really listen to them, not just to the surface of what they are saying, but the themes that come through. You see, oftentimes they are face to face with life and death situations and they are scared. They are searching for ways to deal with their fears and suffering. Being a safe listener is a good place to start"
Zara interrupted her instructor with an urgent question that troubled her.
"But what do I do if the patient asks me about my beliefs? What do I do then? Do I tell them that I am an atheist?"

(Box 4.5) cont.....

The instructor paused for a moment to think about her response before addressing Zara's inquiry.
"I would tell them that I was inexperienced concerning the topic of religion and spirituality, but that I was willing to listen to their views to better understand. That way you do not have to disclose aspects of your private spiritual beliefs. You can maintain professional boundaries but communicate the message that you care about what they believe, and that you are there to listen to them. Does that help?"
Zara looked relieved.
"It helps a lot, but I have one more question? Do I need to research their religious faith before talking to them."
Anticipating that this question may come up, Zara's instructor was ready with a response.
"No, you do not need to be up to date on their religion before speaking to them. However, you can ask them to educate you and to let you know what sort of support they may need. Some faiths have special times of day and directions when it comes to formal prayers or other specific needs. You can also ask if they would like a member of their faith or someone in their family to come and be with them. Also, check and see what sort of supports are offered by the hospital's clergy staff."
Zara, seemed a bit calmer, and her instructor made one more comment before the call ended.
"Zara, just remember to work with the patient and with what they believe. Try not to disclose too much about your own beliefs because this is about them and not about you. Be empathetic and genuinely interested in understanding what they are going through. Do your best to connect them with outside religious support if needed, and do what you did today. Ask for help from others who are more experienced, or who can support you when you feel like you do not know how best to proceed. Remember, all you can do is your best. Does that help?"
Zara felt relieved and glad that she made that call and commented one more time before hanging up.
"Yes, it does. It helps a great deal. Thank-you."

NARRATIVE CASE STUDY ONE: IDENTIFICATION OF THEMES & ANALYSIS

Two key themes were identified from this story.

Theme # 1: Zara felt unprepared to talk to her patient about spiritual matters.

Theme # 1 Analysis: As pointed out earlier, even though the profession of nursing includes spirituality as a part of holistic care it is not always explicitly addressed in all nursing programs when training students. Practicing nurses also do not aways feel adequately educated or prepared to properly address spiritual matters when they arise (Kuven & Giske, 2019; Harrad *et al.*, 2019; Watson, 2008).

Theme # 2: Zara's instructor advised that she be honest with her patient about her lack of knowledge concerning spiritual matters, and to inform them that she was there to listen and help in any way that she could.

Theme # 2 Analysis: These directives were beneficial because being honest and real with our clients/patients about our lack of knowledge about spiritual matters, and meeting them right where they are, increases trust and makes it more likely that they will share their fears and concerns with us (Stephany, 2020). Ray (2016) when referring to transcultural caring and spirituality also points out that maintaining an empathetic, caring, and compassionate attitude and being a safe place, is often exactly what may be needed at the time.

QUESTIONS FOR FURTHER DISCUSSION

1-Discuss the issue of professional boundary setting in nursing, especially regarding when a client/patient asks a nurse to disclose something personal about themselves. What are the best practices regarding this important issue?

2-Is it ever okay for a nurse to disclose their own religious or spiritual views with a client/patient? Why or why not? When answering this question, be sure to consult your Nursing Code of Ethics and your Nursing Regulatory Body's Standards of Practice guidelines or directives concerning this issue.

ADDITIONAL LIFE-ENHANCING RESPONSES TO ADVERSITY

Further life-enhancing responses to adversity that are related to post-traumatic growth are included in the ensuing discussion and consist of the importance of meaning-making, the instillation of hope, and the power of self-compassion.

THE IMPORTANCE OF MEANING-MAKING

The importance of meaning was presented earlier in this current Chapter as an element of PERMA well-being theory (Seligman, 2011). It is re-introduced here because this subject matter is relevant to post-traumatic growth. For instance, as Sowers (2022) points out, for a person to begin and persist through the journey of recovery they need to learn new strategies that can enhance their coping. One way is through meaning-making. **Meaning-making** consists of the way in which a person makes sense from what has happened in their life, while also discovering and pursuing something that gives them purpose and a will to carry on. The likelihood that meaning-making will become a priority in recovery is associated with a high degree of distress experienced during and following the adverse event (Kashdan & Kane, 2011).

The likelihood that meaning-making will become a priority in recovery is associated with a high degree of distress experienced during and following the adverse event (Kashdan & Kane, 2011). The connection between the severity of the trauma and meaning-making is best illustrated by a historical account of someone's experience. Viktor Frankl was a Jewish Austrian Psychiatrist who survived living in Nazi death camps in World War II. After enduring such a horrific experience full of torture, serious abuse, and starvation, and losing every member of his immediate family to the carnage committed in the death camps, Dr. Frankl (2006) wrote a book called *"Man's Search for Meaning."* In his writings, he so poignantly shares his story of how he survived living in a concentration camp by discovering personal meaning. Dr. Frankl described how while imprisoned in a concentration camp he came to a point in time when he lost all will to live, but then something changed for him (Brooks & Goldstein, 2003). After some serious soul-searching Frankl devised a plan that would help him survive the treacherous conditions, he was forced to live in. That strategy consisted of imagining himself getting out of the camp alive and lecturing again, so he could share the story of what he and millions of others had endured and survived. This goal became his will to meaning (Brooks & Goldstein, 2003). Dr. Frankl (2006) described the **will to meaning** in life as a primary motivator, that is unique, valued, and specific to the individual, and can only be fulfilled by them. It is also what assists a person to endure and overcome pain and suffering.

After surviving his horrific experience in World War II, Dr. Frankl (2006) went on to develop **Logotherapy,** which is a type of psychotherapy that focuses on the purpose of human life and man's search for meaning, as a way to help people heal from situations that were traumatic (Lantz, 1992). Through the course of the later years of his life, Frankl used this theoretical premise to help adults who had been sexually assaulted as children (Lantz). The process he used had three key aspects to it. The first action compelled the person to find a vocation, or another means of service to give them purpose. The second strategy was to encourage them to surround themselves with people who support them. The third challenge was to help them understand that, even if the past cannot be changed, the individual who suffered can turn their trauma into triumph by changing themselves and learning how to live a second new life (Frankl; Lantz). The following passage from Dr. Frankl poignantly explains the meaning derived from suffering.

> We must never forget that we may also find meaning in life even when confronted with a hopeless situation when facing a fate that cannot be changed. For what then matters is to bear witness to the uniquely human potential at its best, which is to transform a personal tragedy into triumph, to turn one's predicament into a human achievement (Frankl, 2006, p. 112).

INSTILLATION OF HOPE

"Hope is being able to see that there is light despite all the darkness" Desmond Tutu, South African Theologian, Human Rights Activist, and Nobel Peace Prize Recipient.

Embracing the possibility of change during the journey of post-traumatic growth must be proceeded by the belief that success is attainable and that may involve hope (Sowers, 2022). For Dr. Frankl (2006) it was his hope that he would someday get out of the prison camps to share his story and to help others, that gave him the will to carry on. **Hope** is not something that is mysterious or magical, it is real and consists of the confidence that something better is possible and attainable in the future. But getting to a place where you can trust life enough to feel hopeful is not always easy for people who have lived through dire circumstances. Sometimes you need to lend the other person some of your hope (Stephany, 2012). That may consist of helping them to identify and own their strengths and abilities. Having them listen to the stories of peers who have been in the process for some time can be convincing because a person is more likely to trust those who have been through similar life challenges. It also offers them real examples of what it is like to be living life more fully.

THE POWER OF SELF- COMPASSION AND POST- TRAUMATIC GRO-WTH

"Self-compassion is simply giving the same kindness to ourselves that we would give to others." Christopher Germer, Author & Psychotherapist.

When we experience suffering it can either harden our hearts or it can teach us to be compassionate. **Compassion** enables us to see suffering and to identify with the experience. After experiencing trauma, some people develop compassion and a sincere desire to help others (Poseck *et al.*, 2006). However, becoming compassionate is not limited to identifying with the suffering of others, but involves learning how to be compassionate toward ourselves. **Self-compassion** consists of purposefully viewing yourself with the same degree of empathetic concern that you would offer someone else in a similar situation. It causes you to look at the unfortunate circumstances that you may have endured, and instead of resorting to self-loathing, you offer compassion to yourself. Evidence demonstrates that self-compassion as a specific response to adversity benefits people who have experienced trauma. For example, Bluth *et al.*, (2022) conducted research on youth who had been traumatized. The results revealed that developing an attitude of self-benevolence was associated with enhanced coping, increased personal self-acceptance, enabled healthier perspective-taking, decreased the incidence of psychopathology, and facilitated post-traumatic growth.

Mindful self-compassion combines mindfulness and being fully present, with self-compassion in the form of caring and loving directed at oneself (Shapiro *et al.*, 2018). It consists of using measures that foster self-kindness to improve emotional reactivity and to prevent mental health issues from developing, in persons who have experienced serious adversity and abuse. The following Case Study demonstrates how nurturing mindful self-compassion helped a young teen who had been traumatized as a child. Refer to Box (**4.6**).

Box 4.6. Narrative case study two: nurturing mindful self-compassion through meditation and creative self-visualization.

Annie was a Social Worker who was involved in counselling a teen, named Natalie, who had survived quite significant adversity in her short life, that included terrible abuse while in foster care when she was younger. Annie had been working with Natalie for quite some time, doing her very best to help her to stop feeling shame and blaming herself for what transpired. The goal was to assist Natalie to feel a sense of self-compassion. However, Annie met with considerable resistance from Natalie in most sessions and was almost ready to give up trying when she decided to attempt one more strategy. She would check and see if Natalie was interested in participating in a meditation and creative visualization process with the goal of nurturing mindful self-compassion. Natalie had just arrived for her session and Annie proceeded with her normal check-in.
"Good morning Natalie. It is good to see you here again. How has it been going for you."
Natalie glanced at Annie without any emotional expression and spoke quietly.
"Okay, I guess."
Sensing Natalie's ambiguity, Annie wanted to learn more.
"Okay, in what way?"
Her next response was vague but somewhat informative.
"Well, nothing bad happened. I didn't feel as sad as I sometimes do, and I also did not get into a fight with my new foster mom this week so that is pretty good I think."
Annie paused for a moment to give Natalie a chance to speak again, but she remained quiet, so it was the Social Worker's turn to validate Natalie's success.
"Sounds like that is progress compared to last week, don't you think?"
With a little smile, Natalie nodded in agreement.
"Yeah, not fighting with my foster mom is a big deal. I think it is because you have helped me to not react to everything all the time and to take a minute before lashing out. I think that is helping. In fact, my foster mom told me she noticed that I was a bit better and nicer to her this week."
Jumping at the opportunity to make the best out of Natalie's slightly elevated mood, Annie decided to let her client know what she had planned for this session.
"Natalie, I have decided to do something different today. I think you will enjoy it and that it may help you. What do you think?"
Looking rather skeptical, Natalie replied.
"Well, it depends on what it is. Tell me more first."
Annie proceeded to explain her plan to Natalie.

(Box 4.6) cont.....

"I want to do a creative visualization session with you to help you to go back in time to a place when you were happier. Do you think that would be okay?"
Looking a bit scared, Natalie interjected.
"Why would we do this and what about if I go back to a scarier time? Can you stop it and get me back before I get upset?"
Annie proceeded to reassure Natalie.
"This exercise helps to take you to a time when you were happier with the goal of increasing your sense of peace. I promise that if you consent to us doing this, I will make sure that I will not let you stay in a scary place and will help you to avoid that. Will you trust me with ensuring you are okay?"
Natalie seemed a bit relieved and eager to begin.
"If you think it will help me then let's do it."
Annie proceeded very cautiously and walked Natalie through the meditation process, and she participated fully. They began by performing slow deep breathing exercises to relax Natalie and to help her shut out any intrusive thoughts. Through creative visualization techniques, Annie then proceeded to guide Natalie to return to the memory of a happy place in her past. When she seemed ready, she helped her go back in time to when she was five years old, when her natural mother was still alive. Natalie went there quite naturally, and she initially seemed to still enjoy the process. To ensure she would not be re-traumatized, Annie kept checking in to see if there was anything that was scaring Natalie, and she openly denied experiencing anything frightening so far. However, near the end of the process, Natalie started to softly cry with her eyes still closed. She seemed somewhat okay, but Annie asked her to share with her what she was seeing and feeling. Natalie assured her Social Worker that she was not afraid, but a bit overwhelmed by her feelings and asked that she please bring her back to the present. The session was then carefully ended and followed by a debrief to explore what Natalie had experienced. Natalie explained what transpired while she had been in a trance-like state.
"Don't worry about me. I am okay. I really am okay. I was not really that afraid or anything like that. I just felt some stuff. I was with my mom and felt good for a moment but that changed to sadness because I knew she was dead. I also saw myself as this pretty little girl, playing with a doll-like other children did, sitting with my mom. I seemed so happy then. My mom was happy too and smiling at me. I also felt love for that little girl who was me, because she seemed so little, and a bit frail. She also did not know that her life was going to change. She did not know that bad things were going to happen."
Natalie paused for a minute and was crying a bit more than before. Annie remained quiet so Natalie could process what she was feeling, hoping she would elaborate.
"That little girl who was happy was me. Then I remembered that my mom was gone now, and I felt sad. But instead of feeling angry at myself, I felt sorry for that little girl who was me. I realized that I had been through lots of bad stuff after my mom died, and that it was not my fault that she died, or my fault for being treated badly."
Natalie continued to cry but she seemed okay. Annie noticed that Natalie kept repeating her new realization that she was seeing herself as a child in the imagery and that she was experiencing something quite profound. Then Natalie revealed a revelation.
"You know what, today is the first time that I feel love for that little girl and for what happened to her, and that little girl is me."

(Box 4.6) cont.....

Annie then proceeded to carefully debrief Natalie and to walk her through what she had just experienced, to ensure that she was able to sort through all her feelings associated with this exercise. However, Annie was a bit pleased at the progress made that day because Natalie had experienced self-compassion for the first time. Sure, there would still be challenges to work through in the future, but the hope was that what Natalie has just learned would help her to cope better and love herself a little bit more.

NARRATIVE CASE STUDY TWO: IDENTIFICATION OF THEMES & ANALYSIS

Two key themes were identified from this story.

Theme # 1: Natalie was a youth survivor of childhood adversity and abuse who was prone to feeling shame and blaming herself for what happened to her.

Theme # 1 Analysis: Many survivors of trauma and violence tend to blame themselves for what transpired, even though it was not their fault. On-going and unresolved post-traumatic shame combined with self-blame is unhealthy and can lead to mental health problems (Aakvaag *et al.*, 2016). This is explained by the fact that **shame** occurs when someone believes they have done something wrong and is usually experienced as an unchangeable intrinsically flawed character trait. Subsequently, shame not only causes a person to feel bad but often results in them hating themselves. Alternatively, **guilt** is healthier because when it is experienced after making a mistake, the blame attributed to it is not personalized or internalized but is assumed to be due to less than desirable choices. The takeaway from the theme of caring for someone who is experiencing self-blame and shame is that the healthcare practitioner must ensure that they treat the client/patient with genuine empathy, compassion, and unconditional positive regard, regardless of the particular circumstances (Asley, 2020).

Theme # 2: Meditation and creative visualization was used by a trained Counsellor to nurture mindful self-compassion.

Theme # 2 Analysis: Meditation consists of exercises in the form of either uttering a mantra or using breathing exercises to become calm, to shut out the outside world, and to sustain a heightened level of awareness. **Creative visualization** is a process where you to use your mind's eye to imagine a scenario, with your eyes closed, with the general goal of assisting you to better manage your emotions or problem**s. Mindfulness** is a form of awareness that is increasingly being used to decrease personal suffering and cultivate personal growth (Shapiro *et al.*, 2018). **Mindful self-compassion** is utilized in therapy to help those who suffer, to develop kindness toward themselves as a means to heal from traumatic experiences in the past (Germer & Neff, 2019; Tesh *et al.*, 2015). In this case, Natalie had a positive result from the exercise. She was able to feel compassion and love for the little girl that she once was and stopped blaming herself for what happened in her past. This strategy was therefore successful in instigating a small, but significant change in Natalie's self-concept.

QUESTION FOR FURTHER DISCUSSION

1-How do you feel about the use of mindful self-compassion to assist someone in healing from past traumatizing situations? Are you willing to investigate it further? Do you think it would be something you would want to recommend? Why or why not? Be sure to examine evidence-based information to support your stance.

SELF-CARE STRATEGY: PRACTICING GRATITUDE

Gratitude is a way to focus on what is going well in one's life. It does not necessarily change your set of circumstances but helps you to pay attention to what is still going well, which in turn changes your focus from pessimism to one of possibility. It is about acknowledging blessings rather than burdens (Emmons & McCullough, 2003). Gratitude is also known to enhance adaptability, coping, overall well-being, happiness, and flourishing (Seligman, 2011).

The Self-Care Challenge: Introducing Gratitude into Your Daily Practice

1. After learning about the many benefits of gratitude in this Chapter, would you be willing to make it a daily routine in your life? Will you consider doing at least one of the gratitude strategies that were suggested earlier, like *The Gratitude Journal*, *The Gratitude Visit*, or the *What-Went Exercise*. Try your best to make being grateful a part of your daily routine and see what happens.

Note: Any suggested strategies are not intended to be a substitute for medical or psychological advice from a trained professional. The reader is therefore encouraged to seek medical or other professional help in any matters related to their physical or emotional health.

CONCLUSION

- Chapter Four presents trauma-informed recovery from the viewpoint of Positive Psychology and post-traumatic growth.
- Positive Psychology and trauma-informed care share the common goal of helping people to live better lives. However, Positive Psychology strategies are designed to be used by everyone, including those who have not experienced adversity.

- These three different outcomes of a traumatic stress response were identified and the particular response that a person experiences is somewhat context-dependent. The first is a normal reaction. The second consists of the development of maladaptive functioning, and the third alternative response stimulates post-traumatic growth.
- We learned how neuroplasticity, or the brain's intrinsic ability to develop new neural connections, contributes to positive alterations post-trauma.
- Positive Psychology is the scientific study of human well-being, optimal functioning, and flourishing. Its historical roots stem from the Humanist psychological movement in the 1950s and a disillusionment with Psychology's primary focus on disease and pathology.
- Well-being theory in Positive Psychology consists of elements that are measurable and are comprised of what people are willing to choose as contributing to life satisfaction.
- The five key elements of well-being theory were identified as PERMA, which stands for positive emotions, engagement, relationships, meaning, and accomplishment. Positive emotions were acknowledged as the foundation of life satisfaction.
- PERMA+4 was later added as a framework for work-related well-being in Positive Psychology. It consists of these four additional elements, physical health, mindset, work environment, and economic security.
- Flourishing was acknowledged as a central component of well-being theory and consists of the capacity to be satisfied with our life achievements, and concerns by being involved in something that is meaningful, gives us a sense of purpose, and fosters close social connections with other people.
- Positive emotions, optimal functioning, optimistic thoughts, and healthy supportive relationships, have all been identified as the components to flourishing, yet positive emotions seem to be the foundation for all the other elements.
- Positive Psychology strategies that foster well-being consist of being grateful, possessing a positive attitude, random acts of kindness, and positive psychotherapy.
- Positive psychotherapy is a therapeutic approach based on the premise of creating balance in therapy by focusing on a person's strengths and weaknesses, and by utilizing their strengths as the means to well-being.
- Positive psychotherapy is implemented by applying specific positive exercises that emphasize a person's specifically chosen signature character strengths and incorporating them into treatment.
- Post-traumatic growth consists of positive changes in a person's life following trauma that develop as a direct result of their struggle to work through what happened to them.

- We were informed that post-traumatic growth is different than resilience. Resilience is a personal attribute that involves the capacity to bounce back to normal functioning after experiencing trauma without excessive effort, whereas in post-traumatic growth working through the struggle after trauma is what creates a positive change.
- There are three models, two interpretive stages, and five domains of post-traumatic growth. The three models of post-traumatic growth consist of strengths attained due to suffering, psychological preparedness, and existential reevaluation.
- The two interpretive stages of post-traumatic growth consist of perception of reality, where someone is in a sort of denial about the trauma; and interpretative reality, where they face the facts about what happened.
- The five domains of post-traumatic growth are used to evaluate how a person is progressing through their recovery. They consist of appreciation of life, new possibilities, relating to others, personal strength, and spiritual change.
- An interest in religion and spirituality often occurs as a part of post-traumatic growth, and although these two spiritual pursuits are similar, they also differ. Religion involves the worship of a being or greater power outside of human material existence. It may consist of following sacred texts, books, rules, formal prayers, or engaging in worship. Alternatively, spirituality emphasizes the energy that exists within the person and their connection with a universal source of power and may involve practices of reaching alternative dimensions.
- Participation in religious or spiritual practices may not be appropriate for those who have been abused by members of the clergy, or for persons who believe that their traumatic experiences were a form of abandonment or punishment from God.
- Three additional life-enhancing responses to adversity that facilitate positive outcomes were also explored, the importance of meaning-making, the instillation of hope, and the power of self-compassion.
- Two Narrative Case Studies were reviewed. The first one identified how a student nurse felt unprepared to discuss spiritual issues with her patient. A lack of adequate education in nursing school was identified as one of the key contributing factors to this problem. However, being honest about our knowledge deficit, and offering empathy, care, and compassion in a safe environment is sometimes what is needed.
- The second Narrative Case Study demonstrated how nurturing mindful self-compassion through meditation and creative visualization helped a teen to begin to heal from childhood trauma.

- These three learning activities were recommended (*e.g.*, Debating the Value of Positive Emotions; Understanding the 24 Signature Character Strengths of Positive Psychotherapy; and Lessons Learned from Those who Experienced Post-Traumatic Growth following Adversity).
- At the closing of the Chapter, a self-care strategy recommended making gratitude a daily routine and suggested adopting one of three specific gratitude-enhancing activities.

RECOMMENDED READINGS

Brett, R. (2012). *Be the miracle: 50 lessons for making the impossible possible.* Grand Central Publishing.

Donnelly, D. (2017). *Relentless optimism: How a commitment to positive thinking changes everything.* Shamrock New Media, Inc.

Ferrucci, P. (2006). *The power of kindness: The unexpected benefits of leading a compassionate life.* Jeremy P. Tarcher/Penguin.

Forrest, M. S. (2003). *A short course in kindness: A little book on the importance of love and the relative unimportance of just about everything else.* L. M. Press.

Goleman, D. (2005). *Emotional intelligence: Why it can matter more than IQ.* Bantam Books.

Seligman, M. (2011). *Flourish: A new understanding of happiness and well-being – and how to achieve them.* Nicholas Brealey Publishing.

REFERENCES

Aakvaag, HF, Thoresen, S, Wentzel-Larsen, T, Dyb, G, Røysamb, E & Olff, M (2016) Broken and guilty since it happened: A population study of trauma-related shame and guilt after violence and sexual abuse. *J Affect Disord,* 204, 16-23.
[http://dx.doi.org/10.1016/j.jad.2016.06.004] [PMID: 27318595]

Armenta, CN, Fritz, MM & Lyubomirsky, S (2017) Functions of positive emotions: Gratitude as a motivator of self-improvement and positive change. *Emot Rev,* 9, 183-90.
[http://dx.doi.org/10.1177/1754073916669596]

Ashley, P (2020) *Shame-informed therapy: Treatment strategies to overcome core shame and reconstruct the authentic self.* PESI Publishing & Media.

Balboni, MJ, Puchalski, CM & Peteet, JR (2014) The relationship between medicine, spirituality and religion: three models for integration. *J Relig Health,* 53, 1586-98.
[http://dx.doi.org/10.1007/s10943-014-9901-8] [PMID: 24917445]

Brett, R (2012) *Be the miracle: 50 lessons for making the impossible possible.* Grand Central Publishing.

Brooks, R & Goldstein, S (2003) *The power of resilience: Achieving balance, confidence, and personal strength in your life.* McGraw Hill.

Buchanan, KE & Bardi, A (2010) Acts of kindness and acts of novelty affect life satisfaction. *J Soc Psychol,* 150, 235-7.
[http://dx.doi.org/10.1080/00224540903365554] [PMID: 20575332]

Cabrera, V & Donaldson, SI (2023) PERMA to PERMA+4 building blocks of well-being: A systematic review of the empirical literature. *J Posit Psychol,* 1-20.
[http://dx.doi.org/10.1080/17439760.2023.2208099]

Calhoun, LG & Tedeschi, RG (2000) Early posttraumatic interventions: Facilitating possibilities for growth. In: Violanti, J.M., Patton, D., Dunning, D., (Eds.), *Posttraumatic stress intervention: Challenges, issues, and perspectives* . Charles C. Thomas Publisher, Ltd 135-52.

Calhoun, LG & Tedeschi, RG (2013) *Posttraumatic growth in clinical practice.* Routledge.

Canadian Nurses Association (CNA) (2017) *CNA code of ethics for registered nurses* Available from: https://cna.informz.ca/cna/data/images/Code_of_Ethics_2017_Edition_Secure_Interactive.pdf

Cashwell, CS & Swindle, PJ (2018) When religion hurts: Supervising cases of religious abuse. *Clin Supervisor,* 37, 182-203.
[http://dx.doi.org/10.1080/07325223.2018.1443305]

Christopher, M (2004) A broader view of trauma: A biopsychosocial-evolutionary view of the role of the traumatic stress response in the emergence of pathology and/or growth. *Clin Psychol Rev,* 24, 75-98.
[http://dx.doi.org/10.1016/j.cpr.2003.12.003] [PMID: 14992807]

Collier, L (2016) Growth after trauma: Why some people are more resiliency than others, and can it be taught. *J Trauma Stress,* 9, 455-71.
[http://dx.doi.org/10.1007/BF02103658]

Costandi, M (2016) *Neuroplasticity.* The MIT Press Essential Knowledge Series.
[http://dx.doi.org/10.7551/mitpress/10499.001.0001]

Csikszentmihalyi, M & Seligman, ME (2014) Positive psychology: An introduction. In: Csikszentmihalyi, M., (Ed.), *Flow and the foundations of positive psychology: The collected works of Mihaly Csikszentmihalyi* . Springer 279-98.
[http://dx.doi.org/10.1007/978-94-017-9088-8]

Diener, E & Chan, MY (2011) Happy people live longer: Subjective well-being contributes to health and longevity. *Appl Psychol Health Well-Being,* 3, 1-43.
[http://dx.doi.org/10.1111/j.1758-0854.2010.01045.x] [PMID: 26286968]

Donaldson, SI, van Zyl, LE & Donaldson, SI (2022) PERMA+4: A framework for work-related wellbeing, performance, and positive organizational psychology 2.0. *Front Psychol,* 12, 817244.
[http://dx.doi.org/10.3389/fpsyg.2021.817244] [PMID: 35140667]

Donnelly, D (2017) *Relentless optimism: How a commitment to positive thinking changes everything.* Shamrock New Media, Inc.

Emmons, RA & McCullough, ME (2003) Counting blessings *versus* burdens: An experimental investigation of gratitude and subjective well-being in daily life. *J Pers Soc Psychol,* 84, 377-89.
[http://dx.doi.org/10.1037/0022-3514.84.2.377] [PMID: 12585811]

Ferrucci, P (2006) *The power of kindness: The unexpected benefits of leading a compassionate life.* Penguin Group Inc.

Filipp, SH (1999) A three-sage model of coping with loss and trauma. In: Maercker, A., Schutzwohl, M., Solomon, Z., (Eds.), *Posttraumatic stress disorder: A lifespan development perspective* . Hougrefe & Huber 43-78.

First, J, First, N, Stevens, J, Mieseler, V & Houston, JB (2018) Post-traumatic growth 2.5 years after the 2011 Joplin, Missouri tornado. *J Fam Soc Work,* 21, 5-21.
[http://dx.doi.org/10.1080/10522158.2017.1402529]

Forrest, MS (2003) *A short course in kindness: A little book on the importance of love and the relative unimportance of just about everything else.* L. M. Press.

Frankl, V (2006) *Man's search for meaning.* Beakon Press.

Fredrickson, B (2003) The value of positive emotions: The emerging science of positive psychology is coming to understand why it's good to feel good. *Am Sci,* 91, 330-5.
[http://dx.doi.org/10.1511/2003.26.330]

Fredrickson, BL (2006) Unpacking positive emotions: Investigating the seeds of human flourishing. *J Posit Psychol,* 1, 57-9.
[http://dx.doi.org/10.1080/17439760500510981]

Froh, JJ (2004) The history of positive psychology: Truth be told. *New York State (NYS). Psychologist,* 16, 18-20.

Germer, C & Neff, KD (2019) Mindful self-compassion (MSC). In: Itvzan, I., (Ed.), *The handbook of mindfulness-based programs: Every established intervention, from medicine to education* Routledge 357-61.
[http://dx.doi.org/10.4324/9781315265438-28]

Ginwright, S (2018) The future of healing: Shifting from trauma informed care to healing centered engagement. *Occasional paper,,* 25, 25-32.

Goleman, D (2005) *Emotional intelligence: Why it can matter more than IQ.* Bantam Books.

Gulnar, A, Snowden, M, Wattis, J & Rogers, M (2018) Spirituality in nursing education: Knowledge and practice gaps. *International Journal for Multidisciplinary Comparative Studies,* 5, 27-49.

Haas, M (2015) *Bouncing forward: Transforming bad breaks into breakthroughs.* Atria & Enliven.

Harrad, R, Cosentino, C, Keasley, R & Sulla, F (2019) Spiritual care in nursing: An overview of the measures used to assess spiritual care provision and related factors amongst nurses. *Acta Biomed,* 90, 44-55.
[http://dx.doi.org/10.23750/abm.v90i4-S.8300] [PMID: 30977748]

Henson, C, Truchot, D & Canevello, A (2021) What promotes post traumatic growth? A systematic review. *European Journal of Trauma & Dissociation,* 5, 100195.
[http://dx.doi.org/10.1016/j.ejtd.2020.100195]

Hipolito, E, Samuels-Dennis, JA, Shanmuganandapala, B, Maddoux, J, Paulson, R, Saugh, D & Carnahan, B (2014) Trauma-informed care: Accounting for the interconnected role of spirituality and empowerment in mental health promotion. *J Spiritual Ment Health,* 16, 193-217.
[http://dx.doi.org/10.1080/19349637.2014.925368]

Janoff-Bulman, R (2004) Posttraumatic growth: Three explanatory models. *Psychol Inq,* 15, 30-4.

Jayawickreme, E, Infurna, FJ, Alajak, K, Blackie, LER, Chopik, WJ, Chung, JM, Dorfman, A, Fleeson, W, Forgeard, MJC, Frazier, P, Furr, RM, Grossmann, I, Heller, AS, Laceulle, OM, Lucas, RE, Luhmann, M, Luong, G, Meijer, L, McLean, KC, Park, CL, Roepke, AM, al Sawaf, Z, Tennen, H, White, RMB & Zonneveld, R (2021) Post☐traumatic growth as positive personality change: Challenges, opportunities, and recommendations. *J Pers,* 89, 145-65.
[http://dx.doi.org/10.1111/jopy.12591] [PMID: 32897574]

Kashdan, TB & Kane, JQ (2011) Post-traumatic distress and the presence of post-traumatic growth and meaning in life: Experiential avoidance as a moderator. *Pers Individ Dif,* 50, 84-9.
[http://dx.doi.org/10.1016/j.paid.2010.08.028] [PMID: 21072251]

Kelly, JD, IV (2022) Your best life: In the lowest moments, an opportunity for post-traumatic growth. *Clin Orthop Relat Res,* 480, 33-5.
[http://dx.doi.org/10.1097/CORR.0000000000002070] [PMID: 34812794]

Khaw, D & Kern, ML (2014) A cross-cultural comparison of the PERMA Model of well-being. *Undergraduate Journal of Psychology at Berkeley, University of California,* 8, 10-23.

Kuven, BM & Giske, T (2019) Talking about spiritual matters: First year nursing students' experiences of an

assignment on spiritual conversations. *Nurse Educ Today,* 75, 53-7.
[http://dx.doi.org/10.1016/j.nedt.2019.01.012] [PMID: 30731404]

Leitch, L (2017) Action steps using ACEs and trauma-informed care: a resilience model. *Health Justice,* 5, 5.
[http://dx.doi.org/10.1186/s40352-017-0050-5] [PMID: 28455574]

Linley, A, Joseph, S, Harrington, S & Wood, AM (2006) Positive psychology: Past, present, and (possible) future. *J Posit Psychol,* 1, 3-16.
[http://dx.doi.org/10.1080/17439760500372796]

Lowe, J, Butler, J & Lunn, I (2018) *Essential personal finance: A practical guide for employees.* Taylor and Francis.
[http://dx.doi.org/10.4324/9781351041669]

Macfarlane, J & Carson, J (2019) Positive psychology: an overview for use in mental health nursing. *British Journal of Mental Health Nursing,* 8, 34-8.
[http://dx.doi.org/10.12968/bjmh.2019.8.1.34]

Malhotra, M (2016) Posttraumatic growth: Positive changes following adversity – an overview. *Int J Psychol Behav Sci,* 6, 109-18.
[http://dx.doi.org/10.5923/j.ijpbs.20160603.03]

Martela, F & Steger, MF (2016) The three meanings of meaning in life: Distinguishing coherence, purpose, and significance. *J Posit Psychol,* 11, 531-45.
[http://dx.doi.org/10.1080/17439760.2015.1137623]

Maslow, AH (1954) *Motivational personality.* Harper & Row Publishers.

McEwen, BS (2016) In pursuit of resilience: Stress, epigenetics, and brain plasticity. *Ann N Y Acad Sci,* 1373, 56-64.
[http://dx.doi.org/10.1111/nyas.13020] [PMID: 26919273]

Menschner, C & Maul, A (2016) *Issue Brief: Key ingredients for successful trauma-informed care implementation* Available from: https: //www.samhsa. gov/sites /default /files /programs _campaigns /childrens _mental_ health/ atc-whitepape r-040616 .pdf

Nakamura, J & Csikszentmihalyi, M (2014) *The concept of flow and the foundations of positive psychology.* Springer.
[http://dx.doi.org/10.1007/978-94-017-9088-8_16]

Oral, R, Ramirez, M, Coohey, C, Nakada, S, Walz, A, Kuntz, A, Benoit, J & Peek-Asa, C (2016) Adverse childhood experiences and trauma informed care: the future of health care. *Pediatr Res,* 79, 227-33.
[http://dx.doi.org/10.1038/pr.2015.197] [PMID: 26460523]

National Alliance on Mental Illness (NAMI) (2016) *The mental health benefits of religion & spirituality.* . Available from: https://www.nami.org/Blogs/NAMI-Blog/DEcember-2016/The-Mental-Health-Benef-ts-of-Religion-Spiritual

Pal, R & Elbers, J (2018) Neuroplasticity: The other side of the coin. *Pediatr Neurol,* 84, 3-4.
[http://dx.doi.org/10.1016/j.pediatrneurol.2018.03.009] [PMID: 29685608]

Perlman, HH (1983) *Relationship: The heart of helping people.* The University of Chicago Press.

Peterson, C (2006) *A primer in positive psychology.* Oxford Press.

Peterson, C & Seligman, MEP (2004) *Character strengths and virtues: A handbook and classification.* American Psychological Association & Oxford University Press.

Poseck, BV, Baquero, BC & Jimenez, MLV (2006) The traumatic experience from positive psychology: Resiliency and post-traumatic growth. *Pap Psicol,* 27, 40-9. http://www.cop.es/papeles

Rashid, T & Seligman, MP (2018) *Positive psychotherapy: Clinician manual.* Oxford University Press.

Ray, MA (2016) *Transcultural caring dynamics in nursing and healthcare.* FA Davis.

Rendon, J (2015) *Upside: The new science of post-traumatic growth.* Touchtone Publishing.

Rowland, L & Curry, OS (2019) A range of kindness activities boost happiness. *J Soc Psychol,* 159, 340-3.
[http://dx.doi.org/10.1080/00224545.2018.1469461] [PMID: 29702043]

Seligman, M (2011) *Flourish: A new understanding of happiness and well-being – and how to achieve them.* Nicholas Brealey Publishing.

Shaffer, J (2016) Neuroplasticity and clinical practice: Building brain power for health. *Front Psychol,* 7, 1118.
[http://dx.doi.org/10.3389/fpsyg.2016.01118] [PMID: 27507957]

Shapiro, S, Siegel, R & Neff, KD (2018) Paradoxes of Mindfulness. *Mindfulness,* 9, 1693-701.
[http://dx.doi.org/10.1007/s12671-018-0957-5]

Sowers, WE (2022) Recovery and person-centered care: empowerment, collaboration, and integration. In: Sowers, W.E., McQuistion, H.L., Ranz, J.M., Feldman, J.M., Runnels, P.S., (Eds.), *Textbook of Community Psychiatry* Springer 21-32.
[http://dx.doi.org/10.1007/978-3-031-10239-4_3]

Stanford, P S (2010) *Religion: 50 ideas you really need to know about religion.* Chartwell Books.

Stephany, K (2012) *Each day is a new creation: Guidelines on living a life on purpose.* Balboa Press: A Division of Hay House.

Stephany, K (2020) *The ethic of care: A moral compass for nursing practice.*Bentham Science Publishers Pte. Ltd.

Stephany, K (2022) *Cultivating empathy: Inspiring health professionals to communicate more effectively.* Bentham Science Publishers Pte. Ltd.

Tedeschi, RG & Calhoun, LG (1996) The posttraumatic growth inventory: Measuring the positive legacy of trauma. *J Trauma Stress,* 9, 455-71.
[http://dx.doi.org/10.1002/jts.2490090305] [PMID: 8827649]

Tedeschi, RG & Calhoun, LG (2004) Posttraumatic growth: Conceptual foundations and empirical evidence. *Psychol Inq,* 15, 1-18.
[http://dx.doi.org/10.1207/s15327965pli1501_01]

Tedeschi, RG, Calhoun, LG & Groleau, JM (2015) Clinical applications of posttraumatic growth. In: Joseph, S., (Ed.), *Positive psychology in practice: Promoting human flourishing in health, education, and everyday life* . Wiley Online Books 503-18.
[http://dx.doi.org/10.1002/9781118996874.ch30]

Tesh, M, Learman, J & Pulliam, RM (2015) Mindful self-compassion strategies for survivors of intimate partner abuse. *Mindfulness,* 6, 192-201.
[http://dx.doi.org/10.1007/s12671-013-0244-4]

Values in Action (VIA) Institute on Character (2023) *The 24 Character strengths.* https: //www. viacharacter .org/ charactr strenghts

van der Kolk, B (2014) *The body keeps score: Brain, mind, and body in the healing of trauma.* Viking Penguin.

Walker, V (2010) *The art of comforting: What to say and do for people in distress.* Penguin Group.

Watson, J (2008) *Nursing: The philosophy and science of caring.* University Press of Colorado.

Werdel, MB, Dy-Liacco, GS, Ciarrocchi, JW, Wicks, RJ & Breslford, GM (2014) The unique role of spirituality in the process of growth following stress and trauma. *Pastoral Psychol,* 63, 57-71.
[http://dx.doi.org/10.1007/s11089-013-0538-4]

Wilson, KR, Hansen, DJ & Li, M (2011) The traumatic stress response in child maltreatment and resultant neuropsychological effects. *Aggress Violent Behav,* 16, 87-97.

[http://dx.doi.org/10.1016/j.avb.2010.12.007]

Xiang, Y, Chao, X & Ye, Y (2018) Effect of gratitude on benign and malicious envy: The mediating role of social support. *Front Psychiatry,* 9, 139.
[http://dx.doi.org/10.3389/fpsyt.2018.00139] [PMID: 29867595]

CHAPTER 5

Mitigate the Negative Effects of Secondary Traumatic Stress and Compassion Fatigue by Cultivating a Caring Pedagogy and Resilience

Abstract: Students and practicing nurses are at risk of developing empathy-based stress conditions related to caring for people who have been traumatized. Caring is a known factor in all suggested interventions for empathy-based stress conditions. Therefore, Chapter Five explores ways to mitigate the negative effects of secondary traumatic stress and compassion fatigue through employing a caring pedagogy and resilience. Caring pedagogy in nursing education is important because it incorporates caring components into the delivery of the core curriculum, creates a community of learning that prioritizes students, is inclusive, and engaging, and protects the emotional integrity of student nurses. Noddings' elements of moral education such as modeling, dialogue, practice, and confirmation are identified as essential to a caring learning environment. For example, student nurses can learn what it means to care by observing the behavior of their instructor, by a dynamic exchange of ideas, by prioritizing caring, and by encouraging the best in others. A learning environment that is caring must also be based on civility and is the shared responsibility of both faculty and students. Self-care is identified as a known strategy to reduce the emotional stress experienced by nurses and student nurses. Watson's Caritas processes are subsequently recommended as the basis for self-care and consist of demonstrating sensitivity toward oneself and everyone else, through spiritual practices that support loving, caring relationships. Resilience consists of the ability to quickly return to normal functioning after experiencing adversity. Resilience skills can be learned through the development of protective factors and mechanisms and may prevent empathy-based stress conditions related to trauma, can assist a trauma survivor to bounce back more quickly, and teach people how to deal with the stress of everyday life. The following ways to cultivate resilience in nurses are presented, building positive nurturing relationships and networks; maintaining positivity; developing emotional insight; achieving life balance and spirituality; and becoming more reflective. Three strategies to foster resilience in nursing education include resilience training in the school curriculum; prioritizing role modelling; and enabling generativity. Two Narrative Case Studies are presented. The first one tells the story of how a Psychiatric Nurse developed the signs of secondary traumatic stress after one of her clients ended their life through suicide. The second one describes how a student nurse was unaware that she was experiencing emotional strain. The following four learning activities are proposed, sharing examples of being cared for; exploring ways to enhance learning; nurturing caring experiences in educational settings; and implementing Watson's caring processes and strategies to enhance self-care. The Chapter ends by recommending a self-care challenge that promotes emotional appraisal to manage negative emotions.

Kathleen Stephany

Keywords: Trauma, Trauma-informed care, Secondary traumatic stress (STS), Compassion, Compassion fatigue (CF), Empathy-based stress, Moral disengagement, Relational practice, Burnout, Critical incident debriefing, Safety plan, Pedagogy, Caring pedagogy, Trauma-informed educational processes, Four Core Assumptions of Trauma-informed Care, Potential psychologically traumatic events (PPTEs), Caring, Pedagogy, Caring pedagogy, Student-focused learning, Nodding's Four elements of Moral Education, Role modeling, Dialogue, Caring presence, Confirmation, Emotional strain, Philosophy and Science of Caring, Watson's Caritas Processes, Civility, Incivility, Resilience, Cognitive behavioral therapy, Emotional intelligence, Generativity, Negative emotions, Emotional regulatory process, Emotional suppression, Emotional appraisal.

LEARNING GUIDE

After completing this chapter, the reader should be able to:

- Be reminded that people working in healthcare, including nurses and student nurses, are at risk of being exposed to trauma-related stress and developing empathy-based stress conditions.
- Gain an understanding of the similarities and differences between secondary traumatic stress and compassion fatigue and their risks, signs and symptoms, and measures to reduce their negative effects.
- Identify caring as a key factor in all suggested interventions for empathy-based stress conditions.
- Describe what it means to care, to be cared for, and to be present.
- Identify the 4 Cs of trauma-informed care.
- Recognize that caring relationships are not only essential in nursing but also for nursing education.
- Define the premise of caring pedagogy and its connection to trauma-informed educational processes.
- Describe how learning environments in nursing school can be re-designed to be more student-focused.
- Explain how Noddings' four elements of moral education are essential for a caring learning environment.
- Create a learning atmosphere that is embedded in key components of caring and mutual civility.
- Understand the importance of self-care and its capacity for mitigating the emotional strain experienced by nurses and student nurses.
- Become aware of Watson's Caritas processes as the basis for self-care and how to apply each of her ten Caritas processes in practice.
- Be introduced to some useful personal self-care activities.
- Identify the basic components of resilience.

- Learn strategies that promote personal resilience.
- Point out three specific strategies to foster resilience in nursing education.
- Review two Narrative Case Studies and ensuing Thematic Analysis. The first one explores how a Psychiatric Nurse develops the signs of secondary traumatic stress after one of her clients ends their life through suicide. The second one describes how a student nurse is unaware that she is experiencing the signs of emotional stress.
- Participate in these learning activities (*e.g.*, Sharing Examples of Being Cared For; Exploring Ways to Enhance Learning; Nurturing Caring Experiences in Educational Settings; and Implementing Watson's Caring Processes and Strategies to Enhance Self-care).
- Consider a self-care strategy that challenges nurses to use emotional appraisal to manage negative emotions.

INTRODUCTION TO CHAPTER FIVE

People working in healthcare, including students, and practicing nurses, are at risk of being exposed to trauma related empathy-based stress (Goddard *et al.*, 2021). **Empathy-based stress** is due to trauma exposure and accompanied by an affective reaction that causes a strain in empathetic capacity, where the caregiver is no longer able to identify with the experiences of another person (Rauvola *et al.*, 2019). Because caring is a key component to all suggested interventions for empathy-based stress conditions, Chapter Five explores ways to mitigate the negative effects of secondary traumatic stress and compassion fatigue by employing a caring pedagogy and resilience. Although secondary traumatic stress and compassion fatigue were introduced in Chapter One, in this current Chapter, they are revisited with the specific goal of applying strategies to reduce their negative impact.

Caring pedagogy is promoted because it creates a healthy educational environment where caring is not only prioritized but consistently practiced (Duffy, 2018). For example, caring pedagogy prioritizes human relationships, fosters engagement, and values the subjective, contextual, and objective aspects of learning. It is also important in nursing education because it protects the emotional integrity of student nurses. **Resilience** strategies are recommended to assist in the following ways. They help prevent work-related traumatic conditions, assist someone to bounce back and return to their original functioning after experiencing a trauma, and teach people how to deal with the stress of everyday life. (Collier, 2016). Specific ways to foster resilience in nursing education are also suggested.

SECONDARY TRAUMATIC STRESS AND COMPASSION FATIGUE

Secondary traumatic stress and compassion fatigue develop due to exposure to trauma and human suffering. However, **Secondary traumatic stress (STS)** does not necessarily develop due to actual personal experience with trauma but is an after-effect of being confronted with another person's experience of adversity. For example, secondary traumatic stress quite often manifests over time, after directly observing traumatic events, listening to a detailed account of one, or being exposed to adverse situations (Mottaghi & Poursheikhali, 2020).

Compassion, or the capacity to identify with, and relate to, the suffering of others, is considered a hallmark of caring nursing practice (Fig. **5.1**). However, sometimes a nurse's capacity to feel empathy is thwarted and may lead to compassion fatigue. **Compassion fatigue (CF)** occurs when a caregiver becomes overly preoccupied and emotionally involved with the suffering or trauma experienced by people in their care (Ariapooran, 2014; Figley, 1995). It results in caregiver emotional exhaustion and interferes with their ability to act in empathetic ways to avoid further psychological trauma (Foli & Thompson, 2019: Kearney & Weininger, 2011).

Fig. (5.1). Compassion. Source: www.pixabay.com.

The Similarities and Differences Between Secondary Traumatic Stress and Compassion Fatigue

Secondary traumatic stress and compassion fatigue are both associated with empathy-based stress due to being exposed to other people's trauma. Although they have sometimes been used interchangeably, they also differ in some ways (Hinderer *et al.*, 2014). For example, some believe that secondary traumatic stress disorder is a form of compassion fatigue that occurs over time, due to repetitive exposure to traumatic material. Unfortunately, secondary traumatic stress eventually leads to serious illness in the form of post-traumatic stress disorder

(PTSD). The symptoms a person may experience due to PTSD are quite distressing and include repetitive and recurring bad dreams, fearful thoughts, anger, irritability, difficulty with interpersonal relationships, and an inability to cope (Jenkins *et al.*, 2022; Rauviola *et al.*, 2019).

In contrast, compassion fatigue develops acutely and results in a lack of emotional engagement, and although the symptoms are distressful, they are not as serious as PTSD. They mimic those experienced by the person who has been traumatized and can include hyperarousal, avoidance of situations that are reminders of stressful circumstances, and problems with sleep (Ariapooram, 2014; Hinderer *et al.*, 2014; Figley, 1995). Compassion fatigue may also directly, and adversely affect a nurse's physical and psychological health. Those who develop it are prone to excessive exhaustion, become ill more frequently, complain of physical pain and headaches, and experience increased incidences of anxiety, sadness, loneliness, and depression (Gustafsson & Hemberg, 2022).

Moral disengagement is an additional negative repercussion related to compassion fatigue and consists of a nurse avoiding relational aspects of nursing care, and only performing tasks as a way of shielding themselves from further exposure to human anguish (Stephany, 2020). Moral disengagement rarely occurs on purpose but is more commonly due to unconscious mechanisms that protect the person from being exposed to additional psychological trauma (Kearney & Weininger, 2011). Subsequently, compassion fatigue may negatively affect the nurse's professional life because they feel less satisfied with the work they are doing, and experience remorse due to their inability to care for their clients/patients in a holistic manner.

Compassion fatigue also often co-exists with burnout. **Burnout** is depicted by physical and mental exhaustion due to longstanding exposure to emotionally demanding and stressful working conditions (Figley, 1995). Burnout can result in a decreased interest in one's work including absenteeism. It also causes physical and psychological fatigue, sleep disturbances, depression, anxiety, sleep difficulties, and relationship difficulties with clients/patients and other healthcare professionals (Ariapooram, 2014; Hinderer *et al.*, 2014).

WHEN SECONDARY TRAUMATIC STRESS OR COMPASSION FATIGUE IS SUSPECTED

Recognizing General Susceptibility

One of the first steps in helping those who may be experiencing secondary traumatic stress or compassion fatigue is to recognize and acknowledge specific vulnerabilities (Mangoulia *et al.*, 2015). All healthcare professionals who care for people who have been traumatized are at risk of developing these conditions. However, increased risk is associated with people with unresolved personal trauma, who do not cope well, and who are self-critical (Kerig, 2019). Because empathy is a required prerequisite to care for those who have been traumatized, those with excessive empathetic reactions are also more likely to develop a stress-related condition. (Figley, 1995). For example, Mottaghi *et al.*, (2020) point out that student nurses who have high levels of empathic concern for their clients' suffering, experience greater incidences of secondary traumatic stress and compassion fatigue, than students who are less emotionally affected by human anguish.

Potential Psychologically Traumatic Events

Exposure to **potential psychologically traumatic events (PPTEs)** increases the risk of a healthcare professional developing an empathy-based stress condition. PPTEs consist of any distressing experience like exposure to death, severe injury, or violence (Stelnicki *et al.*, 2020). For example, nursing specific PPTEs may consist of caring for the severely ill, injured, dying, or patients with COVID-19 (Foli & Thompson, 2019; Wedgeworth, 2016). Other quite distressing forms of PPTEs entail dealing with injury or death due to extreme violence; the death of a child; the death of a patient/client after strenuous and lengthy efforts to try and revive them; and the death of someone who resembles a family member (Mayer *et al.*, 2022; Stelnicki *et al.*,).

Enhanced Risk Associated with Specific Work Environments

Although all empathy-based conditions can occur in those who work in a wide variety of work settings, certain specific areas of work where exposure to trauma occurs quite often, are known to pose a higher risk (Kerig, 2019). In the profession of nursing, they include working in the emergency room (ER), intensive care unit (ICU), mental health, hospice, and palliative care. The ER, ICU, and psychiatric settings are especially stressful due to regular exposure to demanding conditions, and the emotionally disturbing nature of the work (Duffy *et al.*, 2015; Mangoulia *et al.*, 2015). For instance, in the ER there can be a regular bombardment of traumatic injuries due to motor vehicle and other accidents, violent physical and sexual assaults, and other crimes. ICU nurses care for clients/patients who are high acuity, critically ill, or injured, and are prone to greater-than-normal rates of morbidity and mortality (Hinderder *et al.*, 2014). In some mental health settings nurses are also exposed to violence, and when aggressive acts are directed toward them it can have serious psychological impacts (Mangoulia *et al.*,).

The Signs & Symptoms of Secondary Traumatic Stress & Compassion Fatigue

Recognizing the signs and symptoms of any empathy-based stress condition is essential for early diagnosis and treatment. In both secondary traumatic stress and compassion fatigue numbing and avoidant reactions are apparent. In secondary traumatic stress the symptoms of PTSD, such as intrusive imagery, recurring nightmares, avoidance, relationship difficulties, and angry outbursts, may be indicators of a need for urgent intervention (Gates & Gillespie, 2008). In compassion fatigue emotional detachment, distancing oneself from all aspects of relational practice, and an inability to offer empathy, are manifestations of this condition (Kearney & Weininger, 2011). In both empathy-based stress conditions difficulty dealing with workload, decreased job performance, disinterest in making a difference, along with a gradual onset of negative feelings or hopelessness, can all be indicators that the person is in trouble (Mangoulia *et al.*, 2015). The following Case Study tells the story of how a Psychiatric Nurse develops some of the signs and symptoms of secondary traumatic stress after one of her clients' ends their life. Refer to Box (**5.1**).

Box 5.1. Narrative case study one: when a psychiatric nurse develops signs of secondary traumatic stress.

Abigail is a new Psychiatric Nurse who has been working in an acute Mental Health Unit for Children and Youth in Crisis. Abigail chose this area for her practice because she had been a troubled youth and felt like she was following her calling. Abigail also did her preceptorship on this unit in her last term as a student nurse and got along well with the whole team, so it seemed like a good decision to begin her career there. However, after six months of working on this unit, Abigail started to feel a bit down after each of her shifts. She also dreaded going back to work after her days off. She suspected that her sad feelings might have something to do with hearing too many sad stories from the kids on the unit. She also felt upset at times that many of the youth went back home to the same abusive situations that contributed to their distress in the first place. Then one day a really bad thing happened that seemed to put Abigail over the edge. Jaya, one of her clients who was only 14 years of age ended her life by suicide while on a weekend pass.

Abigail learned the tragic news during the morning handover on her first day back at work after days off. She immediately broke out into a cold sweat, her heart was racing, and she felt like she was going to cry, so she ran into the bathroom to get herself together. After a few minutes, she was able to contain her emotions, returned to the unit, and proceeded to get through her shift normally, or so she thought. That same night Abigail had a nightmare. In her dream, she saw Jaya crying uncontrollably while screaming out for someone to help her, but no one came to her rescue. It was a horrific dream and Abigail woke up quite suddenly and in considerable distress. She returned to work the next day as scheduled and did her best to show up for work every day. However, Abigail started to have recurring nightmares about Jaya, that got increasingly more graphic and disturbing. Sometimes they even included flashbacks from an earlier time in Abigail's life, when bad things happened to her, situations that Abigail had previously blocked out of her memory.

The dreams were becoming so distressing that Abigail was afraid to fall asleep at night. She still did her best to show up for her scheduled shifts, but only did the bare minimum of what was expected of her. Abigail experienced a numbing and avoidant response, where she refused to emotionally connect with her assigned clients to protect herself from becoming too attached to them. After all, what if they chose to do what Jaya did? Abigail didn't think she could deal with that sort of loss again. She also seemed to be agitated, refused to take care of any clients who had a history of self-harm and was not herself. Abigail's change in behavior was noticed by her colleagues on the unit and several of them reached out to the Manager with their concerns. One day, about three weeks after the tragic death of Jaya, the Unit Manager, Ms. Black, asked to meet with Abigail in her office after her shift ended. Abigail willingly attended but was visibly upset, not knowing why she was being summoned to see her supervisor.
"Am I in any trouble, Ms. Black?"
Sensing Abigail's concern, Ms. Black responded with a degree of sensitivity.
"You are not in trouble Abigail. I just need to talk to you because many of your colleagues are really worried about you and so am I. I made a request for critical incident debriefing to occur for all of us to process the sudden death of Jaya, but it has not happened yet. I apologize for that because if you had been properly debriefed sooner, you might be doing better. You clearly have been struggling with what happened to Jaya and that is to be expected, but now I am worried that you may be affected more than normal, and that you need help. I would very much like it if you would allow me to refer you to our Employee recommended Therapist, so you can be supported, and have a chance to talk about what you have been dealing with. I want to remind you that you are not in trouble, but I also have worked on this unit long enough to know that if you don't get the right type of help you could become sick emotionally. Does that make sense?"
Abigail was doing her best to contain her tears.
"Yes, it does make sense and I feel relieved because I know I have not been coping with what happened and that is scaring me. I am afraid I might never be the same again, and that I will no longer be good at caring for these types of clients. I am scared that I might not be cut out for this type of work, work that I have always wanted to do because I am so afraid that another client will do what Jaya did."
Ms. Black proceeded to do her best to validate what Abigail was feeling.
"Abigail, what you are going through happens to lots of us who work in these high-stress areas in nursing. It happened to me a long time ago, but because I got professional help, I cope better with what goes on, and if I am not coping, I quickly reach out for more help before it gets worse. That is what I want for you and everyone else who works here. If we don't take care of the caregivers there will be no one left to take care of the clients, and they need people like us to remain healthy and strong. I have to say one more thing."
Abigail curiously looked straight into her boss' eyes.
"What is the one more thing you want to tell me?"
After taking a deep breath, Ms. Black proceeded.
"I want you to know that what happened to Jaya was not your fault. We cannot protect everyone from ending their life. We can only do our best to keep them safe long enough to get them more help, and because we do our best, we can save some lives, but not every life. Even the most beneficial interventions, administered by the most qualified in the field sometimes fail. It is not your fault that Jaya died. You need to understand that and not feel guilty. You need to get that first. What happened was not your fault."
Feeling rather emotional and somewhat relieved to hear those words, Abigail started crying.
"Thank you for being there for me, and for telling me that it was not my fault. Please send me to the Therapist. I think I am ready to get some help."

(Box 5.1) cont.....

Ms. Black proceeded to make the Counselling referral and promised Abigail that her door was always open if she needed to talk.

NARRATIVE CASE STUDY ONE: IDENTIFICATION OF THEMES & ANALYSIS

Four key themes were identified from this story.

Theme # 1: Following the death of Jaya by suicide, it became evident that Abigail was experiencing symptoms of secondary traumatic stress.

Theme # 1 Analysis: Following the death of a client by suicide it is not uncommon for a healthcare professional who had cared for them prior to the lethal event to experience feelings of anger and sadness (Ting *et al.*, 2006). However, some of Abigail' symptoms were indicative of secondary traumatic stress. For example, after working with troubled youth for six months, Abigail was feeling a bit sad and emotionally stressed, likely due to being constantly exposed to the sad stories of the youth in her care. Following Jaya's death, Abigail also experienced some signs of PTSD, such as intrusive imagery in the form of repetitive and distressing nightmares, and a numbing and avoidant response, where she refused to emotionally connect with her assigned clients and did not want to care for ones who were suicidal.

Theme # 2: Although Abigail's Manager had made a request for the staff on the unit to receive professional critical incident debriefing. Three weeks after Jaya's death it still had not been implemented.

Theme # 2 Analysis: Critical incident debriefing is conducted by a trained professional after a traumatic event has occurred that is outside of normal human experience. The goal of critical incident de-briefing is to help those who have been exposed to the event to sort through their feelings and other emotional stress. However, for critical incident de-briefing to be effective, it should ideally occur as soon as possible after the adverse event (Mathieu, 2012). A long delay in this essential process may have impeded Abigail's ability to move forward.

Theme # 3: Ms. Black in her wisdom conveyed to Abigail that her client's suicide was not her fault and pointed out that, as caregivers, we cannot prevent everyone from ending their life.

Theme # 3 Analysis: Ms. Black's words of validation were beneficial in helping Abigail understand that we cannot always save everyone from willfully ending their life and that it is not necessarily our fault when suicide does occur. It is normal to initially feel self-blame and guilt following such a tragedy, but personally harmful if these feelings persist over time (Ting *et al.*, 2006). Too many healthcare professionals have inadvertently quit their jobs after the suicide death of a client because they felt they could have done better. But hindsight is always clearer after the fact, and looking back you sometimes can see what was not so obvious in the moment. But nevertheless, as Ms. Black pointed out, all we can do is our best. What we can also do is learn from what transpired, be supported to sort through our loss, and not give up a helping career when these sorts of devastating losses do occur (Stephany, 2017).

Theme # 4: Ms. Black referred Abigail for professional therapy to help her with what she was experiencing.

Theme # 4 Analysis: It is also crucially important that we normalize the experience of seeking professional assistance because oftentimes nurses and others who work in healthcare settings will not reach out for help when they need it, because of the fear of being stigmatized or judged (Gates & Gillespie, 2008). Please refer to Box (**5.2**) for further important information concerning suicide prevention.

Box 5.2. Information about suicide prevention for further reflection (as adapted from Stephany, 2017).

After reviewing this Case Study, some additional education concerning the topic of suicide is worth sharing. In my former role as a Coroner in charge of Special Investigations, I was involved in conducting research into deaths by suicide in the form of Psychological autopsies, to inform measures aimed at prevention of death. In that capacity, and as a member of the International Association for Suicide Prevention, I have gained some insight worth sharing about the ambiguity of assessing for suicide intent. Although there are extensive and reliable tools that have been created to assess suicide risk, none of them is completely infallible.

Sometimes we are not able to prevent someone from ending their life. That is because suicide is a complicated issue, multifaceted, and unique for each person. What we do know is that the most difficult cases to discern actual suicide risk, involve people who have made up their mind to carry through with a premeditated plan. They often willingly hide any indication of their intention from caregivers. These are the people that cause health professionals the most distress when they end their lives, because the caregiver did not foresee what was about to occur, and often feels tremendous guilt for not being able to prevent the death. In other situations, when someone is vacillating about their intent, they are more likely to reach out for help before acting and this disclosure provides the caregiver with an opportunity to intervene. Nevertheless, all we can do is our best to help, and that begins by training gatekeepers in suicide prevention measures. Suicide prevention involves assessing for risk and implementing a comprehensive safety plan. A **safety plan** is designed to assist someone who is suicidal in identifying their warning signs, and ways to keep them safe, establishing anchors for living, and writing down the names and phone numbers of people to call when they are in crisis.

General Measures that May Help Reduce the Negative Effects of Empathy-based Stress Conditions

Different forms of assistance can be helpful in warding off the symptoms of empathy-based stress conditions. The following measures are helpful, educating nurses and other health professionals that these conditions exist, informing them of their specific signs and symptoms, and where to go for support, when and if needed (Gates & Gillespie, 2008). Peer support is especially beneficial because work colleagues can relate to what they are experiencing and are therefore more likely to offer empathy and understanding (Caringi *et al.*, 2017) (Fig. **5.2**).

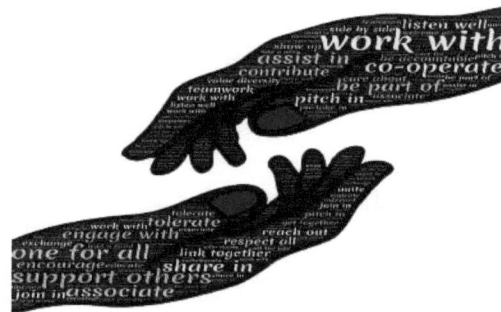

Fig. (5.2). The Importance of Support. Source: www.pixabay.com.

Healthcare Organizations Have a Role to Play in Reducing Risk

Organizations that adopt a trauma-informed system of care also need to ensure that they not only insulate the client/patient from situations that may re-traumatize them but that they also protect staff (Handran, 2015). For example, evidence indicates that health professionals whose role is to care almost exclusively for trauma survivors have a higher risk of developing secondary traumatic stress or compassion fatigue (Handran, 2015). Therefore, it is highly recommended that Employers provide opportunities, when possible, to balance scheduling that allows for alternative work experiences to reduce exposure to trauma (Handran). I witnessed firsthand how this strategy can work. For instance, because of the high attrition and burnout rates of Neonatal Intensive Care Unit (NICU) nurses, a local Health Authority, with the approval of the affected nurses, decided to have them work one week per month in the birthing unit. This was done as a way to give them a break from their exposure to neonatal morbidity and mortality, and to work in a more positive environment. Over time, this policy successfully reduced the incidence of burnout, and those leaving the unit, and increased NICU nurses' emotional well-being.

CARING IS A KEY FACTOR IN INTERVENTION STRATEGIES FOR EMPATHY-BASED STRESS CONDITIONS

Caring is a key component in intervention strategies to mitigate the effects of empathy-based stress conditions. For example, when it comes to nursing education, caring relationships displayed by faculty actually assist in decreasing some of the adverse effects of exposure to trauma in students (Goddard *et al.*, 2021). Therefore, prior to examining the merits of caring pedagogy and resilience an overview of specific aspects of caring are presented, the merits of caring in nursing; the action of being present; applying the 4 Cs of trauma-informed care; and the importance of caring relationships.

The Merits of Caring in Nursing

The need to belong and feel connected to others is an inherent need of all human beings, and caring for others is the essence of everything that nurses do, and (Ray, 2016; Watson, 2008) (Fig. **5.3**). To **care** for someone consists of offering them respect, inclusivity, empathy, emotional warmth, and genuine concern for their well-being (Perlman, 1979, Ray, 2016). It involves doing our very best to understand the other person's perspective, to see through their eyes with the goal of wanting to understand what they are going through, and doing what we can to comfort them and alleviate their suffering (Perlman, 1979; Stephany, 2020).

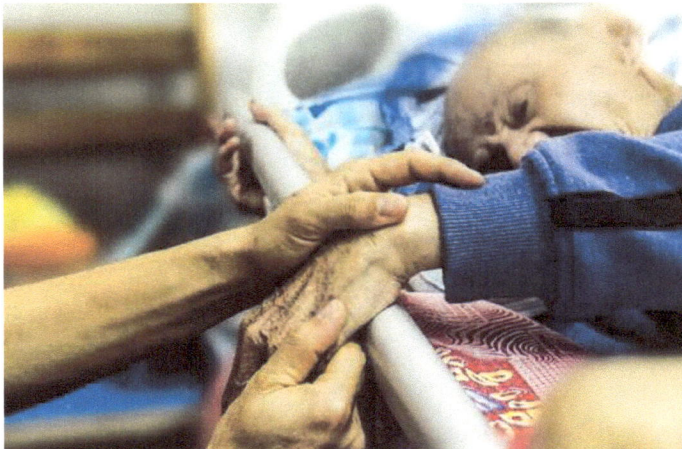

Fig. (5.3). Caring in Nursing. Source: www.pixabay.com.

Caring in nursing can be viewed as a process, where the nurse relates to their client/patient as a fellow human being, and results in a feeling of mutual trust, understanding, and being cared for in all who participate in that intricate relationship (Duffy, 2018); Noddings, 2013).

Being cared for is depicted by the recipient in a myriad of ways, because everyone's experience is subjective and personal, and has been so poignantly illustrated by patients who lived through a serious illness or injury while admitted to an Intensive Care Unit. They described it as living through suffering within a secure and trusting environment and being helped to live a fulfilling life more harmoniously (Locsin & Kongsuwan, 2013). Caring in this holistic fashion is all-encompassing and includes elements of safety and implicit trust, (Noddings, 2013). Subsequently, when clients/patients feel cared for in this fashion, they are more likely to award a higher satisfaction score on the quality of the nursing care provided, because they believe that their well-being and general welfare are a priority for their nurse. More importantly, the feeling of being cared for fosters in its recipient, a collaborative, cooperative, and receptive attitude of engagement in the healthcare being provided, and often results in an increased willingness to participate in healthier life choices (Duffy, 2018). We have just briefly reviewed some aspects of being cared for in nursing. A Learning Activity is included in Box (**5.3**) where you are tasked with the challenge of coming up with additional examples of the experience of being cared for.

Box 5.3. Learning activity: sharing examples of being cared for.

In small groups or as a large class spend time discussing additional examples of being cared for. Try and be as descriptive as you can. If you decide to do the exercise in small groups, reconvene after you have finished the exercise to share your findings with the whole class.
You can include examples from nursing, trauma-informed care, and your personal lived experience. You may refer to your own stories. However, do not reveal details that are traumatizing. Set clear expectations that no one will reveal the content of these narratives or repeat them outside the classroom setting, without the expressed permission of the individual who shared them.

The Action of Being Present

"The greatest gift you can give another is your undivided attention" Dorothy Sander, Freelance Writer.

Being empathetic, compassionate, interested in a person's lived experience, and listening to their story are the actions of a nurse who is genuinely present (Zyblock, 2010). **Being present** is about being fully engaged and engrossed in the one being cared for, with an attitude that demonstrates a heartfelt desire for their well-being and wanting what is best for them (Noddings, 2013; Stephany, 2020). Being present also concerns making ourselves available to them. It is about letting go of our agenda and becoming quiet and still enough to give the other person the opportunity to let us know what they need. Listening to them, without interruption, and with the explicit and genuine intent to understand, is the essence of active listening (Rakel, 2018).

Applying the 4 Cs of Trauma-informed Care

People who have experienced trauma need to experience being cared for, but what they require may be somewhat more challenging for the nurse, not because these people are difficult, but because they have unique needs. For example, merely focusing your attention on the problems they present with may be inadequate, especially if what has occurred to them, and the emotional struggles that they have endured, are ignored or unaddressed (Menschner & Maul, 2016). Emotional excitability, poor self-esteem, and an earned lack of trust in other people may also occur. Therefore, specific and helpful ways to deliver trauma-informed caring concern that are evidence-based consist of applying the 4 Cs of Trauma-informed Care (*e.g.*, Calm, Contain, Care, and Cope) (Kimberg & Wheeler, 2019). **Calm** refers to you as the practitioner. It occurs during your encounter with the person you are caring for, where you adopt measures to calm yourself so that you can transfer that sense of peacefulness to them. This action is based on the notion of biological co-regulation and can be achieved in several ways. One is through intentionally adopting an attitude of patience and understanding. Another means is by paying attention to what you are feeling because if you display anxiety it will interfere with your client/patients sense of calm. Subsequently, to maintain a sense of serenity you should adopt actions that facilitate peacefulness through deep breathing or grounding exercises (Kimberg & Wheeler, 2019).

Contain consists of deliberate protection of the person's physical and emotional well-being by limiting their discloser of trauma details during history taking or other aspects of treatment. It also includes respectfully assisting them if a triggering response does occur by referring them for follow-up support from appropriate community resources (Kimberg & Wheeler, 2019). **Care** involves the caregiver role modelling the importance of self-care in the form of self-compassion and offering compassion to clients/patients and work colleagues. For instance, if a caregiver utilizes self-care measures to keep themselves physically and emotionally well, they can legitimately speak to the benefits that have been derived from them. The client/patient is, therefore, more likely to trust someone who uses those techniques. Cultural humility is another important aspect of care where the caregiver intentionally dismantles the power differentials and acts in ways that make the other person feel like an equal partner in the treatment that is provided (Kimberg & Wheeler, 2019). **Cope** promotes skills that enhance a person's ability to handle stress. It also fosters resilience, and hope, and encourages them to form positive relationships with supportive people. It includes a cultural perspective that emphasizes social connection and may consist of a referral for mental health, substance use, or other treatment modalities when needed (Kimberg & Wheeler, 2019).

The Importance of Caring Relationships in Nursing

Caring relationships are essential to the practice of nursing and healthy caring relationships between caregivers and clients/patients are good for both parties. It can make working in healthcare more meaningful for the nurse, enhance client/patient outcomes, and provide a trusting environment for healthcare delivery to occur (Duffy, 2018). For example, a caring and trustworthy relationship with a nurse may enable the person to feel safe enough to reach out for assistance when they need it. Caring relationships also extend to family members. It is important to be reminded of the fact that clients/patients and their families are often thrust into an unsettling situation where illness or injury threatens their sense of normality and fills them with uncertainty (Duffy, 2018). Furthermore, a hospitalized client/patient who recovers will eventually get sent home and they do not take their nurse with them. That is why clear, and respectful communication with those who will be acting as caregivers not only alleviates their concerns but also provides an opportunity to teach them how best to care for their loved one. When a family is not located locally or someone does not have family, being cared for by a trustworthy, compassionate nurse becomes even more important (Duffy, 2018).

THE ROLE OF CARING PEDAGOGY IN NURSING EDUCATION

Caring relationships and respectful behaviors exhibited by nurse educators toward their students are a necessary component of nursing education that can help mitigate some of the adverse effects of students being exposed to trauma (Goddard *et al.*, 2021). Therefore, this section begins by introducing how a caring pedagogy and its alignment with trauma-informed educational approaches support student nurses. The following ways to ensure that learning environments in nursing school are embedded in caring pedagogy include ensuring that they are student-focused, are imbedded in Noddings key elements of a moral and caring learning environment, and are civil. The importance of teaching self-care strategies is also emphasized which includes applying Watson's ten caritas processes.

However, before proceeding with this discussion it is important to stress what Goddard *et al.*, (2021) have pointed out, that applying a trauma-informed approach or caring pedagogy in nursing education does not mean that teaching expectations should be lowered, or rules obliterated. A healing learning environment in nursing school still requires attention to all the necessities of a superb education. High standards should still be upheld and include setting clear expectations, ensuring that academic and clinical skills requirements for competency are met, and an insistence that academic integrity and professionalism be maintained (Goddard *et al.*, 2021).

Education *Versus* Pedagogy

Education is not the same as pedagogy. **Education** is described as "learning for its own sake," which means that you participate because you want to and not because you are required to (Hinchliffe, 2001, p. 31). In contrast, **pedagogy** refers to the process of teaching and includes specific designs, methods, and teaching strategies that facilitate the acquisition of knowledge A key priority in modern-day pedagogy is its role in higher education and its capacity to influence the social, political, and psychological development of students (Duffy, 2018); Hinchliffe, 2001). Therefore, choice in subject matter and methods of instruction in circles of higher education are crucially important.

Caring Pedagogy & Trauma-informed Educational Practices

Caring pedagogy in nursing education incorporates caring components into the delivery of the core curriculum, creates a community of learning that prioritizes students, is inclusive, engaging, and fosters caring relationships (Duffy, 2018); Ray, 2016; Watson, 2008). Caring pedagogy also protects the emotional and psychological integrity of student nurses, especially in today's stressful clinical work environments. Therefore, the basic premise of a caring pedagogy is closely associated with **trauma-informed educational processes** that value respectful interpersonal relationships, a supportive teaching venue, people's feelings, effective communication skills, and all aspects of genuine caring (Thomas *et al.*, 2019).

ENSURING THAT THE LEARNING ENVIRONMENT IS STUDENT-FOCUSED

"Teaching is more than imparting knowledge; it is inspiring change. Learning is more than absorbing facts; it is acquiring understanding." William Arthur Ward, American Author.

Student-focused learning is a central component of caring pedagogy in nursing education. Therefore, what follows is an overview of these specific strategies, moving away from imparting knowledge, changing the teaching environment, active engagement, and mutual problem-solving.

Moving Away from Imparting Knowledge

Even though evidence indicates that student-focused learning is beneficial and well-received by students, nursing schools still primarily deliver teacher-based methods of imparting knowledge instead of making students active participants in the process (Berg & Lepp, 2023). For example, in teacher-driven methods faculty decide what information is vital, then plan and deliver the content in their preferred manner, often in the form of a lecture. The student nurse's role is to listen and be an impartial receiver of knowledge. Unfortunately, this type of learning is not very collaborative and largely ignores the learning needs of modern-day students (Bankert & Kozel, 2005). In caring pedagogy, students are encouraged to actively participate by asking questions, sharing their thoughts and ideas, and being responsible for their own learning. That is why **student-focused learning** prioritizes an educational experience that is cooperative, creative, sensitive to the learner's needs, and utilizes activities that encourage engagement, critical thinking, discussion, debate, and personal reflection (Bankert & Kozel, 2005).

Student-focused delivery of nursing school content is known to be beneficial in several ways. For instance, Berg and Lepp (2023) conducted a comprehensive and consolidative review of the literature to explore the significance and application of student-focused learning in nursing education. Their findings came up with recommendations by student nurses. The first suggestion was that faculty treat students as equal partners in the learning process and create democratic learning environments. In order to be better prepared for teamwork after graduation, student nurses requested to be taught how to think critically, problem-solve, and work in groups. They also asked to be taught how to become life-long learners and how to maintain competency to practice following graduation (Berg & Lepp, 2023). Another literature review conducted by Ward *et al.*, (2018) revealed additional suggestions to implement student-focused learning in nursing school. Because many nursing students work in jobs outside of their nursing program and extensive at-home preparation was time-consuming and stressful, a recommendation to design pre-class activities that were achievable and helped to consolidate their learning was suggested. Making use of short, pre-recorded videos, internet modules, and online quizzes, was identified as a less labor-intensive way to better prepare them for class. The following classroom learning activities were also proposed to engage them in learning, role plays, case studies, group discussions, and active problem-solving (Ward *et al.*, 2018).

Changing the Teaching Environment

A simple change in the arrangement of a class is another student-focused initiative that can make the learning venue less intimidating (Bankert & Kozel, 2005). For example, the traditional classroom arrangement of the Professor situated at the front of the room as lecturer, and students seated in rows facing the front as passive participants, not only emphasizes a power differential between teacher and learner but is also not that conducive to participatory learning. Alternatively, getting students to sit in small groups for learning activities, with the instructor moving around the room as a facilitator, makes the learning less intimidating, more interactive, and cooperative, and promotes relevant discussion. Student involvement in class presentations also boosts their self-esteem and facilitates knowledge retention (Bankert & Kozel, 2005).

Active Engagement

People are more likely to retain what they have been taught if they can apply what they are learning to real-life scenarios. Therefore, meaningful participation in the learning process is at the heart of student-focused learning. It consists of active student engagement which begins by making sure that everyone participates and is accountable for their learning. It may include reinforcing the need for students to do their best to come to class prepared and may also involve encouraging them to share relevant and personal stories to promote discussion, critical reflection, and knowledge retention (Bankert & Kozel, 2005).

Mutual Problem Solving

Another specific approach to student-focused learning occurs through mutual problem-solving. Although the instructor may have extensive expertise and knowledge, they must resist the temptation to inform and allow their students to actively participate in the process. When the teacher takes a step back before providing the students with information, they create opportunities for them to use their critical thinking skills to make sense of what they are learning. This can also be achieved through interactive brainstorming activities with other students, and back-and-forth active discussion that involves careful feedback from the instructor. For example, helpful constructive feedback by the instructor that promotes student self-confidence includes patience when answering student's questions, correcting errors in a way that helps the student to better understand how to do it right the next time, and acknowledging successes (Bankert & Kozel, 2005; Duffy, 2018). A Learning Activity is included in Box (**5.4**) where you are asked to explore other ways that the learning experience of nursing school can be improved upon.

Box 5.4. Learning activity: explore additional ways to enhance learning.

In small groups or as a large class spend time brainstorming ideas on additional suggestions for improving the learning experience in the classroom or clinical setting.

FOSTERING A CARING LEARNING ENVIRONMENT BY APPLYING NODDINGS ELEMENTS OF A MORAL AND CARING LEARNING ENVIRONMENT

A philosophy of education by Nel Noddings is based on the premise "that caring is an ethical imperative (and a) moral duty that defines the nature of teaching and learning, and shapes what education should be" (Chinn & Falk-Rafael, 2018), p. 687). Her assertion is that education has the capacity and power to affect a person's personal character, values, beliefs, attitudes, and thinking which subsequently influences their actions and behavior. Therefore, according to Noddings, regardless of the discipline of study, caring must be at the center of what is taught to develop morally sound agents of society. The profession of nursing must therefore ensure that caring is included in what is taught by acknowledging the interrelatedness of the relationships between those doing the teaching, students, nurses, and the people being cared for (Chinn & Falk-Rafael, 2018). Noddings (2016) identified modelling, dialogue, practice, and confirmation as the key elements of moral education and essential components of a caring learning environment. These elements and how they can be applied to nursing education will be explained.

Modelling Caring in The Learning Environment

Faculty Displaying Caring Action in the Classroom

Student nurses learn what it means to care through observing the behavior of their instructor, and a classroom environment where caring is lived by the instructor, is not only conducive to learning how to behave, but also reduces student nurses' anxiety (Barbour & Volkert, 2021; Duffy, 2018). Caring in action in the classroom setting can be made apparent through respectful behaviors such as politeness, civility, inclusivity, acceptance, encouraging class participation, and promoting active sharing of experiences. Encouraging students to ask questions showing patience when addressing them and praising them when they come up with good ideas is also very important (Duffy, 2018).

Role Modelling Caring in Clinical Settings

Role modelling requires being a good example for others to follow. Faculty also role model caring in the clinical setting by how they treat students. One way is by being approachable, so students are not afraid to ask questions or to get help when they need it. Another strategy is offering encouragement, giving students enough time to think about answers to questions posed, and using their lack of knowledge as a learning opportunity (Duffy, 2018). Providing feedback presents an instructor with additional opportunities to role model. For example, an instructor who praises their students for a job well done, and offers positive feedback when warranted, demonstrates an act of caring. However, students will make mistakes and errors in judgment and these situations are not easy for the student or the instructor, but they still can be dealt with in a caring fashion. There should be consequences for the error that was made, but the student will still need guidance that may require developing a plan to enhance their nursing competence (Duffy, 2018); Noddings, 2013). For instance, the situation can be used as a learning opportunity for the student, where mistakes are treated as opportunities in disguise on what to do better next time. Addressing the problem in this way supports the student, promotes self-confidence, and motivates them to change (Duffy, 2018).

In the clinical setting, the instructor can role model what it means to care, not only by how they treat students but also by the way that they treat everyone they encounter. For example, the instructor can demonstrate how to honor the worth of each client/patient and their family members unconditionally, by accepting them as they are, especially when they are less than cooperative or angry. This can be made apparent through the faculty member's demeanor, through how they approach the person or group, by verbal and non-verbal cues that convey kindness, and by offering to help.

Role modeling and caring for fellow colleagues in the clinical setting are also important. It is about establishing good relationships with other health professionals and collaborating with them. I have found that when I have a good working affiliation with the management and staff working on a unit, my clinical students are well-received and more fully supported. Another key component of being an example is to demonstrate how conflict can be resolved amicably between professionals through mutual respect, and by taking responsibility for how we behave. This action demonstrates that although disagreements do occur in work settings if they are managed in a caring and professional manner, it is more likely that the difficulties will be amicably resolved. Note that a discussion of how caring can be addressed in a nursing school simulation setting was not included in this current discussion, because it will be explored in Chapter Six under the topic of psychological safety.

Dialogue & Talking About Why We Do What We Do

Dialogue involves a dynamic exchange of opinions and ideas, and faculty can demonstrate caring discourse through the way in which we respectfully communicate with one another. According to Noddings (2010) when we approach our world through an ethic of care we are motivated to listen attentively to the opinions of others. Conversing with one another becomes the way in which we show engaged interest in the other person while displaying empathy, understanding, and appreciation for what they contribute to the conversation. It may also concern exploring the big questions about life in classroom settings, such as why we are here, what makes life worth living, and what is most important to us. For instance, do we have the right to decide what is best for others or not? Dialogue in this fashion also becomes a powerful way for teachers to foster students' moral ideals of what is right or wrong (Noddings, 2016).

Dialogue also values the opinions of everyone, not just those of the teacher, and includes the views of students, by encouraging reflective discussions during each learning opportunity (Chinn & Falk-Rafael, 2018). The teacher may take the lead and initiative on the topic of discussion, but in caring dialogue a student's ideas and views also matter. Learning becomes an active and participatory process of exchange of ideas where discourse is used for the meaning-making of experiences and honors different perspectives (Chinn & Falk-Rafael, 2018). How is this operationalized in nursing education? It plays out in a learning environment where no one is silenced, and where opposing ideas or inquisitive questions are considered, debated, and discussed in a respectful manner (Chinn & Falk-Rafael, 2018).

Caring Practices

In **caring practice,** the nurse prioritizes the one being cared for, by seeking to understand what they need. The nurse may have other duties to perform, but they are willing to set aside some time to be emotionally available to the one they are caring for (Noddings, 2010). In nursing education, helping students to participate in caring activities like valuing a client's/patient's lived experience and life story, treating them with dignity and respect, and practicing unconditional positive regard are excellent ways for them to learn the art of caring (Stephany, 2020).

Providing students opportunities to demonstrate acts of caring for student colleagues through the sharing of resources, and helping through other means, is another explicit way for them to learn to practice caring. Group work provides them with another means to care for each other, especially when the emphasis is placed on how the group can learn to work together in a cooperative fashion, instead of just accomplishing the task at hand (Chin & Falk-Rafael, 2018). For instance, rather than being overly competitive when engaging in group work, students can be encouraged to participate in actions that contribute to everyone's learning. This may include assisting a weaker member of the group by giving them constructive feedback and providing them with strategies and assistance to successfully contribute to the project. In this way, the needs of the weaker student are addressed with care. This is in comparison to just complaining about their lack of involvement or shunning them (Noddings, 2010).

However, to be able to make caring a part of one's lived experience and way of being, involves ongoing practice that extends beyond nursing school. Subsequently, student nurses should be encouraged to practice their caring skills on everyone. They can employ caring actions toward family, friends, strangers, animals, and larger community causes (Chinn & Falk-Rafael, 2018). From the viewpoint of care ethics, the practice of caring must also extend beyond individuals to the larger community, not only because it is the morally right thing to do, but because suffering can be alleviated on a larger scale (Noddings, 2010). That is the essence of nursing advocacy.

Confirmation and Caring

Confirmation consists of acknowledging and inspiring the best in us and in everyone else (Chin & Falk-Rafael, 2018). Confirmation is demonstrated through loving moral gestures where we do not harshly judge another's undesirable behavior, but rather look for the good in them. Confirmation is based on the belief that all people are capable of change. Hence, when someone errs the goal should be to acknowledge what has happened and to focus on the potential learning that can occur from the mistake. In this fashion, the person's experience can be re-shaped into something better (Chinn & Falk-Rafael, 2018). The rationale associated with confirmation assumes that people learn best in a supportive learning venue, and if given the opportunity, they can become their best selves. However, this assumption does acknowledge the difference between good and evil acts and the human capacity for both but also asserts that we should do our best to confirm the best in others before condemning or abandoning them (Noddings, 2010). A Learning Activity is included in Box (**5.5**) where you are encouraged to explore how students can contribute to a learning environment that supports each of Noddings' four elements of moral education.

Box 5.5. Learning activity: nurturing caring experiences in educational settings.

We have just been introduced to Nodding's (2016) four elements of moral education that are imperative to a caring learning environment such as modelling, dialogue, practice, and confirmation. Although instructors are in a position of authority and power, creating a caring learning environment is a shared responsibility for everyone who is involved. Therefore, you are encouraged to break into groups to explore your ideas when answering the following question.
What role can students play in operationalizing these four elements of a caring learning environment? Try to be as specific as possible and use examples to support your assertions.

NURTURING CIVILITY

Creating a Caring Venue for Everyone

Caring pedagogy is not solely the responsibility of faculty in nursing programs because it is based on the premise of a reciprocal, respectful, and genuine relationship between those doing the teaching and the ones who are learning. Therefore, a civil teaching environment must exist for everyone involved in the educational process. **Civility** consists of polite, considerate, and courteous behaviors that are exhibited in all forms of communication (Oxford Languages Dictionary, n. d.). In the educational setting, civility consists of respectful tolerance and acceptance of opinions, values, and views that differ from your own (Gallo, 2012). Civility in nursing education creates a mutually respectful learning setting, promotes well-mannered behavior in nursing students, influences their nursing practice, and results in positive outcomes for clients/patients (Ackerman-Barger *et al.*, 2021; Woodworth, 2015).

Incivility is the direct opposite of civility and consists of disrespecting others through rudeness, condescending attitudes, a blatant disregard for the needs of others, and a refusal to consider views that differ from your own (Gallo, 2012). Incivility in nursing education negatively impacts faculty and students by impeding learning (Woodworth, 2015). Both instructors and students have been known to sometimes exhibit behavior that is disrespectful. For example, students identified the following faculty actions as uncivil, making rude remarks; demonstrating a lack of patience; inadequate ability to communicate which includes not listening to students; being disinterested in teaching; and not being accessible outside of class (Gallo & Springer, 2007). Students also identified the following behaviors by their fellow student nurses as unacceptable, being late for class or leaving early on a regular basis; disrupting the class with cell phone use; using computers for activities not related to class; responding to the instructor or classmates in a disrespectful manner; making rude, belittling, or derogatory comments; and sleeping in class (Gallo & Springer, 2007; Woodworth, 2015).

Setting Clear Expectations Concerning Civility

Although being aware of conduct that is disrespectful is important to understand how not to behave, focusing on what supports civility in the nursing learning environment is even more beneficial because it encourages positive change in behaviors. For example, it is highly recommended that Instructors create clear guidelines of what is acceptable and unacceptable class conduct, encourage students to also develop a civility code of conduct, and have both included in the course syllabus (Woodworth, 2015). On the first day of class, I have the students create their list of what is considered acceptable behaviors as a class exercise.

They write the rules they have all agreed upon on the whiteboard, and then these agreed upon rules of conduct are posted in the course announcements. The students are then required to respectfully communicate when they think that their fellow students are disregarding the rules as a way to hold each other accountable. I have found this process to work quite well. Another mechanism I use is to make it clear to the students, that if they find my conduct or communication unacceptable in any way, that they approach me in person, to make me aware of their observations, so I can change my behavior. A specific example occurred concerning language usage, when I uttered a cliché in class that someone found offensive. I immediately apologized for the indiscretion and gave them my word that I would refrain from using that phrase in the future.

The following are additional ways for instructors to ensure that they act with civility in a consistent manner. They should readily and directly address any unacceptable behaviors when they arise. They can also role model civility by living it through their own actions by treating students with respect; praising them when they do a good job; refraining from providing negative feedback in front of others; and showing empathy when a student fails (Henderson *et al.*, 2020).

PRIORITIZING SELF-CARE

Nursing as a profession can be stressful and the demands associated with this career often begin in nursing school. For instance, student nurses experience elevated levels of anxiety in their programs related to the difficulties associated with their studies, and working in clinical settings where they are exposed to the suffering, injury, illness, trauma, and death of clients/patients (Wedgeworth, 2016). These stressors are often combined with the additional pressures associated with having to balance school with other work and home life commitments, and financial difficulties. When combined, the accumulation of a considerable number of stressors can contribute to emotional strain (Stubin, 2017). **Emotional strain** is a concept that refers to emotional exhaustion and related responses due to prolonged exposure to stressful situations that result in an inability to cope. It not only occurs in nursing but is also seen in lay persons who care for ailing relatives, in those who work in the business sector and is known to happen in academic settings (Stubin, 2017).

Emotional strain belongs in the category of other conditions due to work-related stress, which includes empathy-based stress conditions. However, the symptoms of emotional strain are specifically associated with low-stress tolerance to disturbing events, and result in irritability, anger, anxiety, and fear, which may inevitably lead to emotional detachment, physical and mental illness, burnout, and choosing to leave the profession (Potter *et al.*, 2010). Student nurses are at risk of developing the following specific responses of emotional strain such as anger, fear, anxiety, irritability, indecisiveness, and impatience. These symptoms are also known to be exacerbated by the inability to cope and are worsened by conflicts in relationships with clients/patients, clinical instructors, and other student nurses (Arieli, 2013). The following Case Study tells the story of a nursing student who is experiencing emotional strain. Refer to Box (**5.6**).

Box 5.6. Narrative case study two: when a student nurse experiences emotional strain.

Elizabeth is in her 3rd year of a Psychiatric Nursing Program. She has been doing well academically and in the clinical setting. However, lately, she has noticed that she is feeling more tired than usual. She has been drinking excessive amounts of coffee and even resorted to drinking power soft drinks loaded with sugar and caffeine, just so she can stay awake at night to catch up with her workload. Elizabeth has also noted that she sometimes feels sad when she hears the stories of some of the clients she is caring for in Psychiatry. Money has also become an issue. Even though Elizabeth has student loans, the cost of living has been going up lately due to inflation, so she has had to rely on Foodbanks from time to time because she runs out of money. Elizabeth usually prides herself on being quite levelheaded emotionally, but of late she has noticed that she has a rather short temper and gets angry when things do not go her way. Her emotional reactivity has even caused her to have problems doing group work with other students because she is impatient with them. Earlier today, Elizabeth's instructor asked to speak with her in private after class, because she was concerned about her recent changes in behavior.
When the instructor asked Elizabeth how she was doing, she burst into tears.
"I am not sure what is wrong with me. Everything seems to be getting to me these days. I know something is wrong, but I am not sure what to do about it."
Sensing Elizabeth's distress, the instructor chose her words carefully.
"Elizabeth, I think you are under a great deal of stress and that you may benefit by getting some help. Would you be willing to be referred for help?"
Looking worried, Elizabeth responded to her instructor's suggestion.
"What kind of help would I need and would getting help affect my chances of graduating."
Sensing Elizabeth's anxiety, the instructor offered her reassurance.
"The help would be in the form of a self-referral to the Student Services Counselling Department. Your referral to them and what you talk about will not be shared with anyone in the University because the sessions are confidential. I would highly recommend going to see them. Would you be willing to go?"
Elizabeth looked a bit more relieved but proceeded to ask one more question.
"I will make sure I refer myself. Could you advise me what to ask them specifically when I ask for help?"
The instructor responded.
"I would suggest that you ask them to suggest some self-care strategies to help you cope better. I know that they have helped other students to devise a personally designed self-care plan. That has proven to be useful in reducing their anxiety and increasing their ability to handle stress better."
Elizabeth smiled at her instructor.
"Sounds like a good plan. Thank you for taking the time to talk to me and for suggesting that I get some help. I really needed this."

NARRATIVE CASE STUDY TWO: IDENTIFICATION OF THEMES & ANALYSIS

Two key themes were identified from this story.

Theme # 1: Elizabeth experienced symptoms of emotional strain but she was not openly aware of what was going on for her.

Theme # 1 Analysis: Being aware of one's stressors and emotional needs is an important first step in getting help when someone is experiencing the symptoms of emotional strain. However, nursing students are not always able to readily recognize what is happening to them when they are feeling stressed out, and this is sometimes related to their younger age (Tharani *et al.*, 2017). However, self-awareness is the first step in their understanding that they may need assistance (Green, 2019). Elizabeth's instructor served the role of caringly pointing out her concerns to Elizabeth which resulted in her agreeing to a self-referral for counseling.

Theme # 2: Counselling with a focus on self-care was recommended by Elizabeth's instructor. Meaningful self-care strategies have been known to help nursing students to deal with emotional strain.

Theme # 2 Analysis: Counselling is sometimes needed to assist students with what they are experiencing, to help them express their emotions, and to develop an action plan to take better care of themselves (Tharani *et al.*, 2017). Self-care behaviors when implemented, not only reduce stress, but also serve to protect students from becoming more despondent, anxious, or depressed (Tharani *et al.*, 2017). The type of self-care initiatives that work well initially are ones that are easy to implement, like getting more sleep, eating better, reducing caffeine intake, and journaling (Green, 2019).

NARRATIVE CASE STUDY TWO: GROUP DISCUSSION & ROLE PLAY

1-If you were one of Elizabeth's nursing student colleagues and you noticed the changes in her behavior, would you feel brave enough to approach her to tell her what you observed? If not, why not?

2-If you did find the courage to share your observations with Elizabeth, how exactly would you go about doing that in a manner that would be well received? You may want to participate in role-playing to practice giving a student colleague this type of feedback.

Watson's Philosophy and Science of Caring as the Foundation for All Caring

Watson's Philosophy and Science of Caring has been identified as the foundation for all caring, professing the unity among all things and "the great circle of life, such as change, illness, suffering., death, and rebirth" (Watson, 2008, p. 17). There are many basic assumptions of this caring science. It asserts that caring is demonstrated best when practiced, and that caring can transcend normal channels of direct communication because it can be felt. It is comprised of the many ways of knowing such as through, being, doing, personal experience, ethics, intuition, science, aesthetics, metaphysics, and spirituality. It intersects with disciplines associated with Clinical Science, the Humanities and Arts, and processes that situate caring as a principal component of nursing's professional, social, and moral commitment to society (Watson, 2008).

WATSON'S CARITAS PROCESSES AS THE BASIS OF CARING FOR SELF AND OTHERS

Self-care is often neglected by nurses because they view it as selfish, but nothing is further from the truth. For instance, caring for oneself is a moral obligation for nurses because if they are not well, they cannot care for others, and they are also obligated to model health promotion for their clients/patients (Linton & Koonmen, 2020). Watson proposed that caring in nursing consists of **Caritas processes** that demonstrate sensitivity toward oneself and everyone else by fostering spiritual practices that support loving, caring relationships (Sitzman, 2017). They are based on the premise that we must learn how to treat ourselves with lovingkindness, forgiveness, and compassion before we can genuinely and authentically care for others (Linton & Koonmen, 2020). Therefore, it is vitally important that a philosophy of caring be prioritized and integrated into the nursing school curriculum so that nursing students learn how to better care for themselves, which in turn results in them doing a better job of genuinely caring for their clients/ patients (Devi *et al*., 2022). A Learning Activity is recommended to explore and implement each of Watson's ten Caritas processes as a way to enhance self-care. Refer to Box (**5.7**). Be prepared that some of these ideas may challenge your preconceived ideas, and you may want to consider journaling to sort through what seems counterintuitive or daunting. You may also find some of the practical personal self-care activities suggested in Box (**5.8**) to be useful in your everyday life.

Box 5.7. Learning Activity: Implementing Watson's caritas processes and strategies to enhance self-care (as adapted from Linton & Koonmen, 2020; Sitzman, 2017; Sitzman & Watson, 2014; Watson, 2008; watson caring science institute, 2023).

Assignment: Plan how you will apply each of the following strategies for self-care in your life.
1- Embrace (Lovingkindness)
Self-love is the foundation for being able to care for others and involves the practice of loving-kindness, compassion, and equanimity for self and others. **Strategy for Self-care:** To increase your resilience, or your ability to bounce back after adversity, consider reaching out for support from others, such as nursing colleagues and people outside of work.
2- Inspire (Faith & Hope)
Concerns being fully present, honoring the inner life of self and others, and fostering hope and faith. **Strategy for Self-care:** Consider practicing mindfulness and paying attention to how you are feeling through breathing techniques, becoming aware of your thoughts and feelings, and being present during interactions with clients/patients.
3- Trust (Transpersonal)
Involves being sensitive to self and others by applying personally chosen spiritual practices to transcend ego. It is about cultivating spirituality. **Strategy for Self-care:** Think about the potential benefits of adopting some sort of spiritual practice that is specific to you and your unique needs.
4- Nurture (Relationship)
This is about developing and fostering trusting, caring relationships with yourself and others as the basis of a sense of connection and belonging, that begins with how you think and treat yourself. **Strategy for Self-care:** Adopt some strategies associated with cognitive behavioral therapy (CBT) that teach you how to recognize negative beliefs, challenge those ideas with the truth, and think of yourself in a more positive way.
5- Forgive (All)
You need to forgive yourself and others for their imperfections. Try not to be judgmental. Be willing to listen to your own and other's stories. **Strategy for Self-care:** Consider emotional regulation to better manage your responses and emotional reactions to stress, trauma, or loss. Journalling is useful, as is talking it out with someone supportive, or reaching out for professional help.
6- Deepen (Creative Self)
Caring is used as the means for creative problem solving, is solution focused, and makes use of healing practices that use all ways of knowing/being/doing/becoming. **Strategy for Self-care:** If you make a mistake do not be so hard on yourself. Focus on what you have learned from the error.
7- Balance (Learning)
Engaging in teaching and learning occurs within a meaningful context of caring relationships with others. These learning opportunities facilitate growth, fulfillment, and joy. **Strategy for Self-care:** Purposefully pursue opportunities to gain experience through new things in areas of interest. They may help you feel more fulfilled and even bring you joy.
8- Co-create (Carita Field Healing Environment)

(Box 5.7) cont.....

Consists of creating an environment of healing at all levels to foster a genuine energetic caring presence. Involves valuing and caring for oneself as much as you do for others. **Strategy for Self-care:** Consider making your surroundings more conducive to peacefulness. If you cannot control the noise and business of your nursing workplace, do your best to make your home surroundings quiet and serene.
9- Minister (Humanity)
Demonstrates a reverence for the basic needs of the body as a part of the sacred acts. It is about appreciating the magnificence of what your body does for you. **Strategy for Self-care:** Take better care of your body and your basic needs, through efforts that support good nutrition, exercise, and sleep. Also plan some leisure time, even if it is short, with an activity that connects you with the goodness of life.
10- Open (Infinity)
Being open to things spiritual, mysterious, and unknown, like miracles. It may consist of feeling gratitude for the possibilities that still exist. **Strategy for Self-care:** Be more willing to notice the hidden blessings in everyday life that you usually take for granted. Also, be open to derive some greater meaning from challenges when they present themselves.

Box 5.8. Personal self-care activities worth considering (as adapted from Sitzman, 2017; Stephany, 2015).

1-Do your best to make sure you prioritize your basic human needs (*e.g.*, good nutrition, exercise, and adequate sleep). These measures may seem like common sense, but when they are regularly neglected, they can lead to illness. Do what you can to eat foods that are healthy. Get some exercise by taking the stairs instead of the elevator, walking instead of using transportation, and plan so you can get at least 6 – 8 hours of sleep in a 24-hour period.
2-Develop a healthy sense of humor. Laughing is good for the soul.
3-Spend even just a little bit of time doing what you love. It will revitalize you.
4-Avoid procrastination because it increases anxiety. The best way to do that is to plan to get stuff done in a scheduled time and to stay on schedule. If you do not know how to stop procrastinating, get help from student support services.
5-Spend time in nature because it will help you to re-focus on aspects of life that are refreshing. If time is an issue, going for a walk outdoors will suffice.
6-Devote some quality time to spend with the people who love and support you. If you cannot be with them physically, use other means to connect (*e.g.*, social media).
7-Be kind to yourself especially when you make mistakes. Some of the best learning comes from what does not work. So, try not to judge yourself so harshly. Admit what went wrong, identify what you learned from it, and move on.
8-Before beginning your day, think about what you would like to do that day that involves serving others. That is a wonderful way to begin clinical or just any day because it reminds you that what you contribute, can and does help.

BEING RESILIENT

"Resilience has been described as the capacity for positive outcomes despite challenging or threatening circumstances" Byron Egeland, Professor of Child Development at the University of Minnesota.

Being **resilient** consists of the ability to quickly return to normal functioning after experiencing adversity and is made possible because a person's belief system remains intact, through their ability to regulate their emotions and thoughts (Kerig, 2019) (Fig. **5.4**). It consists of constructive attributes of endurance, strength, and the will and motivation to move forward, despite what has occurred (Collier, 2016). The topic of resilience was formally introduced in Chapter Three of this textbook with an emphasis on resilience-based strategies that can be adopted by clients/patients. It is re-introduced here with special attention to the development of resilience skills in practicing nurses and nursing students.

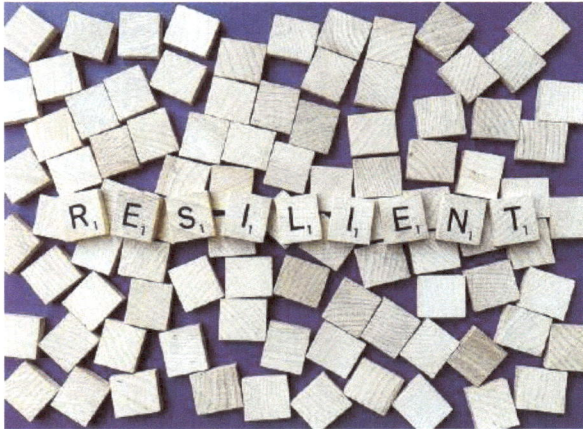

Fig. (5.4). Being resilient. Source: www.pixabay.com.

THE BASIC COMPONENTS OF RESILIENCE AND STRATEGIES TO IMPLEMENT THEM

Resilience skills can be learned through the development of protective factors and mechanisms, which may prevent empathy-based stress conditions related to trauma, can assist a trauma survivor to bounce back more quickly, and teach people how to deal with everyday life stress. Therefore, recommended ways to cultivate resilience in nurses that were developed by Jackson *et al.*, (2007) will be presented and consist of building positive nurturing relationships and networks; maintaining positivity; developing emotional insight; achieving life balance and spirituality; and becoming more reflective (Jackson *et al.*, 2007).

Building Positive Nurturing Relationships and Networks

Building caring relationships that are positive fosters resilience because feeling connected to others is a tremendous contributor to emotional well-being (Brooks & Goldstein, 2003). Seligman (2011) points out that being around other people who have a positive outlook on life is good for your overall health, and hanging out with negative people has the opposite effect. No matter how strong you may think you are, when you are experiencing excessive stress, having people around you who love and support you and who are hopeful, can provide you with the strength you need to get through it (Brooks & Goldstein, 2003). Receiving support and encouragement from others ensures that you are not alone in your experience, and makes you less likely to buckle under duress (Denz-Penhey & Murdoch, 2008).

As nurses, creating trusting professional relationships with colleagues is also important because you may need to lean on others for help, guidance, and support when needed in work-related matters (Jackson *et al.*, 2007). Furthermore, the type of support offered should be reciprocal with both parties being committed to being there for each other when required. However, creating trusting relationships in a work or a school setting may require effort and an investment in others in order to feel safe enough to be vulnerable without the fear of judgment or retaliation. (Brooks & Goldstein, 2003). Another point is worth making. Student nurses who work in a caring clinical setting and experience positive relationships with staff, are more content with their learning environment and demonstrate increased resilience (Cleary *et al.*, 2018).

Questions for Further Consideration

1-Identify someone in your life who has been supportive in the past. What are some of their character traits?

2-If you need support right now, who would you turn to and why? Who would you NOT turn to for help and why?

3-We know that support works best when it is shared and reciprocated between people. Think about your current relationships and ways to make them more meaningful.

Maintaining Positivity

Developing and sustaining a cheerful outlook can help you weather the storms of life, and positive emotions like humor, joy, gratitude, and love contribute to life satisfaction and happiness. They are also associated with well-being and post-traumatic growth (Fredrickson, 2003; Seligman, 2011). Furthermore, people who are naturally resilient often exhibit a positive outlook on life. Even when difficulties arise, they do not become negative. They view obstacles as opportunities and remain optimistic about the future (Fredrickson). The good news is that you do not need to be a natural optimist to assume an attitude of positivity because being optimistic entails making a conscious choice to think differently. It is about changing your mindset from one that is negative to one that is positive (Brooks & Goldstein, 2003). But even if you feel too defeated to change your thinking on your own, there is professional help in the form of **cognitive behavioral therapy (CBT)** to help you. CBT can teach you how to recognize negative beliefs, challenge those ideas with the truth, and think of yourself in a more positive way. Utilizing CBT techniques, if practiced devoutly will change your way of thinking, which in turn impacts your behavior too.

Strategies for Consideration

1-Do something every day that brings you joy.

2-Limit your exposure to negative content in the news or on social media.

3-Stay away from negative people and make friends with people who are genuinely optimistic.

4-Consider writing in a gratitude journal daily to help you focus on what is going well in your life.

5-Watch your self-talk. When you are tempted to put yourself down, stop and deliberately affirm something good about you.

Developing Emotional Insight

Resilience is closely aligned with personal insight which is a component of emotional intelligence. **Emotional intelligence** is the capacity to be able to monitor your own emotions and to effectively assess and understand the feelings of other people (Goleman, 2005). Emotional intelligence provides you with self-awareness concerning negative emotions when they arise (Goleman, 2005). For example, feeling sad after being exposed to other people's trauma at work, and understanding why you feel that way is the first step in changing how you feel. You embrace your emotions and acknowledge their source, but you do not allow your negative feelings to linger indefinitely. In this fashion, emotional insight motivates you to consider beneficial ways of coping rather than becoming despondent or hopeless. This in turn makes you stronger and more capable of overcoming obstacles in the future, which is the essence of resilience (Jackson *et* *al.*, 2007). Emotional insight also fosters resilience by making someone aware of their personal risk for developing empathy-based stress conditions, and the need for adopting protective mechanisms like enhanced self-care to prevent them (McAllister & McKinnon, 2009).

Strategies for Consideration

1-Consider writing in a journal to increase self-awareness and emotional insight.

2-Practice observing how you are feeling. If you are feeling bad, ask yourself why.

3-Be more self-forgiving when you make mistakes.

4-Celebrate the positive.

Achieving Life Balance and Spirituality

Actively pursuing a work-life balance and spirituality are important for fostering resilience because they give life meaning and purpose (McAllister & McKinnon, 2009). Your work should not be your whole life. In your off-work time, you need to be able to participate in an array of activities that bring you joy, but also ones that enhance your physical and emotional well-being. In fact, you should prioritize them. Similarly, having a purpose for getting up in the morning, having an appreciation for life itself, being of service to others, and pursuing answers through spirituality are all associated with a high degree of resilience (Jackson *et al.*, 2007). For example, we know that people who experience loss are quite often comforted by adopting some sort of spiritual explanation, even if they were not previously interested in religion (Stephany, 2020). Furthermore, although spirituality is not for everyone, Watson (2008) maintains that cultivating our spiritual growth assists us in being more compassionate, caring, and kind to ourselves and others, and helps to buffer us from negativity.

Questions for Further Consideration

1 What is keeping you from creating a work-life balance?

2-List one activity that you used to do that brought you joy. How can you set aside some time to re-introduce that activity into your life?

3-Studies demonstrate that helping others increases your well-being. Have you considered being of service to others in some way?

4-What are some minor changes you can make in your life that will support your physical and emotional health?

Becoming More Reflective

Personal reflection serves the purpose of helping us to transcend our present situation or anguish (McAllister & McKinnon, 2009). We learn a great deal about ourselves, and our motives through reflection, because when we examine our thoughts and behaviors retrospectively, we can often ascertain what went well, what went wrong, and why. Subsequently, reflection is an excellent way to increase insight into our experiences and can help us to make better choices in similar circumstances, which is the essence of resilience (Jackson *et al.*, 2007). Journalling is an excellent way for nurses and student nurses to reflect. Journalling not only facilitates self-awareness, but also helps you to explore ways to adopt more optimistic responses to specific occurrences, people, or situations (Jackson *et al.*, 2007).

Questions for Further Consideration

Brooks and Goldstein (2003) recommend making time every day to do exercises that help you become resilient. The following five questions are specifically designed by him for use in reflection.

1 Have I truly listened and attempted to understand the viewpoints of others today?

2-How have I related to others?

3-Have I practiced empathy and respect?

4-How have I responded to stress, mistakes, and setbacks?

5-If I am not happy with my response, what will I do differently next time?

6-In what areas did I do well? How do I maintain or reproduce these positive behaviors? (Brooks & Goldstein, 2003, p. 265).

RECOMMENDED STRATEGIES TO FOSTER RESILIENCE IN NURSING EDUCATION

Our exploration of resilience ends with recommendations for how to foster it through educational endeavors. Resilience training of student nurses is highly suggested because these skills can help mitigate their vulnerability to trauma, increase their overall well-being, improve the atmosphere of the healthcare setting, and decrease a tendency to prematurely leave the profession due to stress (Jackson *et al.*, 2007). Therefore, three recommendations as proposed by McAllister & McKinnon (2009) are presented to foster resilience in nursing education.

Recommendation # 1: Resilience Training

The first recommendation is to formally include resilience training in the school curriculum. Discussions should ideally explore the relationship of resilience to personal well-being, and identification of the personal traits associated with resilience such as adaptability, enhanced coping, spirituality, and meaning-making. Cultivating one's capacity to be strength-focused, to develop a resilient mindset, and how to effectively deal with change, should also be highlighted (Brooks & Goldstein, 2003; McAllister & McKinnon, 2009).

Recommendation # 2: Prioritize Role Modelling

The second recommendation prioritizes formal role modelling in the clinical setting. What we now know is that learning that is derived from behaviors observed in actual practice is an influential component of learning, especially when practitioners demonstrate the skills associated with resilience and post-traumatic growth. Subsequently, exposure to positive mentors such as instructors and staff who thrive and cope in times of stress, can serve as excellent examples for students (McAllister & McKinnon, 2009).

Recommendation # 3: Enable Generativity

The third recommendation is to enable **generativity**, which is about investing in the well-being and future of members of the profession. Suggestions to promote generativity include having others set a good example, mentor, lead, and coach students. Professional storytelling where resilient, and experienced practitioners share their stories of how they were able to persevere in less than desirable circumstances can be inspiring. Providing forums where final-year students share their experiences of how they dealt with the pressures and challenges associated with work and school, is another way for generativity to be fostered (McAllister and McKinnon, 2009).

SOMETHING TO REFLECT UPON

Are you resilient? Try and remember a time when you experienced something stressful. Were you able to bounce back afterwards or were you negativley impacted for quite sometime? Knowing what you know now, would you consider applying at least one of the suggested strategies to move forward?

SELF-CARE STRATEGY: MAKING PEACE WITH NEGATIVE EMOTIONS

"When embraced and accepted, negative emotions can be a powerful catalyst to positive change in one's life and can lead to deeper feelings, meaning and authenticity." Paul T. P. Wong, Canadian Clinical Psychologist.

Negative emotions are feelings that cause you to feel distressed or uncomfortable and may decrease life satisfaction. Fear, anger, disgust, and sadness are some common examples. (Forgas, 2014). Additional displays of negative affect include frustration, envy, jealousy, shame, guilt, regret, and anxiety (Hutson, 2015). The expression of all emotions is a normal human experience, including the ones we label as negative because they serve a purpose (Hallis, 2017). For example, historically anger has helped humans to survive by fighting when threatened, and sadness and depression have been known to inspire creativity in some people (Forgas). Additional evidence indicates that anger motivates people to pursue actions to end social injustice and can serve as a catalyst for someone to pursue their goals. Openly displaying sadness is also important because it sends the message to others that you are in trouble, and may serve as a signal for you to take action to change what you are currently doing (Hutson, 2015).

Emotional Suppression *Versus* Emotional Appraisal

One way to facilitate positive change in yourself, especially if you may be at risk of empathy-based stress, is for you to learn how to accept and sort through negative emotions when they occur. A misconception exists that negative emotions should be avoided, but the evidence indicates that this can actually be harmful (Forgas, 2014). For example, a study was conducted that compared individual differences between these two emotional regulatory processes, emotional suppression, and emotional appraisal. **Emotional suppression** consists of avoiding all displays of negative emotions, whereas **emotional appraisal** is restructuring the meaning associated with a situation, to view its outcome more optimistically. The results revealed that people who suppress their negative emotions experienced less positive affect and more pronounced negative feelings. They also exhibited a decreased capacity in interpersonal functioning and reduced well-being. In comparison, those who resorted to emotional appraisal experienced more positive emotions, better interpersonal functioning, and enhanced well-being (Gross & John, 2003).

The Self-Care Challenge: Making Use of Emotional Appraisal to Manage Negative Emotions

The following are a few evidence-based strategies to help you to sort through negative emotions by making use of emotional reappraisal. They have been adapted from the book by Tina Hallis (2017) entitled, *Sharpen Your Positive Edge*. I strongly encourage you to consider adopting some or all of them.

1-Make it your intention not to suppress your feelings. Instead, openly acknowledge your emotions.

2-Try your best to gain an understanding of why you are feeling the way that you are. What is going on in your life right now? Is there anything you should be doing differently?

3-Do not stay in a place of discouragement or defeat. Reach out for help if you feel like these feelings are taking you to a dark place.

4-Do your absolute best to stay away from negativity (*e.g.*, negative people or overexposure to negative media).

5-Try not to worry about things that are out of your control.

6-Think of a time when you felt angry, sad, or anxious. Did you suppress or express what you were feeling at the time? If not, why not? Consider journalling to sort through your rationale (Hallis, 2017).

Note: Any suggested strategies are not intended to be a substitute for medical or psychological advice from a trained professional. The reader is therefore encouraged to seek medical or other professional help in any matters related to their physical or emotional health.

CONCLUSION

• People who work in healthcare, including nurses and student nurses are at risk of developing empathy-based stress conditions, such as secondary traumatic stress and compassion fatigue, which are related to caring for people who have been traumatized.

- Caring is a key factor in all suggested interventions for empathy-based stress conditions. Subsequently, Chapter Five explores ways to mitigate the negative effects of these specific stress reactions through employing a caring pedagogy and resilience.

- Secondary traumatic stress (STS) develops as an after-effect of being confronted with another person's experience of adversity.

- Compassion fatigue (CF) occurs when a caregiver becomes overly preoccupied and emotionally involved with the suffering or trauma experienced by people in their care.

- Similarities and differences exist between these two conditions. For instance, both occur due to being exposed to other people's trauma. However, STS occurs over time due to repetitive exposure to traumatic material and can lead to PTSD. In contrast, CF is acute in onset and results in a lack of emotional engagement, and although the symptoms associated with CF are distressful, they are not as serious as PTSD.

- We learned that people working in healthcare, including student nurses, are at risk of being exposed to on-gong trauma. Those with a history of trauma, who do not cope well, are self-critical, or overly empathetic, are at an increased risk for developing STS, CF, or other empathy-based stress conditions.

- Specific areas of work where exposure to trauma is common are known to pose a higher risk and include working in the emergency room (ER), intensive care unit (ICU), mental health, hospice, and palliative care.

- Identification of the signs and symptoms of decreased coping is imperative for early diagnosis and treatment. In both STS and CF numbing and avoidant reactions are apparent. In STS the symptoms of PTSD, such as intrusive imagery, recurring nightmares, avoidance, relationship difficulties, and angry outbursts, may indicate a need for urgent intervention. In CF emotional detachment, distancing oneself from all aspects of relational practice, and an inability to offer empathy, are manifestations of this condition.

- Measures to reduce their negative effects consist of educating nurses and other health professionals that these conditions exist, informing them of their specific signs and symptoms, and where to go for support.

- The merits of caring were presented as the basis for all suggested intervention strategies because caring is a fundamental focus of nursing practice and nursing education.

- To care for someone consists of offering them respect, inclusivity, empathy, emotional warmth, and genuine concern for their well-being.

- Caring in nursing was identified as a process where the nurse relates to their client/patient as a fellow human being, and results in a feeling of mutual trust, understanding, and being cared for in both participants.
- We learned that delivering sensitive trauma-informed care concerns can be accomplished through applying the 4 Cs of Trauma-informed Care: Calm, Contain, Care, and Cope.
- We were made to realize that caring relationships are not only essential in nursing but also for nursing education.
- Caring pedagogy in nursing education is important because it incorporates caring components into the delivery of the core curriculum, creates a community of learning that prioritizes students, is inclusive, and engaging, fosters caring relationships, and protects the emotional integrity of student nurses.
- Caring pedagogy is connected to trauma-informed educational processes because they both value respectful interpersonal relationships, a supportive teaching venue, people's feelings, effective communication skills, and all aspects of genuine caring.
- Learning environments in nursing school can be re-designed to be more student-focused by moving away from merely imparting knowledge; changing the teaching environment; actively engaging students; and through mutual problem-solving.
- These four elements of Noddings' moral education were declared to be essential for a caring learning environment, modelling, dialogue, practice, and confirmation. For example, student nurses learn what it means to care through the following means, observing the behavior of their instructor, a dynamic exchange of ideas, prioritizing caring, and encouraging the best in others.
- It was pointed out that a learning environment that is caring and based on civility is the shared responsibility of both faculty and students.
- Self-care was identified as a known strategy to mitigate the emotional strain experienced by both nurses and student nurses.
- Watson's ten Caritas processes were recommended as the basis for self-care through the action of demonstrating sensitivity toward oneself and everyone else by adopting spiritual practices that support loving, caring relationships.
- Resilience consists of the ability to quickly return to normal functioning after experiencing adversity. We were made aware that resilience skills can be learned through the development of protective factors and mechanisms that serve several purposes. They may prevent empathy-based stress conditions related to trauma, assist a trauma survivor to bounce back more quickly, and teach people how to deal with the stress of everyday life.

- The following ways to cultivate resilience in nurses were presented: building positive nurturing relationships and networks; maintaining positivity; developing emotional insight; achieving life balance and spirituality; and becoming more reflective.
- These three strategies to foster resilience in nursing education were also recommended, formally including resilience training in the school curriculum; prioritizing role modelling; and enabling generativity.
- Two Narrative Case Studies were presented. The first explored how a Psychiatric Nurse developed the signs of secondary traumatic stress after one of her clients ended their life through suicide. We learned that it is not uncommon for a healthcare professional to experience a range of emotional reactions after their client commits suicide. Critical incident debriefing is therefore highly recommended, and a referral for professional help may also sometimes be necessary. It is important for healthcare professionals to understand that they may not always be able to prevent everyone from ending their life. It is, however, good practice to be trained in suicide prevention measures that assess for risk, warning signs, and how to implement a comprehensive safety plan.
- The Second Narrative Case Study revealed how a student nurse was unaware that the symptoms that she was experiencing were related to emotional strain. Her instructor reached out to this student with her concerns, which resulted in the student agreeing to see a counsellor to help deal with her stress and to develop a self-care plan.
- These learning activities were recommended (*e.g.*, Sharing Examples of Being Cared For; Exploring Ways to Enhance Learning; Nurturing Caring Experiences in Educational settings; and Implementing Watson's Caring Processes and Strategies to Enhance Self-care).
- At the closing of the Chapter a self-care strategy was recommended that utilized emotional appraisal to manage negative emotions.

RECOMMENDED READINGS

Cori, J.L. Healing for trauma: A survivors guide to understanding your signs and symptoms and reclaiming your life. Marlowe & Company, 2008.

Parrott, W.G., Ed. The positive side of negative emotion. The Guildford Press, 2014.

van der Kolk, B. The body keeps score: Brain, mind, and body in the healing of trauma. Viking Penguin, 2014.

Walker, V. The art of comforting: What to say and do for people in distress. Jeremy P. Tarcher/Penguin, 2010.

REFERENCES

Ackerman-Barger, K, Dickinson, JK & Martin, LD (2021) Promoting a culture of civility in learning environments. *Nurse Educ, 46,* 234-8.
[http://dx.doi.org/10.1097/NNE.0000000000000929] [PMID: 33093348]

Ariapooran, S (2014) Compassion fatigue and burnout in Iranian nurses: The role of perceived social support. *Iran J Nurs Midwifery Res, 19,* 279-84.
[PMID: 24949067]

Arieli, D (2013) Emotional work and diversity in clinical placements of nursing students. *J Nurs Scholarsh, 45,* 192-201.
[http://dx.doi.org/10.1111/jnu.12020] [PMID: 23462103]

Bankert, EG & Kozel, VV (2005) Transforming pedagogy in nursing education: A caring learning environment for adult students. *Nurs Educ Perspect, 26,* 227-9. [National League for Nursing].
[PMID: 16175914]

Barbour, C & Volkert, D (2021) Nursing students' perspective of faculty caring using Duffy's quality caring model: A Q-methodology study. *Int J Caring Sci, 14,* 18-28.

Berg, E & Lepp, M (2023) The meaning and application of student-centered learning in nursing education: An integrative review of the literature. *Nurse Educ Pract, 69,* 103622.
[http://dx.doi.org/10.1016/j.nepr.2023.103622] [PMID: 37054488]

Brooks, R & Goldstein, S (2003) *The power of resilience: Achieving balance, confidence, and personal strength in your life.* McGraw Hill.

Caringi, JC, Hardiman, ER, Weldon, P, Fletcher, S, Devlin, M & Stanick, C (2017) Secondary traumatic stress and licensed clinical social workers. *Traumatology, 23,* 186-95.
[http://dx.doi.org/10.1037/trm0000061]

Chinn, PL & Falk-Rafael, A (2018) Embracing the focus of the discipline of nursing: Critical caring pedagogy. *J Nurs Scholarsh, 50,* 687-94.
[http://dx.doi.org/10.1111/jnu.12426] [PMID: 30230200]

Cleary, M, Visentin, D, West, S, Lopez, V & Kornhaber, R (2018) Promoting emotional intelligence and resilience in undergraduate nursing students: An integrative review. *Nurse Educ Today, 68,* 112-20.
[http://dx.doi.org/10.1016/j.nedt.2018.05.018] [PMID: 29902740]

Collier, L (2016) Growth after trauma: Why some people are more resiliency than others, and can it be taught. *J Trauma Stress, 9,* 455-71.
[http://dx.doi.org/10.1007/BF02103658]

Denz-Penhey, H & Murdoch, C (2008) Personal resiliency: serious diagnosis and prognosis with unexpected quality outcomes. *Qual Health Res, 18,* 391-404.
[http://dx.doi.org/10.1177/1049732307313431] [PMID: 18235162]

Devi, B, Pradhan, S, Giri, D & Lepcha, N (2022) Watson's theory of caring in nursing education: Challenges to integrate in into nursing practice. *J Posit Psychol, 6,* 1464-71.http://journalppw.com

Duffy, E, Avalos, G & Dowling, M (2015) Secondary traumatic stress among emergency nurses: A cross-sectional study. *Int Emerg Nurs, 23,* 53-8.
[http://dx.doi.org/10.1016/j.ienj.2014.05.001] [PMID: 24927978]

Duffy, JR (2018) *Quality caring in nursing and health systems: Implications for clinicians, educators, and leaders.* Springer Publishing Company.
[http://dx.doi.org/10.1891/9780826181251]

Figley, CR (1995) Compassion fatigue: Toward a new understanding of the costs of caring. In: Stamm, H., (Ed.), *Secondary traumatic stress: Self-care issues for clinicians, researchers, and educators* . The Sidran Press 3-28.

Forgas, JP (2014) Can sadness be good for you? On the cognitive, motivational, and interpersonal benefits of negative emotions. In: Parrott, W.G., (Ed.), *The positive side of negative emotions* The Guildford Press 3-36.

Foli, K & Thompson, JR (2019) *The influence of psychological trauma in nursing.* Sigma Theta Tau International.

Fredrickson, B (2003) The value of positive emotions: The emerging science of positive psychology is coming to understand why it's good to feel good. *Am Sci,* 91, 330-5.https://www.jstor.org/stable/27858244 [http://dx.doi.org/10.1511/2003.26.330]

Clark, CM & Springer, PJ (2007) Thoughts on incivility: Student and faculty perceptions of uncivil behavior in nursing education. *Nurs Educ Perspect,* 28, 93-7. [PMID: 17486799]

Gallo, VJ (2012) Incivility in nursing education: A review of the literature. *Teach Learn Nurs,* 7, 62-6. [http://dx.doi.org/10.1016/j.teln.2011.11.006]

Gates, DM & Gillespie, GL (2008) Secondary traumatic stress in nurses who care for traumatized women. *J Obstet Gynecol Neonatal Nurs,* 37, 243-9. [http://dx.doi.org/10.1111/j.1552-6909.2008.00228.x] [PMID: 18336450]

Goddard, A, Jones, RW, Esposito, D & Janicek, E (2021) Trauma informed education in nursing: A call for action. *Nurse Educ Today,* 101, 104880. [http://dx.doi.org/10.1016/j.nedt.2021.104880] [PMID: 33798984]

Goleman, D (2005) *Emotional intelligence: Why it can matter more than IQ.* Bantam Books.

Green, C (2020) Teaching accelerated nursing students' self-care: A pilot project. *Nurs Open,* 7, 225-34. [http://dx.doi.org/10.1002/nop2.384] [PMID: 31871706]

Gustafsson, T & Hemberg, J (2022) Compassion fatigue as bruises in the soul: A qualitative study on nurses. *Nurs Ethics,* 29, 157-70. [http://dx.doi.org/10.1177/09697330211003215] [PMID: 34282669]

Hallis, T (2017) *Sharpen your positive edge: Shifting your thoughts for more positivity & success.* The Positive Edge, LLC.

Henderson, D, Sewell, KA & Wei, H (2020) The impacts of faculty caring on nursing students' intent to graduate: A systematic literature review. *Int J Nurs Sci,* 7, 105-11. [http://dx.doi.org/10.1016/j.ijnss.2019.12.009] [PMID: 32099867]

Hinchliffe, G (2000) Education or Pedagogy? *J Philos Educ,* 35, 31-45. [http://dx.doi.org/10.1111/1467-9752.00208]

Hinderer, K A (2014) compassion fatigue, compassion satisfaction, and secondary traumatic stress in trauma nurses. *J Trauma Nurs,* 21, 160-9. [http://dx.doi.org/10.1097/JTN.0000000000000055]

Hutson, M (2015) Beyond happiness: The upside of feeling down. *Psychol Today,* 48, 44-82.

Jackson, D, Firtko, A & Edenborough, M (2007) Personal resilience as a strategy for surviving and thriving in the face of workplace adversity: A literature review. *J Adv Nurs,* 60, 1-9. [http://dx.doi.org/10.1111/j.1365-2648.2007.04412.x] [PMID: 17824934]

Jenkins, E, Slemon, A, Bilsker, D & Goldner, EM (2022) *A concise introduction to mental health in Canada* Canadian Scholars.

Kearney, M & Weininger, R (2011) Whole person self-care: Self-care from the inside out. In: Hutchinson, T.A., (Ed.), *Whole person care: A new paradigm for the 21st century,* Springer Science & Business Media 109-25. [http://dx.doi.org/10.1007/978-1-4419-9440-0_10]

Kerig, PK (2019) Enhancing resilience among providers of trauma-informed are: A curriculum for protection against secondary traumatic stress among non-mental health professionals. *J Aggress Maltreat Trauma,* 28, 613-30.

[http://dx.doi.org/10.1080/10926771.2018.1468373]

Kimberg, L & Wheeler, M (2019) Trauma and trauma informed care. In: Gerber, M.R., (Ed.), *Trauma-informed healthcare approaches: A guide for primary care,* Springer 25-56.
[http://dx.doi.org/10.1007/978-3-030-04342-1_2]

Linton, M & Koonmen, J (2020) Self-care as an ethical obligation for nurses. *Nurs Ethics,* 27, 1694-702.
[http://dx.doi.org/10.1177/0969733020940371] [PMID: 32720570]

Locsin, RC & Kongsuwan, W (2013) Lived experience of patients *being cared for* in ICUS in Southern Thailand. *Nurs Crit Care,* 18, 200-11.
[http://dx.doi.org/10.1111/nicc.12025] [PMID: 23782114]

Mangoulia, P, Koukia, E, Alevizopoulos, G, Fildissis, G & Katostaras, T (2015) Prevalence of secondary traumatic stress among psychiatric nurses in Greece. *Arch Psychiatr Nurs,* 29, 333-8.
[http://dx.doi.org/10.1016/j.apnu.2015.06.001] [PMID: 26397438]

Mathieu, F (2012) *The compassion fatigue workbook: Creative tools for transforming compassion fatigue and vicarious traumatization.* Routledge.
[http://dx.doi.org/10.4324/9780203803349]

Mayer, KA, Linehan, KJ & MacMillan, NK (2022) Student perspectives on potential sources of trauma exposure during nursing school. *Nurs Forum,* 57, 833-42.
[http://dx.doi.org/10.1111/nuf.12728] [PMID: 35485449]

McAllister, M & McKinnon, J (2009) The importance of teaching and learning resilience in the health disciplines: A critical review of the literature. *Nurse Educ Today,* 29, 371-9.
[http://dx.doi.org/10.1016/j.nedt.2008.10.011] [PMID: 19056153]

Menschner, C & Maul, A (2016) *Issue Brief: Key ingredients for successful trauma-informed care implementation* Available from: https://www.samhsa.gov/sites/default/files/programs_campaigns/childrens_mental_health/atc-whitepaper-040616.pdf

Mottaghi, S, Poursheikhali, H & Shameli, L (2020) Empathy, compassion fatigue, guilt and secondary traumatic stress in nurses. *Nurs Ethics,* 27, 494-504.
[http://dx.doi.org/10.1177/0969733019851548] [PMID: 31284826]

Noddings, N (2010) Moral education and caring. *Theory Res Educ,* 8, 145-51.
[http://dx.doi.org/10.1177/1477878510368617]

Noddings, N (2013) *Caring: A relational approach to ethics and moral education.* University of California Press..

Noddings, N (2016) *Philosophy of Education.* Westview Press.

Oxford Language Dictionary n.d. Available from: www.oxfordreference.com

Perlman, HH (1983) *Relationship: The heart of helping people.* The University of Chicago Press.

Potter, P, Deshields, T, Divanbeigi, J, Berger, J, Cipriano, D, Norris, L, Olsen, S & Olsen, S (2010) Compassion fatigue and burnout: Prevalence among oncology nurses. *Clin J Oncol Nurs,* 14, E56-62.
[http://dx.doi.org/10.1188/10.CJON.E56-E62] [PMID: 20880809]

Rakel, D (2018) *The compassionate connection: The healing power of empathy and mindful listening.* W. W. Norton & Company.

Rauvola, RS, Vega, DM & Lavigne, KN (2019) Compassion Fatigue, secondary traumatic stress, and vicarious traumatization: A qualitative review and research agenda. *Occup Health Sci,* 3, 297-336.
[http://dx.doi.org/10.1007/s41542-019-00045-1]

Ray, MA (2016) *Transcultural caring dynamics in nursing and health care.* F. A. Davis Company.

Ting, L, Sanders, S, Jacobson, JM & Power, JR (2006) Dealing with the aftermath: A qualitative analysis of mental health social workers' reactions after a client suicide. *Soc Work,* 51, 329-41.

[http://dx.doi.org/10.1093/sw/51.4.329] [PMID: 17152631]

Seligman, M (2011) *Flourish: A new understanding of happiness and well-being – and how to achieve them.* Nicholas Brealey Publishing.

Sitzman, K (2017) Theory-guided self-care for mitigating emotional strain in nursing: Watson's caring science. *Int J Hum Caring,* 21, 66-76.
[http://dx.doi.org/10.20467/HumanCaring-D-17-00009.1]

Sitzman, K & Watson, J (2014) *Caring science, mindful practice: Implementing Jean Watson's human caring theory.* Springer Publishing.

Stephany, K (2015) *Cultivating empathy: Inspiring health professionals to communicate more effectively.* Bentham Science Publishers Pte. Ltd..

Stephany, K (2017) *How to help the suicidal person to choose life: The ethic of care and empathy as indispensable tools for intervention.* Bentham Science Publishers Pte. Ltd..

Stephany, K (2020) *The ethic of care: A moral compass for Canadian Nursing practice.* Bentham Science Publishers Pte. Ltd..

Stubin, CA (2017) Emotional strain: A concept analysis for nursing. *Int J Hum Caring,* 21, 59-90.
[http://dx.doi.org/10.20467/HumanCaring-D-16-00027.1]

Substance Abuse and Mental Health Services Administration (2014) Available from: https://store.samhsa.gov/sites/default/files/d7/priv/sma14-4816.pdf

Tharani, A, Husain, Y & Warwick, I (2017) Learning environment and emotional well-being: A qualitative study of undergraduate nursing students. *Nurse Educ Today,* 59, 82-7.
[http://dx.doi.org/10.1016/j.nedt.2017.09.008] [PMID: 28961508]

Thomas, MS, Crosby, S & Vanderhaar, J (2019) Trauma-informed practices in schools across two decades: An interdisciplinary review of research. *Rev Res Educ,* 43, 422-52.
[http://dx.doi.org/10.3102/0091732X18821123]

Ting, L, Sanders, S, Jacobson, JM & Power, JR (2006) Dealing with the aftermath: A qualitative analysis of mental health social workers' reactions after a client suicide. *Soc Work,* 51, 329-41.
[http://dx.doi.org/10.1093/sw/51.4.329] [PMID: 17152631]

Ward, M, Knowlton, MC & Laney, CW (2018) The flip side of traditional nursing education: A literature review. *Nurse Educ Pract,* 29, 163-71.
[http://dx.doi.org/10.1016/j.nepr.2018.01.003] [PMID: 29414110]

Watson, J (2008) *Nursing: The philosophy and science of caring.* University Press of Colorado.

Watson's Caring Science Institute (2023) Ten caritas processes. Available from: https://www. wat son car ing scien ce. org

Wedgeworth, M (2016) Anxiety and education: An examination of anxiety across a nursing program. *J Nurs Educ Pract,* 6, 23-6.
[http://dx.doi.org/10.5430/jnep.v6n10p23]

Woodworth, JA (2016) Promotion of nursing student civility in nursing education: A concept analysis. *Nurs Forum,* 51, 196-203.
[http://dx.doi.org/10.1111/nuf.12138] [PMID: 26488502]

Zyblock, DM (2010) Nursing presence in contemporary nursing practice. *Nurs Forum,* 45, 120-4.
[http://dx.doi.org/10.1111/j.1744-6198.2010.00173.x] [PMID: 20536761]

CHAPTER 6

Augment Nursing School and Workplace Experience by Promoting Psychological Safety, Compassion Satisfaction and Joy in Work

Abstract: Chapter Six presents an overview of how trauma-informed educational processes ensure that student nurses feel safe and supported in an ideal learning environment. Strategies that promote psychological safety are recommended followed by measures to foster compassion satisfaction and joy in work. Psychological safety consists of a civil and respectful place for learning to occur. Compassion satisfaction is derived from the gratification experienced by caregivers when caring for others, and joy in work consists of positive components in the work environment. Nursing students are a risk group for trauma, and they identify the following situations as sources of trauma, individual-related interpersonal experiences; those related to their role as students; trauma related to institutional and organizational exposure; and stressors associated with the community. *The Four Core Assumptions of Trauma-informed Care* are used as a guide to implementing psychological safety in nursing school and include specific measures for the classroom, simulation, and clinical settings. Those directly related to high-fidelity simulation include actions to make students feel safe before, during, and after each session. The positive feelings and six core assumptions associated with compassion satisfaction, and the role that self-compassion and work-life balance play are featured. Key aspects of the work environment that have the greatest impact on the well-being of nurses working in critical care consist of adequate staffing, meaningful recognition, and effective decision-making. Student nurses with a history of trauma can experience compassion satisfaction if they are able to identify with some of the positive aspects associated with being a trauma survivor. If new nurses are adequately supported by their employers they experience less stress, and increased fulfillment in their jobs. There are valuable justifications for creating joy in work. A focus on joy enhances the work experience, increases employee engagement, benefits the organization, and improves patient outcomes. Making the workplace happy is a shared responsibility, where everyone is expected to do their best work. Meaningful connection to other people is important where teamwork, cooperation, and a sense of camaraderie are ideal. Two specific forms of governance that promote joy in work are participatory and servant leadership. Psychological personal protective equipment (PPE) consists of individual and system-wide measures that support and safeguard the mental health of employees. Two Narrative Case Studies were presented.

In the first one, a student nurse became re-traumatized when listening to a detailed story of someone's traumatic experience. The second Narrative Case Study revealed how a new nurse considered leaving his high-acuity job because of a lack of appreciation. The following five learning activities were proposed, exploring assumptions about constructive feedback; ways to professionally express appreciation; understanding how you handle mistakes; creating a self-inventory to assess work-life balance; and incorporating the ten characteristics of servant leadership into practice. At the end of the Chapter, specific strategies were recommended to build college students' self-confidence.

Keywords: Trauma, Trauma-informed care, Psychological safety, Compassion satisfaction, Joy in work, Trauma-informed educational processes, Empathy-based stress conditions, *The Four Core Assumptions of Trauma-informed Care*, Appreciation, Constructive feedback, High-fidelity patient simulation (HFPS), Self-compassion, Mindful self-compassion, Work-life balance, Mental health, International Nursing Association for Clinical Simulation and Learning (INACSL), Participatory leadership, Servant leadership, Psychological personal protective equipment (PPE), Self-confidence.

LEARNING GUIDE

After completing this chapter, the reader should be able to:

- Gain an understanding of the similarities and differences between compassion satisfaction and joy in work.
- Define trauma-informed educational processes and psychological safety and what they share.
- Describe psychological trauma.
- Point out specific situations that student nurses find traumatizing.
- Understand how *The Four Core Assumptions of Trauma-informed Care* contribute to psychological safety when applied in a nursing school teaching environment.
- Learn how to ensure psychological safety during simulation sessions.
- Identify the six key assumptions of compassion satisfaction.
- Understand how self-compassion and work-life balance can be implemented.
- Review specific aspects of a critical care unit (CCU) that promote compassion satisfaction.
- Recognize some of the positive features associated with being a student nurse and trauma survivor.
- Recognize the importance of supporting new nurses.
- Ascertain how each of the following components specifically contribute to joy in work, sharing the responsibility; interpersonal connection; leadership; and making use of psychological personal protective equipment (PPE).
- Review two Narrative Case Studies and ensuing Thematic Analysis. The first one reveals how a student nurse becomes re-traumatized while listening to an uncensored story of another person's trauma. The second one describes how a

student nurse contemplated leaving his high-acuity job because of a lack of support and appreciation.
- Participate in these five learning activities (*e.g.*, Exploring Assumptions About Constructive Feedback; Ways to Express Appreciation in a Professional Manner; Understanding How You Handle Mistakes; Creating a Self-Inventory to Assess Work-life Balance; and Incorporating the Ten Characteristics of Servant Leadership into Practice).
- Consider specific recommended self-care strategies to build self-confidence.

INTRODUCTION TO CHAPTER SIX

Trauma-informed care recognizes the prevalence of trauma, its negative impacts, and aims to decrease re-traumatization. Many of today's nursing students have experienced trauma and are exposed to further trauma and stress during their training. Subsequently, Goddard *et al.*, (2021) assert that trauma-informed education be implemented in nursing education to ensure that students consistently feel safe, are supported in all learning contexts, and that an ideal learning environment is fostered where kindness, sensitivity, and nonjudgment are paramount. Therefore, Chapter Six explores highly recommended trauma-informed educational processes that foster psychological safety, followed by measures that promote compassion satisfaction, and joy in work.

Trauma-informed educational processes value respectful interpersonal relationships, encourage a supportive teaching environment, foster effective communication skills, and incorporate aspects of genuine caring into learning (Thomas *et al.*, 2019). **Psychological safety** creates a positive, civil, and respectful atmosphere for learning to occur without fear of retaliation (O'Donovan & McAuliffe, 2020). Psychological safety is closely aligned with trauma-informed educational processes because they both have the goal of ensuring that the learning environment is safe. **Compassion satisfaction** refers to the gratification experienced by caregivers from doing a good job of caring for others, and **joy in work** consists of positive components in the work environment that contribute to happy employees (Institute for Healthcare Improvement (IHI), 2023; Mangoulia *et al.*, 2015; Perlo *et al.*, 2017).). Compassion satisfaction and joy in work have similar goals in that they both improve the overall work experience for a nurse. However, they also differ somewhat. For instance, **compassion satisfaction** refers to the gratification experienced by a caregiver from doing a good job of taking care of people, whereas joy in work is about positive aspects of the work environment that contribute to their happiness.

The Chapter begins by reviewing sources of trauma and stress experienced by student nurses. *The Four Core Assumptions of Trauma-informed Care* are presented as the premise of psychological safety, followed by measures that can be used in the classroom, simulation, and clinical settings. The remainder of the discussion is concerned with the positive ways to insulate student and practicing nurses from some of the negative effects of trauma, including specific strategies to increase their overall job satisfaction and help them to feel joy in their work.

POTENTIAL SOURCES OF TRAUMA AND STRESS FOR NURSING STUDENTS

Psychological trauma occurs because of exposure to an adverse or stressful event that is experienced by the person as harmful and has lasting negative effects on their emotional well-being (SAMHSA, 2014). Some students have a history of trauma before entering nursing school and may even choose a career in healthcare because their suffering motivated them to want to help others. Nevertheless, as stated in the introduction to the Chapter, a history of trauma predisposes nursing students to be re-traumatized during their training (Wolf, 2019).

Nursing students are also known to experience higher levels of stress when compared to other post-secondary students. Some of the pressure is related to situations that occur in the clinical setting such as caring for the seriously ill, injured, or dying, especially if they involve children (Wedgeworth, 2016). Additional contributing factors to student nurses' stress levels are unrelated to clinical. For example, Salvarani *et al.*, (2020) conducted a study involving nursing undergraduate nursing students to examine predictors of psychological distress. Their findings demonstrated that senior students coped better than junior students, yet 70% of the participants, reported significant psychological distress due to pressures associated with their academic studies. Those who expressed the greatest distress exhibited difficulty with emotional regulation, decreased self-awareness, and poor coping (Salvarani *et al.*,).

Specific Situations that Nursing Students Identify as Traumatizing

Nursing students possess risk factors for trauma and re-traumatization related to situations in their lives that occur inside and outside of their educational experiences (Bosse *et al.*, 2021). In a study conducted by Mayer *et al.*, (2022) nursing students identified four themes as contributing sources of trauma. They consist of individual-related interpersonal experiences; those related to their role as nursing students; trauma from institutional and organizational exposure; and stressors associated with the community.

Theme One: Individual-Related Interpersonal Sources of Trauma

The first theme relates to interpersonal sources of trauma experienced by students in their capacity as a family member, friends, or significant others. Being raised in a home where there was violence was declared as traumatizing, as was witnessing someone close to them being assaulted. Becoming aware of nursing student colleagues who were contemplating suicide or intentionally self-harming, were declared as quite distressful. Breaking up with a significant other during nursing school also left them feeling vulnerable (Mayer *et al.*, 2022).

Theme Two: Potential Sources of Trauma as Nursing Students

The second theme concerns the experiences of nursing students deemed as traumatic in their capacity as students. Blaming and shaming by an instructor was upsetting, as was the perception that their concerns were being ignored by a teacher. Being assigned to a preceptor who is overly critical reduced their confidence. Looking after difficult and disrespectful clients, and caring for clients who were seriously ill, and died were quite upsetting (Mayer *et al.*, 2022).

Theme Three: Potential Sources of Trauma from Institutional and Organizational Exposure

Student nurses revealed additional potential sources of trauma related to being a student. The cost of tuition caused financial concerns, as did the added costs and stress associated with having to repeat parts of their program due to failure. The stress associated with demanding course requirements to get a passing grade was worrisome. The content of the curriculum being based on studying people's suffering, disease, mental illness, and death was declared to be too focussed on the negative aspects of nursing (Mayer *et al.*, 2022).

Theme Four: Potential Sources of Community Trauma Exposure

Additional stressors experienced by nursing students were related to their role as a member of the larger community. For instance, one description that was quite alarming involved a student who went missing. Other participants spoke about broader global issues such as those related to the COVID-19 pandemic, lockdown, and having to learn online (Mayer *et al.*, 2022). The authors of this study highly recommended that trauma-informed healthcare strategies be implemented that promote the academic and career success of future student nurses (Mayer *et al.*, 2022). This recommendation is a perfect segway into our next discussion concerning psychological safety in nursing education.

THE IMPORTANCE OF PSYCHOLOGICAL SAFETY

"Psychological safety emerges when those in power persistently praise, reward, and promote people who have the courage to act, talk about their doubts, successes, and failures, and work doggedly to do things better the next time." Robert I. Sutton, Psychologist, and Author.

Psychological safety ensures that the educational experience occurs in a safe and respectful manner (Fig. **6.1**). It consists of a positive atmosphere for learning without fear of retaliation, by demonstrating a shared belief that it is okay to take personal risks, to speak up when concerns arise, and to freely ask questions and share ideas (O'Donovan & McAuliffe, 2020; Turner & Harder, 2018). It is, therefore, highly recommended that Nursing Schools prioritize therapeutic communication skills, civility, respect, and an atmosphere of non-judgment as essential components of trauma-informed strategies that prioritize psychological safety (Pfeiffer & Grabbe, 2022).

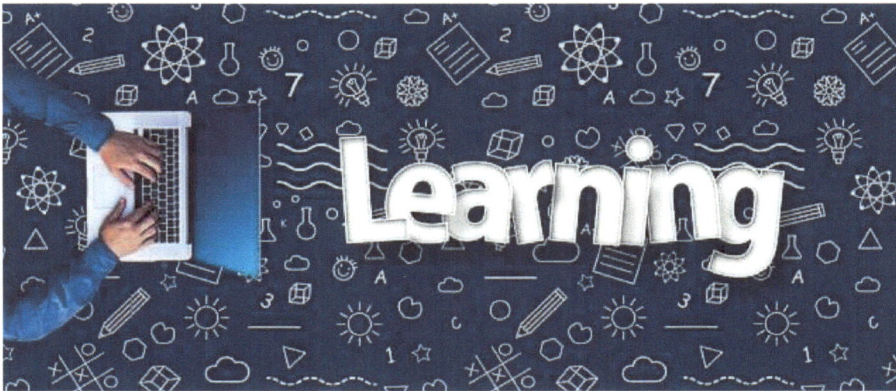

Fig. (6.1). A Safe Place for Learning. Source: www.pixabay.com.

PSYCHOLOGICAL SAFETY AND THE FOUR CORE ASSUMPTIONS OF TRAUMA-INFORMED CARE

Goddard *et al.*, (2021) assert that trauma-informed education be implemented in nursing education to ensure that our students consistently feel safe, and are supported in all learning contexts and that an ideal learning environment is fostered where kindness, sensitivity, and nonjudgment are paramount. They highly recommend using *The Four Core Assumptions of Trauma-informed Care* as the guide to the implementation of a trauma-informed, empathetic, and supportive teaching environment. The core assumptions of trauma-informed care consist of (*e.g.*, realize, recognize, respond, and resist re-traumatization) (SAMHSA), 2014a). Note that although these four core assumptions were introduced in Chapter One, they were presented in relation to caring for traumatized clients/patients in a clinical environment. In this current Chapter, the focus is on how they apply to nursing students.

Realization Consists of Trauma Awareness

The word 'realize' stands for awareness that trauma is prevalent in nursing students and that educators must be sensitive to this fact (Goddard *et al.*, 2021). For instance, Fowler and Wholeben (2020) point out that nursing students may have had prior traumatic experiences during the course of their life. Some student nurses may themselves be survivors of adverse childhood experiences (ACEs) and be reluctant to complete their studies because of increased anxiety. Those who have experienced ACEs and remain in the program may experience a loss of emotional control, feelings of hopelessness, and decreased self-confidence, which may result in declining performance (Fowler & Wholeben, 2020).

Aim to Reduce Harm Through Reducing Power Differentials & Fostering Connection

Decreasing power differentials and cultivating human connection are two recommended ways to reduce student nurses' duress (Foli & Thompson, 2019). Nursing faculty can address the power imbalances between them and students, by avoiding a top-down authoritarian way of teaching, encouraging active student participation through dynamic learning activities, and encouraging safe connections between fellow students (Duffy, 2018; Goddard *et al.*, 2021). Connection is needed because many of our students feel all alone in their experiences, especially after having some of their education taught online due to COVID-19 school closures. Co-operation and connection with other students may help them to feel that they belong to a bigger group who do care for them (Stephany, 2020). Therefore, instructors may consider allowing some degree of class time for students to communicate with each other and may consider encouraging students to form study groups as a way for them to bond while learning (Goddard *et al.*, 2021).

Promote Increased Self-awareness & Self-compassion

Other suggestions to reduce harm include altering course design and assignments to align more cohesively with better self-awareness and to increase self-compassion. Journalling is highly recommended, as are learning activities that have a reflective component. Increased self-awareness can help student nurses identify their negative emotions and help them recognize symptoms associated with empathy-based stress conditions. For example, if they develop a tendency to emotionally withdraw from relational practice, it may be due to feeling overwhelmed by exposure to human suffering (Goddard *et al.*, 2021). If this is the case, the instructor can encourage the student to self-refer to counselling.

Self-compassion assists student nurses in refraining from self-deprecating behaviors and being kinder to themselves. Instructors can recommend that students develop their own self-care plan to offset compassion fatigue through activities that support physical and emotional well-being like exercising, getting enough sleep, eating healthier, connecting with friends and family, and spending time in nature (Stephany, 2020).

Recognizing Signs of Trauma in Students

Recognition is about being able to identify the signs and symptoms of trauma in nursing students. However, it is important to be aware that not every student is courageous enough or willing to reach out for help when they need it, especially if they are feeling insecure and afraid of being judged. It is therefore crucially important for the faculty to consciously look for indications that a student may be struggling. Avoidance is a key symptom associated with trauma so the instructor should watch for clues that this may be occurring (Goddard *et al.*, 2021). A high level of anxiety concerning the expectations of coursework, consistently handing in assignments late, defensiveness, considerable decline in course engagement, and decreased overall performance, may all be indicative that the student is not coping (Sanderson *et al.*, 2020). If one or more of these issues becomes apparent the instructor may consider contacting the student directly, conveying their concern in a caring way, and possibly referring them for additional support at a learning center. When feasible, a faculty could consider negotiating an extension of the assignment due date (Sanderson *et al.*, 2020). However, Goddard *et al.*, (2021) warn that applying trauma-informed care to education does not mean being soft or not enforcing competencies in learning. Professionalism and academic integrity must be upheld. However, applying reasonable consideration and flexibility when possible is still highly recommended.

Responding with Caring Teaching Strategies

Responding also specifically consists of using caring teaching strategies with students, especially when they are not doing well. This may consist of acknowledging their struggle, communicating genuine care, and normalizing the process of reaching out for professional support. Student nurses readily report that faculty caring traits make a difference in how well they do and their overall motivation to succeed is related to their instructor's caring behaviours. Faculty caring attributes have even been described as a driving force for student nurses' intention to complete their program and graduate (Fifer, 2019; Henderson *et al.*, 2020).

The type of caring behaviour expressed by their instructor also matters. Student nurses gave a high rating to faculty who demonstrated civility, respect, and understanding which are pillars of trauma-informed care and boost their self-confidence (Henderson *et al.*, 2020). They also identified creating a compassionate learning environment, using caring communication skills, and offering encouragement as particularly important especially when they are facing difficulties (Henderson *et al.*, 2020). Being approachable also affects a student's willingness to communicate their distress and to seek help when needed (Sanderson *et al.*, 2020).

Providing Constructive Feedback to Students

Constructive feedback is a form of criticism with the goal of a positive outcome and is also referred to as positive criticism or substantive critique. It consists of an unbiased critique of performance and includes correcting any errors. Regardless of whether the feedback is positive or negative, it should ideally be impartial. (Altmiller, 2016; Altmiller *et al.*, 2018; Omer & Abdularhim, 2017). Ideally, constructive criticism should consist of a two-way communication process between the one offering the appraisal and the one receiving it. Providing constructive criticism can be challenging for the person who is tasked with giving it, but if done right can enhance learning, and motivate the person on the receiving end to want to do better next time (Omer & Abdularhim, 2017). Laskowski-Jones (2018) highly recommends that the teacher begin with empathy to connect with the student and communicate care because this sends the message that you have the student's best interest in mind. Inform the student that the feedback is intended to help them to learn and grow. Seek clarification that the student heard and understood what was said and address questions and concerns (Laskowski-Jones, 2018). Feedback that is strength-based builds confidence which makes it more likely that the student will be able to handle criticism (Brooks & Goldstein, 2003). Therefore, what is suggested is beginning with pointing out the person's strengths and good achievements, followed by what needs to be improved upon. A remedial action plan is also a good idea (Omer & Abdularhim, 2017).

However, what if the student responds to the constructive criticism in an emotionally reactive way? What should the instructor do? Altmiller (2016) recommends that the faculty members model the professional behavior they want the student to copy. Utilizing civil responses by speaking calmly and concisely, and staying focused on the task at hand is beneficial. Another good idea is to try and prevent a reaction by the way that you deliver criticism. A learning activity is included in Box (**6.1**) where students are required to explore some of their assumptions about constructive feedback.

Box 6.1. Learning activity: exploring your assumptions about constructive feedback (as adapted from altmiller *et al.*, 2018).

This activity can be done on your own through reflective journalling or in a class discussion or small group exercise. Review the following statements and related questions and your responses to them. Do your best to try and back up what you say.
1-**Feedback is a bridge from undesirable to desirable behavior.** What does that mean to you and why?
2-**There is no such thing as a perfect nurse.** Is that true? Why or why not? How does this question relate to receiving constructive feedback on performance?
3-**Respect is the key to good communication and meaningful feedback.** How exactly is this operationalized in practice?

> ## SOMETHING TO REFLECT UPON
>
> Think of a time when someone gave you constructive criticism. In your opinion, what did they do well? What did they not do well? Also examine your response to their criticism. Did you react with self-loathing? Knowing what you know now, how would you respond differently?

Create a Safe Place for Dialogue to Occur

When students feel safe, they are more likely to reach out for help and support. It is important for the faculty member to do their best to alleviate some student apprehension by responding to questions and concerns when they occur, and by creating a respectful place for dialogue to occur outside of the classroom or clinical setting. That may involve scheduling regular office hours or meetings by appointment (Henderson *et al.*, 2020). It is helpful to do regular check-ins to help students navigate through uncertainties when they arise. When possible, communicating with them through their preferred venue is also highly recommended (Henderson *et al.*, 2020; Sanderson *et al.*, 2020).

The Importance of Expressing Appreciation

"Appreciation can make a day, even change a life. Your willingness to put it into words is all that is necessary" Margaret E. Cousins, Irish Indian Educationist

Expressing genuine appreciation is another important trait that should ideally be evident in the behaviors of faculty and students alike. **Appreciation** involves recognizing or admiring someone's good qualities or noble actions. Appreciation, however, is only beneficial when it is given freely without expecting anything in return and when it is offered as a form of celebration of how our lives have been enriched by the other person (Rosenberg, 2003). Too often we withhold our inclination to praise someone for a job well done because we may have been taught that it may cause them to become conceited. Another reason we withhold compliments is because we think the other person already knows that we value them when they may be unaware of our admiration.

We must not only learn to offer appreciation. We need to be able to receive it graciously too (Rosenberg, 2003). A simple, *"Thank you"* will suffice. Unfortunately, we sometimes feel uncomfortable when someone compliments us, perhaps because we do not believe that we deserve it. But if we shrug off or reject their praise, we have refused their gift to us and that is insulting and may be hurtful to them. I recall doing just that and it was a lesson in how not to behave in the future. A cherished friend of mine had leaned on me during a time of crisis in her life. Once she got through it, she showed up at my doorstep with a bouquet of long-stem white roses. I gasped with astonishment when I saw the roses, but because I was worried about her financial situation, I quickly said something I later regretted. *"You can't give me those roses; they must have cost you a fortune."* My friend immediately started to cry. I knew I had done her a great disservice. Lucky for me, we sat down and had a good cry together and she forgave me. What my friend taught me that day was life-enhancing. I learned the importance of accepting a token of appreciation gracefully. A Learning Activity is included in Box (**6.2**) where you are required to explore ways to professionally express appreciation to others.

Box 6.2. Learning activity: ways to express appreciation in a professional manner

Break into small groups. Half the class is tasked with the role of describing inappropriate ways to demonstrate professional appreciation and why they are not suitable. The second half of the class is required to do the opposite. They are asked to identify how to show professional appreciation and must back up their assertions with evidence. When done, reconvene as a whole class to discuss what you learned.

Resist Re-traumatization

Resisting the re-traumatization of students is essential because persons who have a history of trauma can be emotionally triggered and react if they are exposed to situations that remind them of their adversity. Therefore, it is highly advised that nurse educators be aware of the signs of symptoms of post-traumatic stress disorder (PTSD) (Foli & Thompson, 2019). Some of the symptoms associated with PTSD include reliving the incident in nightmares or flashbacks, experiencing frightening thoughts, anger, fear, irritability, and depression, and avoiding situations that closely resemble their previous trauma (Jenkins *et al.*, 2022). A discussion of how to avoid re-traumatization of student nurses during simulation is presented after the Narrative Case Study exercise. The following Case Study tells the story of how a Student Nurse becomes triggered while listening to a guest speaker's story in class. Refer to Box (**6.3**).

Box 6.3. Narrative case study one: a student nurse becomes re-traumatized while listening to a traumatic story.

Mr. Campbell is an instructor in an Arts and Science class in the 3rd year of a Bachelor of Science in Nursing (BSN) Program. A key focus in this class is on caring for special populations. This week Mr. Campbell booked a guest, Amy Bains to talk about her lived experience of being a victim of human trafficking. Mr. Campbell was excited about this guest speaker because he read about them online, and they received good ratings. However, before asking Amy Bains to attend his class Mr. Campbell had not listened to any of her previous Podcasts or presentations on YouTube. On the day that Amy Bains was scheduled to speak she arrived on time. Mr. Campbell introduced her to the class, and she proceeded with her presentation. Mr. Campbell sat back to listen to her speak and to watch his nursing students' reactions. The guest speaker began her talk by disclosing in detail what happened to her when she was abducted by human traffickers at the age of ten at a refugee camp. She went on to explain in graphic detail, all the horrors she experienced. Mr. Campbell had recently completed a short four-hour Webinar course on trauma-informed care. He became concerned that some of his students may be negatively affected by what they were hearing. He subsequently carefully watched to see if any of the students were distressed during the presentation. Mr. Campbell became aware of one of his students, Michelle, looking downcast with visible tears in her eyes. Before he was able to approach Michelle, she abruptly ran out of the classroom. Mr. Campbell stood up quickly, approached the speaker, and discreetly and quietly asked Ms. Bains to refrain from any further disclosure of her traumatic experiences and to talk about the recovery portion of her journey. He then excused himself, left the classroom, and closed the door behind him. Mr. Campbell noticed Michele sitting on a hallway couch and crying. He rushed to her side, but before he could speak, Michelle yelled at him.
"How could you have someone tell us a story like that? She talked about such horrible things."
Mr. Campbell wanted to apologize and console Michelle, but she was having none of it. Michelle shouted at him again.
"Leave me alone! Some of us in your class have been through stuff that you know nothing about."
Mr. Campbell felt awful about what happened, but he did not know what to do to make the situation better.

NARRATIVE CASE STUDY ONE: IDENTIFICATION OF THEMES & ANALYSIS

Two key themes were identified from this story.

Theme # 1: Michelle was re-traumatized when the guest speaker disclosed details of her own traumatic experiences.

Theme # 1 Analysis: Resisting re-traumatization is one of *The Four Core Assumptions of Trauma-informed Care* (SAMHSA, 2014a). Student nurses may have a history of trauma. It is therefore crucially important to avoid situations that may trigger them and may involve planning for this to occur. In this Case Study, the guest speaker should have been advised by Mr. Campbell before she gave her presentation not to share any details of her trauma. Unfortunately, that did not occur, and the result was that Michelle became distressed. Her reaction was quite intense even though there was no actual imminent threat of harm to her at the time. But her response was not abnormal, because previous trauma leaves a lasting imprint in the brain, and when triggered a whole array of defenses are activated (Cori, 2008).

Theme # 2: Although Mr. Campbell has recently taken a short Webinar Course on trauma-informed care, this was likely not adequate training.

Theme # 2 Analysis : Wheeler and Phillips (2019) point out that, in general, there is a lack of trauma-specific training in nursing programs even though trauma is pervasive and prevalent. More comprehensive formal training in trauma-informed educational practices would have likely enabled Mr. Campbell to be more prepared when planning to have a guest speaker present in his class. Ideally, the speaker should have been informed ahead of time not to disclose any details of her trauma, and Mr. Campbell may have been better prepared to address student distress when it occurred.

QUESTIONS FOR FURTHER DISCUSSIONS

1 What do you think was the instructor's first error in judgment?

2-What would you have done differently?

3 What would you do to help to alleviate some of the student's emotional distress?

4-What type of support or training do you think you and your colleagues may need to be better equipped to address potential issues related to trauma that may arise in the student nursing population?

CREATING A PSYCHOLOGICAL SAFE LEARNING ENVIRONMENT IN HIGH-FIDELITY SIMULATIONS

Simulation imitates real-life clinical scenarios and provides an opportunity for nursing students to safely apply their knowledge and skills and learn from it. Many labs in modern-day nursing schools now have the capacity to offer various forms of simulation opportunities such as using life actors, life-like stationary models, or high-fidelity patient simulations (Lavoie & Clarke, 2017). **High-fidelity patient simulation (HFPS)** in nursing utilizes human resembling manikins to create life-like simulations for learning (Fig. **6.2**).

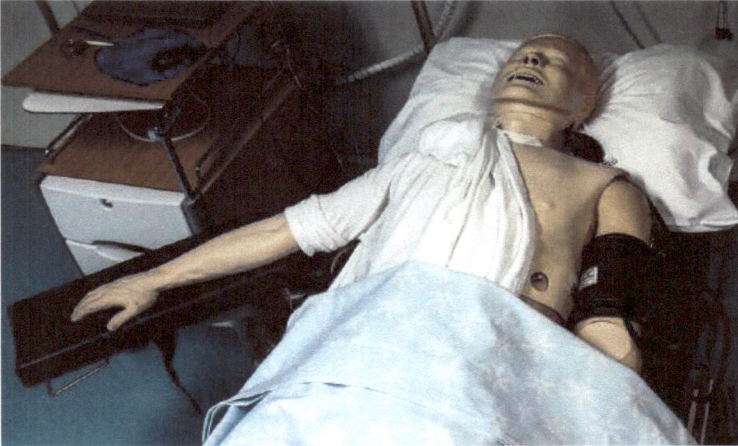

Fig. (6.2). Manikin for simulation. Source: www.pixabay.com.

Research has demonstrated that excessive stress and anxiety during simulations can impede knowledge retention and impair nursing students' performance. Whereas the opposite is also true because a psychologically safe learning venue enhances their learning (Ignacio *et al.*, 2015).

What can an instructor do to offset the likelihood of re-traumatizing the student nurse in a high-fidelity simulation? They can take deliberate actions to make students feel safe, before, during and after simulation (Foli & Thompson, 2019). Specific evidence-based strategies are therefore suggested. They consist of the foundational pre-simulation preparation; qualities of the facilitator; the ability to make mistakes; opportunities for skills acquisition; and the role of de-briefing (Turner & Harder, 2018).

Foundational Pre-simulation Preparation

Foundational pre-simulation preparation activities in high-fidelity simulation consist of orientation, preparation, objectives, and expectations (Turner & Harder, 2018, p. 47). Orientation refers to preparing the students before the simulation starts and consists of getting them to see the area where the simulation will take place, view the mannikin, and if appropriate, be provided with an opportunity to touch some of the equipment (Fey *et al.*, 2014). Preparation involves having the tools to feel ready for the simulation which reduces students' anxiety and includes activities such as readings, videos, and questions assigned ahead of time. Objectives when clearly set allow for clear identification of learning goals and contribute to a psychologically safer learning environment (Turner & Harder, 2018). Faculty can warn students before starting that the simulation may contain content that is disturbing.

The Qualities of the Facilitator

The qualities of the facilitator can have a significant impact on the integrity of a safe learning setting for simulation (Turner & Harder, 2018). Being accessible and available to the learners is the key, as is responding to queries, misunderstandings, or challenging assumptions in a respectful manner, and inviting feedback. Furthermore, a facilitator who is well prepared and organized, who is aware of possible triggers, and willing to warn the students about them before the simulation begins, are all deemed by students to be helpful (Fey *et al.*, 2014). Being approachable, honest, accessible, admitting when you are wrong, and encouraging feedback are also all deemed supportive features of a simulation facilitator (Turner & Harder, 2018).

The Ability to Make Mistakes During the Simulation

During the simulation, the student should feel supported to take risks and make mistakes without harsh penalties because they are being exposed to make-believe emergency crisis scenarios that require a high level of problem-solving and critical thinking, all without harm occurring to an actual person (Fig. **6.3**). This in turn facilitates a stimulating and significant educational experience and creates a great opportunity to learn from what went wrong, with no devasting or enduring consequences for the student or a patient (Turner & Harder, 2018; Rudolf *et al.*, 2014). For example, when students are made aware that they or their colleagues will not be harshly judged, they are more willing to share their views when they notice mistakes. However, the opposite is also true. Fear of being ridiculed or receiving a failing grade for making a wrong decision may impede learning, because the student may be too afraid to step out of their comfort zone (Nielson & Harder, 2013).

Fig. (6.3). Mistakes are Not Failures. They are Lessons. Source: www.pixabay.com.

A Personal Learning Activity is included in Box (**6.4**) where you are asked to reflect on how you handle mistakes. The goal of this exercise is to assist you in examining your approach to dealing with errors in judgment, and to enable you to change ways of thinking and behaving that may no longer be beneficial.

Box 6.4. Learning activity: understanding how you handle mistakes (as adapted from brooks & goldstein, 2003, pp. 186-187 & 300).

This is a personal learning assignment that you are meant to do on your own. It is about exploring how you respond to mistakes. The rationale for this exercise is to help you to gain a better understanding of the negative beliefs that affect how you think and act. You may want to consider journalling to gain further insight into your behavior.
1-List three times in the past year when you made a mistake or failed to successfully complete a task.
2-Before you attempted these tasks, how confident were you that you would be successful?
3-When you failed did you blame yourself as though it was due to some kind of personality flaw?
4-After reflecting, would you respond differently to those situations if they happened today? If yes, explain why. If not, explain why not. (This question assists you to begin exploring different ways of coping with mistakes).
5 What was the worst thing that happened to you when you made a mistake or failed at something? How did you react? Were you devastated? Was your reaction equal to the severity of the error or was it magnified out of proportion? (These questions may help you to look more realistically at what happened and to catastrophize less).
6-What memories do you have about how your parents or other significant people in your life reacted when you made a mistake? (This question addresses where you learned to respond the way that you do).
7-How do you think you will manage mistakes when you make them in the future? Are you ready to challenge your self-critical beliefs? Are you willing to learn something from what transpired?
8-Make it your intention to react differently to mistakes when they occur in the future.

Knowing What to Do When Students Become Distressed During the Session

Sometimes, despite all of the efforts to prepare students some of them may still be triggered during a simulation session and the instructor needs to know how to intervene. For example, they must be also willing to terminate the simulation if a student feels unsafe or distressed and allows them to leave the simulation without consequences if they experience emotional distress, is a good idea. It is highly recommended that the instructor re-emphasizes that confidentiality will be honoured in all group discussions and that personal sharing is not a required component of the learning process. Providing information on internal and external resources for the students to access if they need support is also important (Foli & Thompson, 2019).

Opportunities for Skills Acquisition

Necessary nursing skills acquisition in the areas of performing specific procedures and therapeutic communication is one of the purposes of high-fidelity simulation. When practiced in a safe learning environment, this way of mastering essential skills needed for practice enables student nurses to feel more confident and be better able to apply what they have learned in actual clinical settings. Simulation may even provide an opportunity to re-enact a particular scene to learn how to improve their decision-making and ability to solve problems (Turner & Harder, 2018).

The Role of De-briefing

De-briefing students after the session is also crucially important for the purpose of reflection and additional learning and should preferably begin with acknowledging what went well before discussing errors that were made. To foster a feeling of safety students can be encouraged to openly speak and ask questions without any fear of embarrassment, humiliation, or retaliation. Post-simulation de-brief also provides an opportunity for faculty to assist anyone who may have been disturbed by something that occurred during the scenario. When feasible, the instructors should make themselves available to students who need a little extra help to process the experience (Kolbe *et al.*, 2020). In Box (**6.5**), a summary of positive and negative behaviors that influence a psychologically safe simulation environment are shared.

Box 6.5. Summary of positive & negative behaviors that affect psychological safety in simulation (Turner & Harder, 2018, p. 51).

Positive Behaviors
1-Learners are provided orientation to the simulation room/equipment.
2-Leaners are provided pre-learning activities and clear objectives before the simulation.
3-Pre-briefing is provided.
4-Time limits are provided.
5-Learners are reminded about the ability to make mistakes in simulation.
6-Formative assessment is provided.
Negative Behaviors
7-No pre-learning activities or clear objectives are provided.
8-Debriefing focuses on mistakes made in simulation.
9-No orientation to the simulation room/equipment is provided.
10-Summative evaluation is used cautiously.
11-Facilitator does not respect learner confidentiality.

(Box 6.5) cont.....

Note: The International Nursing Association for Clinical Simulation and Learning (INACSL) provides tremendous resources to enhance the science of simulation.

KEY FACTORS OF COMPASSION SATISFACTION

We learned about empathy-based stress conditions like secondary traumatic stress and compassion fatigue in Chapter Five that are related to the demands placed on nurses, and exposure to other people's suffering, that interferes with their ability to be empathetic (Hinderer *et al*., 2015). Despite the risks associated with their work, most nurses are still able to offer empathy to their patients because of the positive feelings they derive from taking good care of them. This is what is referred to as compassion satisfaction (Sacco & Copel, 2018). **Compassion satisfaction** involves taking pride in one's work, doing a good job, and feeling good about what you do to help others (Kerig, 2019; Mangoulia *et al*., 2015). Key factors associated with compassion satisfaction that will be reviewed are positive feelings, core assumptions, measures that promote care for the caregiver, aspects of the environment, student nurses' role as healers, and new graduates' need for appreciation.

The Positive Feelings Associated with Compassion Satisfaction

Distinct positive feelings are often associated with compassion, and satisfaction that not only contribute to a nurse's overall job satisfaction but also lead to enhanced coping in times of distress (Cheung *et al*., 2020). They also enrich many aspects of a nurse's professional and personal life. For example, deep fulfillment, a sense of award, and an overall sense of caring accomplishment can be derived from the meaning they feel from the work that they do. They may experience an overall enhancement in their general well-being like joy, enrichment, invigoration, inspiration, revitalization, gratitude, and hope (Sacco & Copel, 2018, p. 79). Many of these optimistic affective emotional experiences are a direct result of a nurse's personal positive attitude; an engaging relationship with the client/patient and their families; making a notable contribution to another person's health and welfare; and contribution to the workplace and the profession (Duffy, 2018; Sacco & Copel, 2017; Seligman, 2011).

Six Core Assumptions of Compassion Satisfaction

Sacco and Copel (2018) have identified six assumptions that must occur for a nurse to experience compassion satisfaction. The first involves the nurse's desire to nurture their relationships with their client/patients, and what we now know is that a healthy caring relationship between a nurse, patient, and their families is good for everyone. It can make working in healthcare more satisfying because the nurse feels they are making a difference in people's lives. It also enhances clients/patient and their families' experiences by making them more personal (Duffy, 2018).

The second assumption is that meeting the needs of clients/patients and their families leads to feelings of fulfillment, optimism, appreciation, and a sense of worthiness in the nurse (Sacco & Copel, 2018). For example, the intentional compassion that a nurse feels when connecting with and caring for those who suffer, and helping to alleviate their anguish, is what contributes the most to their job satisfaction (Dunn & Rivas, 2014).

The third supposition is that working in a positive environment is necessary (Sacco & Copel, 2018). For example, there is evidence to indicate that some nurses who care for seriously ill trauma patients report high levels of satisfaction if they feel adequately supported in a positive work environment. For instance, in a study conducted by Hinderer *et al.*, (2014), nurses with specialized training in trauma experienced high prevalence rates of compassion satisfaction and low rates of burnout and secondary traumatic stress related to adequate social support; working fewer hours per week; experiencing good working relationships with colleagues; and being employed in a positive work environment (Hinderer *et al.*,). Kelly *et al.*, (2015) also identified meaningful recognition from supervisors as an additional contributing factor to job satisfaction while working in stressful settings.

The fourth assumption consists of experiencing an empathetic connection with clients/patients which leads to enhanced levels of compassion, understanding, and altruism in the nurse (Sacco & Copel, 2018). However, nurses who readily identify with the good that they do for others, also often possess an attitude of optimism, and prioritize their own self-care, which somewhat buffers them from negativity and from developing compassion fatigue (Radney & Figley, 2007).

Positive emotions are associated with caring concern for another person and negative emotions are linked to feeling the distress of other people's suffering. A fifth postulation involves the nurse's ability to create a balance between concern for another's suffering, and the compassionate energy felt for them. In this manner, compassion is seen to offset negative emotions (Dunn & Rivas, 2014; Sacco & Copel, 2018). The sixth and last assumption is a prerequisite for the fifth assumption and asserts that positive aspects related to caring must be fully experienced by nurses to counteract the negative (Sacco & Copel, 2018). Compassion when fully felt by the nurse, propels the positive energy needed to create a balance between the two energies, and results in an increased sense of fulfillment in the nurse. The nurse compassionately nurtures the patient, which leads to the experience of compassion satisfaction (Dunn & Rivas, 2014; Sacco & Copel, 2018).

CARE FOR THE CAREGIVER: SPECIFIC MEASURES THAT PRO-MOTE COMPASSION SATISFACTION

We are now going to review two specific ways to encourage compassion satisfaction in nurses related to care for the caregiver. They consist of self-compassion and creating a work-life balance.

Self-compassion

Taking care of yourself as a nurse is not optional, it is necessary, and self-compassion contributes to a nurse's well-being and work fulfillment. **Self-compassion** consists of treating yourself with the same degree of empathetic concern that you would offer someone else in a similar situation, especially when it comes to making a mistake. It is a way to demonstrate caring concern toward yourself rather than resorting to self-criticism (Delaney, 2018). **Mindful self-compassion** combines mindfulness and being fully present, with self-compassion in the form of caring and loving directed at oneself that fosters self-kindness. It consists of learning how to place painful feelings and distorted negative thinking into perspective. For example, instead of merely avoiding what is unpleasant, or over-emphasizing the significance of what you feel or think, you consider the facts and a more feasible and helpful explanation to explain your experience (Delaney, 2018).

Research evidence supports the benefits of self-compassion over the detrimental effects of self-criticism. For instance, when nurses judge themselves harshly, they are less likely to be empathetic with clients/patients and are prone to developing compassion fatigue and burnout. However, nurses who are self-compassionate tend to demonstrate increased empathy when caring for others. Furthermore, when self-compassion or mindful self-compassion is practiced, they also provide protection from developing empathy-based stress conditions, enhance resilience, and increase compassion satisfaction (Beaumont *et al.*, 2016; Delaney, 2018; Durante *et al.*, 2016).

> ### SOMETHING TO REFLECT UPON
> How do you feel about introducing self-compassion into your life and getting rid of negative self-talk? Are you willing to give it a try? If not, what is holding you back? You really do not have anything to lose by acting with self-compassion and a great deal to gain.

Creating Work-life Balance

Nursing is a stressful job complicated by many factors such as shift work, working too many hours of overtime, staffing shortages, and caring for very sick patients. These pressures can result in dissatisfaction with work, physical and emotional exhaustion, feelings of loneliness, negativity, pessimism, depression, and anxiety (Simmons, 2012). A specific way to prevent some of these symptoms is through prioritizing work-life balance (Durante *et al.*, 2016; Mulen, 2015). **Work-life balance** entails doing your best to create an equilibrium between work commitments and personal lifestyles. This entails ensuring that employment achievement and leisure time are treated with equal priority so that you can live a harmonious life (Mullen, 2015; Simons, 2012).

How do nurses improve their personal situation to attain work-life balance? They begin by admitting that a problem exists and needs addressing, followed by identifying priorities, creating an action plan, and modifying the plan when needed. Creating a work-life inventory prioritizes what needs to be done first and ensures that any goals that are set are achievable (Mullen, 2015). For example, the best intentions of creating lifestyle changes are often thwarted by setting goals that are almost impossible to achieve. Learning activity is included in Box (**6.6**) where you are asked to create a self-inventory to assess work-life balance. If you are a student nurse, you may still find the exercise to be somewhat useful. Just substitute the word *"work"* with *"school."*

Box 6.6. Learning activity: creating a self-inventory to assess work-life balance (as adapted from Mullen, 2015, p. 97).

1-List role models who have an acceptable balance between demands at home and work. What can you learn from them?
2-What is stopping you from the happiness you deserve in your life at work and at home? What is one thing you think you can change?

(Box 6.6) cont.....

3-Reflect on the events of today and describe how you dealt with the stress you experienced. What did you do well and what could you do differently?
4-Name one of the smallest things on your list that, if it were done, would feel like a weight had been lifted from you. How about another small thing? Can you name three small things that are waiting for you to address? What would it be like to tackle them one at a time?
5-Your situation is unique, but others share similar experiences of feeling stressed. Who might you turn to for support to begin to apply the self-kindness that change requires?
6-How do you experience stress in your mind/body/spirit? What is one small healthy intervention that you can implement to help you to alleviate that stress?

Administrative Measures that Contribute to Work-life Balance

The full onus for increasing work-life balance must not only rest with the individual nurse but should ideally include measures that improve work-organizational culture. Varma *et al.*, (2016) developed a model that can be adopted to promote work-life balance at the administrative level. The first idea addresses work-related stressors like replacing inadequate equipment and ensuring safety; reducing high patient loads; encouraging nurses to take designated breaks; and allowing for some flexibility in scheduling. The second focus ensures that nurses have adequate support systems in place from family, co-workers, and management to buffer them from work-related duress. A third approach is to provide training to help nurses deal more effectively with the emotionally draining aspects of their job, to improve their well-being, and to better manage potential stressors before they get worse. Mindfulness, yoga, and psychosocial interventions are three suggested strategies (Varma *et al.*, 2016). A fourth recommendation made by Mullen (2015) is for management to create in-service educational sessions to improve staff's ability to cope with hospital-based situations involving patient loss and suffering such as serious illness, death, dying, child abuse, and other forms of violence and trauma. A fifth suggestion is for confidential counselling to be made available through employee assistance programs (Mullen, 2015).

Aspects of a Critical Care Unit (CCU) Environment That Promotes Compassion Satisfaction

Key aspects of the work environment that have the greatest impact on the well-being of nurses working in a critical care unit (CCU) consist of adequate staffing, meaningful recognition, and effective decision-making (Kelly *et al.*, 2021, p. 118). Staffing levels matter in CCU because nurses find their work to be more enriching if their workload enables them to properly care for high-acuity patients. For example, insufficient staff working on critical care leads to high levels of burnout, whereas appropriate staffing that adequately addresses the needs of patients is associated with increased compassion satisfaction. Meaningful recognition and collegial support in an intensely stressful environment also contribute to nurses feeling appreciated and finding what they do to be more enjoyable. Effective and cooperative decision-making increases nurses' job satisfaction especially if the perspectives of key stakeholders such as interdisciplinary health professionals, the patient, and their families are considered in the process (Kelly *et al.*, 2021).

Student Nurses as Healers

"To be an effective healer you must always work on your own healing, physical, emotional, spiritual." Donna Cardillo, RN.

Student nurses with a history of trauma can experience compassion satisfaction if they are able to identify with some of the positive aspects associated with being a trauma survivor. For example, Goddard *et al.*, (2021) stress the importance of teaching them that although they may refer to themselves as the walking wounded, they are healers who have learned a great deal about surviving trauma, becoming resilient, empathetic, and compassionate. All these skills are extremely beneficial when caring for clients/patients and their families. Student nurses may also benefit from being reminded that the sense of fulfillment and meaning that they feel from helping to relieve the suffering of others is what will keep them in the profession in the long term. However, they must ensure that they stay well by prioritizing their own well-being through self-care, self-compassion, gratitude, and reaching out for support when required.

New Graduates & The Importance of Feeling Appreciated

Many new nurse graduates feel excessive pressure to do a good job but also experience increased stress and performance anxiety because they do not always feel ready to adequately meet the demands placed upon them (Phillips *et al.*, 2015). However, if new nurses are adequately supported by their employers through the transition process to acquire the knowledge and skills to succeed, they experience less stress, and increased fulfillment in their job. Specific actions that help include formal orientation, explicit clarity of role expectations, and acceptance and recognition from senior nurses (Phillips *et al.*, 2015). For new nurses who are employed in high acuity units, appreciation and meaningful recognition from supervisors is an additional beneficial factor known to offset some of the risks of developing empathy-based stress conditions (Kelly *et al.*, 2015). However, decreased job satisfaction and feeling unappreciated are known to have the opposite effect and even contribute to new nurses leaving the profession (Phillips *et al.*, 2015; Tucker *et al.*, 2014). Subsequently, the following

Narrative Case Study tells the story of how a new nurse considers leaving his job because he no longer feels supported or valued by management. Refer to Box (**6.7**).

Box 6.7. Narrative case study two: a new nurse contemplates to leave his career because of a lack of appreciation.

Austin is a 24-year-old registered nurse who has been working in his dream job for almost a year now. Austin graduated from nursing school at the top of his class and had wanted to be a nurse since he was six years old. His desire to become a nurse stemmed from his own experience with a serious illness at the age of five where he was hospitalized for almost six months. He admired the caring nurses who made his hospital stay bearable. Following completion of his basic nursing training, Austin specialized in a Pediatric Intensive Care Unit (ICU) because he wanted to make a difference in Leaving of the most ill children. At first, Austin loved what he did. He felt challenged by the work but more importantly he felt like he was making a difference in the lives of the children he cared for and their families. In fact, other than his competent intensive care skills, Austin believed that his biggest asset was his capacity to be empathetic.
However, in the past two months, Austin has become dissatisfied with his job. At first, he attributed his discontent to the fact that he cared for sick children, but after a great deal of soul searching and discussing his feelings extensively with a therapist, he realized that the impetus for his dismay with work was also strongly related to a feeling of not being appreciated by his Managers and Administration. In the past few months, he and his ICU nursing colleagues have had to work harder and be required to do excessive overtime, with less staff, due to budget issues and staffing shortages. Even though the nurses on this unit did their best to provide good care often under dire circumstances, most of them never got any sort of recognition or praise from their supervisors. In fact, they were often scolded for not doing enough. Austin decided he didn't want to work like this anymore. Last weekend he informed his parents that he thinks he picked the wrong career and was seriously thinking of leaving the nursing profession and doing something else.

NARRATIVE CASE STUDY TWO: IDENTIFICATION OF THEMES & ANALYSIS

Two key themes were identified from this story.

Theme # 1: Austin was contemplating leaving the profession that he loved after only working as a nurse for less than a year, because he was overworked and did not feel appreciated by his supervisors.

Theme # 1 Analysis: Evidence indicates that one in five nurses leave the profession in the first year of their practice, and an unsupportive work environment influences their willingness to leave the profession (Kelly *et al.*, 2015; Tucker *et al.*, 2014). The reasons given for leaving nursing are a lack of support from managers, uncooperative relationships with nursing colleagues, and a healthcare administration that puts business above personnel and refuses to prioritize job dissatisfaction (Tucker *et al.*, 2014).

Theme # 2: Meaningful recognition of a job well done can ward off compassion fatigue and foster compassion satisfaction in nurses.

Theme # 2 Analysis: Research evidence indicates that meaningful recognition and an increased feeling of being valued for the work that nurses do can lead to compassion satisfaction. Additional strategies to prevent empathy-based stress conditions and that encourage compassion satisfaction include educational efforts that warn nurses about problematic condition associated with their work, formal debriefing, and promoting self-care. Self-awareness was also deemed important so nurses could recognize when they needed help (Kelly *et al.*, 2015). In fact, creating and implementing a self-care plan and implementing it have been known to help nurses become more resilient and improved their ability to provide compassionate care to their clients/patients (Mongoulia *et al.*, 2015).

QUESTIONS FOR FURTHER DISCUSSION

1-In addition to what has already been suggested what else do you think would help a nurse to feel more appreciated in the work that they do?

2-In your opinion, what can be done to help keep new nurses in the profession?

JOY IN WORK

"The only way to do great work is to love what you do." Steve Jobs, American Businessman & Cofounder of Apple Computer Inc.

Joy in work is all about loving what you do and consists of components in the work environment that contribute to a happy, highly industrious, and enthusiastic workforce (Perlo *et al.*, 2017) (Fig. **6.4**). Subsequently, in order to create a joyful work environment necessitates more effort than merely adopting strategies that reduce the risk of staff developing empathy-based stress conditions. It requires a hands-on strategy that begins by making staff feel supported and appreciated (Jalilianhasanpour *et al.*, 2021). We will now proceed with a brief explanation as to why a joyful workplace matters followed by an examination of components that contribute to joy in work. However, to avoid unnecessary repetition of information that overlaps with what has already been discussed, the ensuing dialogue will be limited to these specific topics, shared responsibility; the importance of interpersonal connection; the role of participatory and servant leadership; and making use of psychological personal protective equipment (PPE).

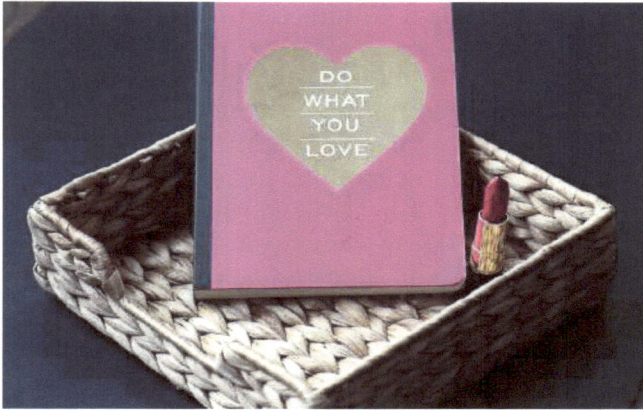

Fig. (6.4). Do What You Love and Love What You Do. Source: www.pixabay.com.

Reasons Why Creating a Joyful Workplace Matters

There are many valuable explanations for providing a work atmosphere that improves joy in work. It creates a safe environment, where respect, support, and autonomy are prioritized, and increases employee commitment, improves patient outcomes, and benefits the organization (Perlo *et al.*, 2017). For example, engaged employees are more inclined to view the organization that they work in a positive light, which ultimately leads to heightened performance (Joy & Sinosh, 2016). Employees who are fully engaged in what they do, experience enhanced psychological well-being, and a sense of purpose. Compassion, empathetic care, and the dedication that nurses feel about their work can also add to the effectiveness of a healthcare setting, and results in higher levels of patient satisfaction (Perlo *et al.*, 2017; Sallas-Vallina *et al.*, 2017).

Creating a Joyful Workplace is a Shared Responsibility

Management should never bear the sole burden of making the workplace happy because it is a shared responsibility. Every individual can intentionally choose to be supportive of others, and role model respect, civility, and inclusivity. They can commit to doing their best work, be fully aware of their role in making things better, and be accountable for their well-being (Perlo *et al.*, 2017). Furthermore, employees can also choose to intentionally contribute to optimism in their workplace by adopting an attitude of gratitude, appreciation, humor, hope, and celebration of achievement. The role of humor, planning fun activities, and other community events outside of work are also beneficial for improving joy (Jalilianhasanpour *et al.*, 2021).

The Importance of Interpersonal Connection

We spend a great deal of our waking life at work and therefore meaningful connection to colleagues is important, and there are many benefits of forming strong collegial relationships with co-workers. Having friends at work makes people more invested in their occupation. Interpersonal caring helps staff feel connected and happy with what they do, and increases productivity (Jalilianhasanpour *et al.*, 2021). However, satisfying interpersonal work relationships do not just happen, they have to be nurtured, and teamwork, cooperation, and a sense of camaraderie are ideal goals. Subsequently, a unified collaborative social working environment is best cultivated through mutual trust, understanding, support, fellowship, and companionship. Strong interpersonal bonds between healthcare professionals also involve a commitment to support each other. For example, when we are struggling it is comforting not to be afraid to reach out to the people we work with for assistance and advice, knowing that they have our best interests at heart. Sometimes we also all need other people to tell us that we are doing a good job (Perlo *et al.*, 2017).

The Role of Leadership

"True leadership, whether personal or corporate, makes a positive difference." Azim Jamal, Author.

Nursing leaders do not have an easy job. They face many expectations and a variety of complex responsibilities. They have to supervise and manage their employees, deal with staffing shortages, address client/patient and families' issues, and attend to the day-to-day problems and stressors associated with healthcare delivery (Chunta, 2020). They also have the added responsibility of creating an environment that fosters joy in work. Leadership style matters and strong supportive supervisors who are fair and respectful actually contribute to employee commitment and job satisfaction (Varma *et al.*, 2016). Two specific forms of governance that promote joy in work are participatory leadership and servant leadership.

Participatory Leadership

A **participatory leadership** style is cooperative in approach, transparent, and builds consensus. It is an environment that honors voice and choice, where people feel that they have some say in how to conduct their duties, as well as the freedom to speak up about their concerns without fear of reprimand. In participatory leadership people who are in charge listen to understand and seek input from staff into big decisions that may affect them directly or impact the quality of patient care (Perlo *et al.*, 2017). Subsequently, this form of shared governance involves three key steps, engage, inform, and listen. Engaging personnel before acting allows for input and buy-in before major changes are implemented. Informing staff keeps them appraised of any decisions that may directly affect them. Listening entails encouraging open dialogue and discourse so employees can communicate their ideas, and also consider the views and perspectives of people working at different levels in the establishment (Perlo *et al.*, 2017).

Servant Leadership

Servant leadership has also been proposed as a way to establish a work atmosphere that promotes the mental wellness of employees and contributes to their joy (Jalilianhasanpour *et al.*, 2021). **Servant leadership** is an altruistic stewardship and caring style of leadership that invests in followers' professional and personal development and well-being (Eva *et al.*, 2019). According to Sherman (2019), it is a leadership philosophy that leads to employee engagement because staff believe that their leader really does care about them. In Box (**6.8**) ten critical aspects of servant leadership are described. A Learning Activity is included for you to discuss ways that each of these attributes can be operationalized in practice.

Box 6.8. Learning activity: applying the ten characteristics of servant leadership (as adapted from Sherman, 2019, p. 86).

As a class or in small groups discuss specific ways that each of Sherman's (2019) characteristics of servant leadership can be applied in practice. When feasible give actual examples.
1-**Listening:** the servant leader actively listens to the needs of staff and assists them in decision making.
2-**Empathy:** the servant leader seeks first to understand and then empathize with the needs of others.
3-**Healing:** the servant leader helps staff to resolve their problems, negotiates to resolve conflict, and encourages a healing environment.
4-**Awareness:** the servant leader has a high degree of emotional intelligence and self-awareness. They view the situation from a holistic and systems perspective.
5-**Persuasion:** the servant leader does not use coercive power to influence but instead uses their powers of persuasion.
6-**Concepulization:** the servant leader sees beyond the day-to-day operations of their unit or department. They can focus on the bigger picture and build a personal vision.
7-**Foresight:** the servant leader can envision the likely outcome of a situation and is proactive in attempts to create the best consequences.
8-**Stewardship:** the servant leader is a good steward of the resources and staff that they are given. They feel an obligation to help and serve others without focusing on their own rewards.
9-**Commitment to the growth of people:** the servant leader is inclusive of all staff and sees value in everyone. They attempt to maximize the strengths of all who work with them.

(Box 6.8) cont.....
10-**Building community:** the servant leader recognizes the importance of building a sense of community among staff.
Making Use of Psychological Personal Protective Equipment (PPE)

The COVID-19 pandemic saw nurses and other health professionals having to wear physical protective gear to ensure that they did not contract the virus while caring for those who were infected. Although physical safety was the initial priority, there was significant evidence to indicate that health professionals also needed actions that would protect their psychological well-being. For example, working excessively long hours and overtime while wearing protective garments and N95 masks, and constantly dealing with human suffering and death, created mental distress for many healthcare workers, especially nurses (Spoorthy *et al.*, 2020). Subsequently, after an extensive review of the literature, the Institute for Healthcare Improvement (IHI) (2020) came up with ways to protect employees psychologically by developing **psychological personal protective equipment (PPE).** PPE consists of individual and system-wide measures that support and safeguard the mental health of employees. These strategies are designed to be applied before and after work. Although they were designed for COVID-19, most of the suggested ideas may still be useful today as a way to prevent emotional duress related to other challenging circumstances. Box (**6.9**) lists individual and team leader actions.

Box 6.9. Psychological PPE (as adapted from IHI, 2020).

Individual Measures
1-Take a day off to create space between work and home life
2-Avoid publicity and negative media coverage
3-Receive mental health support during and after a crisis
4-Facilitate opportunities to show gratitude
5-Reframe negative experiences as positive and reclaim agency
Team Leader Measures
1-Limit staff time on site/shift
2-Design clear roles and leadership
3-Make peer support services available to staff
4-Pair workers together to serve as peer support in a "buddy system"

SELF-CARE STRATEGY: SPECIFIC WAYS FOR COLLEGE STUDENTS TO INCREASE THEIR SELF-CONFIDENCE

"Have the self-confidence to trust that you know what's best for you." Author Unknown.

Self-confidence consists of the self-assurance in your inherent abilities to acquire personal and professional ambitions and goals (Psychology Dictionary, n.d.). It is an important trait for students of higher education to possess. For instance, someone who is self-confident is more likely to succeed with the completion of their academic goals because they possess the courage and poise to persevere when faced with obstacles. Therefore, three specific methods are recommended to enhance personal self-confidence. Refer to Box (**6.10**).

Box 6.10. Three methods to increase self-confidence (as adapted from arizona state university (ASU), 2021; Brooks & Goldstein, 2003).

1- Adopt a Holistic Approach to Self-Confidence
Choose to be stress hardy rather than stressed out. Prioritizing your health and well-being will enable you to develop the physical and mental fortitude to be better equipped to persevere with your academic studies when issues arise.
Develop self-control. Allow yourself to feel your emotions when they arise and choose to manage your feelings so that they do not rule your behavior.
Learn something new every day. Whenever you challenge yourself to learn something new you keep your brain sharp, and you get excited about the variety of opportunities that may await you.
Build Connections with Others. Make relationships with others a priority in your life and learn how to nurture them. Life is meant to be shared with other people.
2- Overcome Your Self-doubt
Setbacks happen. When things do not turn out the way you expected them to, do not allow negative self-talk to take over. Sometimes setbacks provide you with a learning opportunity to try something new. Be a problem solver. Select a new strategy with the greatest probability for success and plan for how to carry it out.
3- Participate in The Following Confidence-Building Activities
Get enough Sleep. It will help you stay well and focus on your studies. Go to bed at the same time every evening and try to get 8-9 hours of rest. Put your phone far away from your bedroom. Avoid using technology just before bedtime.
Make Nutrition a Priority. What you eat matters to your overall health physically and mentally so do your best to eat wholesome and nutritious food.
Get Moving. Get some regular physical exercise every day. Walking and taking the stairs is a good place to start.
Set Goals. Setting clear goals and a way to achieve them makes it more likely that you will succeed. Therefore, make sure that your goals are specific, attainable, relevant, and time bound.

(Box 6.10) cont.....

Practice Mindfulness. Mindfulness is about paying attention to the present moment and being open to everything that life has to offer you. It will also enhance your ability to focus on your studies and be more thankful.

Note: Any suggested strategies are not intended to be a substitute for medical or psychological advice from a trained professional. The reader is therefore encouraged to seek medical or other professional help in any matters related to their physical or emotional health.

CONCLUSION

- In Chapter Six, trauma-informed nursing education approaches were recommended to ensure that students feel safe and supported in an ideal learning environment. Subsequently, educational processes that promote psychological safety were recommended followed by measures to foster compassion satisfaction, and joy in work.
- Compassion satisfaction is derived from the gratification experienced by caregivers from doing a good job of caring for others, and joy in work consists of positive components in the work environment.
- Psychological safety creates a positive, civil, and respectful atmosphere for learning to occur without fear of retaliation. It is closely aligned with trauma-informed educational processes because they both have the goal of ensuring that the learning environment is safe.
- Psychological trauma occurs because of exposure to an adverse event that is experienced by the person as harmful and has lasting negative effects on their well-being.
- Nursing students are a risk group for trauma. They specifically identified the following sources as traumatizing, individual-related interpersonal experiences; those related to their role as nursing students; trauma from institutional and organizational exposure; and stressors associated with the community.
- *The Four Core Assumptions of Trauma-informed Care* were used as a guide to implementing psychological safety in nursing school. *Realize* stands for awareness that trauma is prevalent in nursing students and that educators must be sensitive to this fact. *Recognition* is about being able to identify the signs and symptoms of trauma in nursing students. *Responding* consists of using caring teaching strategies with students. *Resisting re-traumatization* of students is essential because persons who have a history of trauma can be re-traumatized.
- Specific measures that promote psychological safety were recommended to be used in classroom, simulation, and clinical settings. Strategies directly related to high-fidelity simulation include actions to make students feel safe before, during, and after the session. They include a pre-brief to state outcomes, supporting students during the session to take risks and make mistakes without

negative consequences; warning them that the content may be disturbing; re-emphasizing confidentiality; and de-briefing them without any fear of retaliation.

- We learned that there are distinct positive feelings associated with compassion satisfaction such as well-being, fulfillment, reward, accomplishment, joy, enrichment, invigoration, inspiration, revitalization, gratitude, and hope.

- The following six core assumptions of compassion satisfaction were presented. The first involves the nurse's desire to create caring relationships with the people they are caring for. The second concerns the satisfaction derived from being able to meet their needs. The third supposition is that working in a positive environment is necessary and the fourth involves experiencing an empathetic connection with clients/patients. A fifth postulation includes the nurse's ability to create a balance between concern for another's suffering, and the compassionate energy felt for them. The sixth asserts that positive aspects related to caring must be fully experienced by the nurse for compassion satisfaction to occur.

- We learned that self-compassion and work-life balance are important aspects of compassion satisfaction.

- Key aspects of the work environment that have the greatest impact on the well-being of nurses working in critical care were identified as adequate staffing, meaningful recognition, and effective decision-making.

- Student nurses with a history of trauma can experience compassion satisfaction if they are able to identify with some of the positive aspects associated with being a trauma-survivor.

- If new nurses are adequately supported by their employers through the transition process to acquire the knowledge and skills to succeed, they experience less stress, and increased fulfillment in their job.

- We were made aware of the many valuable explanations for providing a work atmosphere that improves joy in work. Key essential reasons include the fact that a focus on joy enhances the work experience, increases employee engagement and work performance, benefits the organization, and improves patient outcomes.

- Making the workplace happy is a shared responsibility, where everyone is expected to do their best work, be fully aware of their role in making things better, and be accountable for their wellbeing.

- We spend a great deal of our waking life at work and therefore meaningful connection to other people is important where teamwork, cooperation, and a sense of camaraderie is ideal.

- Two specific forms of governance that promote joy in work are participatory leadership and servant leadership.

- Psychological personal protective equipment (PPE) consists of individual and system-wide measures that support and safeguard the mental health of employees.

- Two Narrative Case Studies were presented. In the first one, a student nurse becomes re-traumatized in class when listening to details of an uncensored story of someone's traumatic experience. This could have been prevented if the speaker had been informed of the rule of not discussing any details of her trauma. Furthermore, the instructor was not sufficiently trained in trauma-informed care and was therefore unaware of how to prevent re-traumatization.

- The Second Narrative Case Study revealed how a new nurse considered leaving his high-acuity job and the profession of nursing because of a lack of support and appreciation. We learned that meaningful recognition of a job well done can ward off compassion fatigue and foster compassion satisfaction in nurses.

- Five learning activities were recommended (*e.g.*, Exploring Assumptions About Constructive Feedback; Ways to Express Appreciation in a Professional Manner; Understanding How You Handle Mistakes; Creating a Self-Inventory to Assess Work-life Balance; and Incorporating the Ten Characteristics of Servant Leadership into Practice).

- At the end of the Chapter specific strategies were recommended to build college students' self-confidence.

CONCLUDING REMARKS TO THE BOOK

Today's nurse educators are challenged with educating students that may have been traumatized or are presently exposed to human suffering while training in a healthcare field that is riddled with adverse situations. This may leave instructors in peril but also is a call to action to implement trauma-informed care into a nursing curriculum that may lead to many positive outcomes (Goddard *et al.*, 2021). In the short term, students feel supported, more motivated to learn and happier with their learning experience. In the long-term they are more likely to stay in their program, graduate, and remain as practitioners in the field of nursing for a longer period of time (Goddard *et al.*, 2021). The investment in trauma-informed education is also important because these student nurses are our future caregivers, and we will need to do our best to ensure that they acquire the necessary skills and support to be resilient, stay physically and mentally well, and find meaning and joy in their work.

RECOMMENDED READINGS

Bernock, D. (2014). Emerging wings: A true story of lies, pain, and the love that heals. 4F Media.

Hallis, T. (2017). Sharpen your positive edge: Shifting your thoughts for more positivity & success. The Positive Edge, LLC.

Jamal, A., & McKinnon, H. (2008). The power of giving. Penguin Group.

Maté, G. (2022). The myth of normal: Trauma, illness, and healing in a toxic culture. Avery, Penguin Random House.

Stutz, P., & Michels, B. (2013). The tools: 5 tools to help you find courage, creativity, and willpower - and inspire you to live in forward motion. Random House.

REFERENCES

Altmiller, G (2016) Strategies for providing constructive feedback to students. *Nurse Educ,* 41, 118-9.
[http://dx.doi.org/10.1097/NNE.0000000000000227] [PMID: 26418835]

Altmiller, G, Deal, B, Ebersole, N, Flexner, R, Jordan, J, Jowell, V, Norris, T, Risetter, MJ, Schuler, M, Szymanski, K, Vottero, B & Walker, D (2018) Constructive feedback teaching strategy: A multisite study of its effectiveness. *Nurs Educ Perspect,* 39, 291-6.
[http://dx.doi.org/10.1097/01.NEP.0000000000000385] [PMID: 30096111]

Arizona State University (ASU) (2021) *Three ways college students can build self-confidence.* https:// asuonline. asu.edu/ newsroom /online-learning -tips/3-ways- college- students- build-self- confidence/

Beaumont, E, Durkin, M, Hollins Martin, CJ & Carson, J (2016) Compassion for others, self-compassion, quality of life and mental well-being measures and their association with compassion fatigue and burnout in student midwives: A quantitative survey. *Midwifery,* 34, 239-44.
[http://dx.doi.org/10.1016/j.midw.2015.11.002] [PMID: 26628352]

Bosse, JD, Clark, KD & Arnold, S (2021) Implementing trauma-informed educational practices in undergraduate mental health nursing education. *J Nurs Educ,* 60, 707-11.
[http://dx.doi.org/10.3928/01484834-20211103-02] [PMID: 34870506]

Brooks, R & Goldstein, S (2003) *The power of resilience: Achieving balance, confidence, and personal strength in your life.* McGraw Hill.

Cheung, EO, Hernandez, A, Herold, E & Moskowitz, JT (2020) Positive emotion skills intervention to address burnout and in critical care nurses. *AACN Adv Crit Care,* 31, 167-78.
[http://dx.doi.org/10.4037/aacnacc2020287] [PMID: 32526000]

Chunta, KS (2020) New nurse leaders: Creating a work-life balance and finding joy in work. *J Radiol Nurs,* 39, 86-8.
[http://dx.doi.org/10.1016/j.jradnu.2019.12.007]

Cori, JL (2008) *Healing for trauma: A survivors guide to understanding your signs and symptoms and reclaiming your life.* Marlow & Company.

Delaney, MC (2018) Caring for the caregivers: Evaluation of the effect of an eight-week pilot mindful self-compassion (MSC) training program on nurses' compassion fatigue and resilience. *PLoS One,* 13, e0207261.
[http://dx.doi.org/10.1371/journal.pone.0207261] [PMID: 30462717]

Duffy, JR (2018) *Quality caring in nursing and health systems: Implications for clinicians, educators, and leaders.* Springer Publishing Company.
[http://dx.doi.org/10.1891/9780826181251]

Dunn, DJ & Rivas, D (2014) Transforming compassion satisfaction. *Int J Hum Caring,* 18, 45-50.
[http://dx.doi.org/10.20467/1091-5710.18.1.45]

Duarte, J, Pinto-Gouveia, J & Cruz, B (2016) Relationships between nurses' empathy, self-compassion and dimensions of professional quality of life: A cross-sectional study. *Int J Nurs Stud,* 60, 1-11.
[http://dx.doi.org/10.1016/j.ijnurstu.2016.02.015] [PMID: 27297364]

Eva, N, Robin, M, Sendjaya, S, van Dierendonck, D & Liden, RC (2019) Servant Leadership: A systematic review and call for future research. *Leadersh Q,* 30, 111-32.
[http://dx.doi.org/10.1016/j.leaqua.2018.07.004]

Fey, MK, Scrandis, D, Daniels, A & Haut, C (2014) Learning through debriefing: Students' perspectives. *Clin Simul Nurs,* 10, e249-56.
[http://dx.doi.org/10.1016/j.ecns.2013.12.009]

Fifer, P (2019) Associate degree nursing students' perceptions of instructor caring. *Teach Learn Nurs,* 14, 103-10.
[http://dx.doi.org/10.1016/j.teln.2018.12.006]

Foli, K & Thompson, JR (2019) *The influence of psychological trauma in nursing.* Sigma Theta Tau International.

Fowler, K & Wholeben, M (2020) COVID-19: Outcomes for trauma-impacted nurses and nursing students. *Nurse Educ Today,* 93, 104525.
[http://dx.doi.org/10.1016/j.nedt.2020.104525]

Goddard, A, Jones, RW, Esposito, D & Janicek, E (2021) Trauma informed education in nursing: A call for action. *Nurse Educ Today,* 101, 104880.
[http://dx.doi.org/10.1016/j.nedt.2021.104880] [PMID: 33798984]

Henderson, D, Sewell, KA & Wei, H (2020) The impacts of faculty caring on nursing students' intent to graduate: A systematic literature review. *Int J Nurs Sci,* 7, 105-11.
[http://dx.doi.org/10.1016/j.ijnss.2019.12.009] [PMID: 32099867]

Hinderer, K A (2014) compassion fatigue, compassion satisfaction, and secondary traumatic stress in trauma nurses. *J Trauma Nurs,* 21, 160-9.
[http://dx.doi.org/10.1097/JTN.0000000000000055]

Ignacio, J, Dolmans, D, Scherpbier, A, Rethans, JJ, Chan, S & Liaw, SY (2015) Comparison of standardized patients with high-fidelity simulators for managing stress and improving performance in clinical deterioration: A mixed methods study. *Nurse Educ Today,* 35, 1161-8.
[http://dx.doi.org/10.1016/j.nedt.2015.05.009] [PMID: 26047602]

Institute for Healthcare Improvement (IHI) (2020) *Psychological PPE: Promote health care workforce mental health and well-being.* Available from: https://www.ihi.org/resources/Pages/Tools/psychological-PPE-promote-health-care-workforce-mental-health-and-well-being.aspx

Institute for Healthcare Improvement (IHI) (2023) *Joy in work and workforce well-being.* Available from: https://www.ihi.org/Topics/Joy-Work/Pages/default.aspx

Jalilianhasanpour, R, Asadollahi, S & Yousem, DM (2021) Creating joy in the workplace. *Eur J Radiol,* 145, 110019.
[http://dx.doi.org/10.1016/j.ejrad.2021.110019] [PMID: 34798537]

Jenkins, E, Slemon, A, Bilsker, D & Goldner, EM (2022) *A concise introduction to mental health in Canada.* Canadian Scholars.

Joy, MM & Sinosh, PK (2016) Employee engagement in an empirical study on implications for psychological well being. *Int J Manag,* 7, 183-7.

Kelly, L, Runge, J & Spencer, C (2015) Predictors of compassion fatigue and compassion satisfaction in acute care nurses. *J Nurs Scholarsh,* 47, 522-8.
[http://dx.doi.org/10.1111/jnu.12162] [PMID: 26287741]

Kelly, LA, Johnson, KL, Bay, RC & Todd, M (2021) Key elements of the critical care work environment associated with burnout and compassion satisfaction. *Am J Crit Care,* 30, 113-20.

[http://dx.doi.org/10.4037/ajcc2021775] [PMID: 33644798]

Kerig, PK (2019) Enhancing resilience among providers of trauma-informed care: A curriculum for protection against secondary traumatic stress among non-mental health professionals. *J Aggress Maltreat Trauma,* 28, 613-30.
[http://dx.doi.org/10.1080/10926771.2018.1468373]

Kolbe, M, Eppich, W, Rudolph, J, Meguerdichian, M, Catena, H, Cripps, A, Grant, V & Cheng, A (2020) Managing psychological safety in debriefings: A dynamic balancing act. *BMJ Simul Technol Enhanc Learn,* 6, 164-71.
[http://dx.doi.org/10.1136/bmjstel-2019-000470] [PMID: 35518370]

Laskowski-Jones, L (2018) Giving constructive feedback-constructively. *Nursing,* 48, 6.
[http://dx.doi.org/10.1097/01.NURSE.0000545027.50545.9f] [PMID: 29757866]

Lavoie, P & Clarke, SP (2017) Simulation in nursing education. *Nursing,* 47, 18-20.
[http://dx.doi.org/10.1097/01.NURSE.0000520520.99696.9a] [PMID: 28640045]

O'donovan, R & Mcauliffe, E (2020) A systematic review of factors that enable psychological safety in healthcare teams. *Int J Qual Health Care,* 32, 240-50.
[http://dx.doi.org/10.1093/intqhc/mzaa025] [PMID: 32232323]

Omer, AA & Abdularhim, M (2017) The criteria of constructive feedback: The feedback that counts. *Journal of Health Specialties,* 5, 45.
[http://dx.doi.org/10.4103/2468-6360.198798]

Mangoulia, P, Koukia, E, Alevizopoulos, G, Fildissis, G & Katostaras, T (2015) Prevalence of secondary traumatic stress among psychiatric nurses in Greece. *Arch Psychiatr Nurs,* 29, 333-8.
[http://dx.doi.org/10.1016/j.apnu.2015.06.001] [PMID: 26397438]

Mayer, KA, Linehan, KJ & MacMillan, NK (2022) Student perspectives on potential sources of trauma exposure during nursing school. *Nurs Forum,* 57, 833-42.
[http://dx.doi.org/10.1111/nuf.12728] [PMID: 35485449]

Mullen, K (2015) Barriers to work-life balance for hospital nurses. *Workplace Health Saf,* 63, 96-9.
[http://dx.doi.org/10.1177/2165079914565355] [PMID: 25994973]

Nielsen, B & Harder, N (2013) Causes of student anxiety during simulation: What the literature says. *Clin Simul Nurs,* 9, e507-12.
[http://dx.doi.org/10.1016/j.ecns.2013.03.003]

Perlo, J, Balik, B, Swensen, S, Kabeenell, A, Landsman, J & Feeley, D (2017) Available from: https://www.ihi.org

Pfeiffer, K & Grabbe, L (2022) An approach to trauma-informed education in prelicensure nursing curricula. *Nurs Forum,* 57, 658-64.
[http://dx.doi.org/10.1111/nuf.12726]

Phillips, C, Esterman, A & Kenny, A (2015) The theory of organisational socialisation and its potential for improving transition experiences for new graduate nurses. *Nurse Educ Today,* 35, 118-24.
[http://dx.doi.org/10.1016/j.nedt.2014.07.011] [PMID: 25149106]

Psychology Dictionary. Available from: https://psychologydictionary.org/self-confidence/

Radey, M & Figley, CR (2007) The social psychology of compassion. *Clin Soc Work J,* 35, 207-14.
[http://dx.doi.org/10.1007/s10615-007-0087-3]

Dunn, DJ & Rivas, D (2014) Transforming compassion satisfaction. *Int J Hum Caring,* 18, 45-50.
[http://dx.doi.org/10.20467/1091-5710.18.1.45]

Rosenberg, MB (2003) *Nonviolent communication: A language of life.* Puddle Dancer Press.

Rudolph, JW, Raemer, DB & Simon, R (2014) Establishing a safe container for learning in simulation: The role of the presimulation briefing. *Simul Healthc,* 9, 339-49.

[http://dx.doi.org/10.1097/SIH.0000000000000047] [PMID: 25188485]

Sacco, TL, Ciurzynski, SM, Harvey, ME & Ingersoll, GL (2015) Compassion satisfaction and compassion fatigue among critical care nurses. *Crit Care Nurse,* 35, 32-42.
[http://dx.doi.org/10.4037/ccn2015392] [PMID: 26232800]

Sacco, TL & Copel, LC (2018) Compassion satisfaction: A concept analysis in nursing. *Nurs Forum,* 53, 76-83.
[http://dx.doi.org/10.1111/nuf.12213] [PMID: 28662300]

Salas-Vallina, A, López-Cabrales, Á, Alegre, J & Fernández, R (2017) On the road to happiness at work (HAW). *Person Rev,* 46, 314-38.
[http://dx.doi.org/10.1108/PR-06-2015-0186]

Salvarani, V, Ardenghi, S, Rampoldi, G, Bani, M, Cannata, P, Ausili, D, Di Mauro, S & Strepparava, MG (2020) Predictors of psychological distress amongst nursing students: A multicenter cross-sectional study. *Nurse Educ Pract,* 44, 102758.
[http://dx.doi.org/10.1016/j.nepr.2020.102758] [PMID: 32234667]

Sanderson, CD, Cox, K & Disch, J (2020) Virtual nursing, virtual learning. *Nurse Lead,* 18, 142-6.
[http://dx.doi.org/10.1016/j.mnl.2019.12.005]

Seligman, M (2011) *Flourish: A new understanding of happiness and well-being – and how to achieve them.* Nicholas Brealey Publishing.

Simmons, S (2012) Striving for work-life balance. *Nursing,* 42 (Suppl Career), 25-6.
[http://dx.doi.org/10.1097/01.NURSE.0000408207.06032.96] [PMID: 22157905]

Somerville, SG, Harrison, NM & Lewis, SA (2023) Twelve tips for the pre-brief to promote psychological safety in simulation-based education. *Med Teach,* 1-8.
[http://dx.doi.org/10.1080/0142159X.2023.2214305] [PMID: 37210674]

Spoorthy, MS, Pratapa, SK & Mahant, S (2020) Mental health problems faced by healthcare workers due to the COVID-19 pandemic–A review. *Asian J Psychiatr,* 51, 102119.
[http://dx.doi.org/10.1016/j.ajp.2020.102119] [PMID: 32339895]

Stephany, K (2020) *The ethic of care: A moral compass for Canadian Nursing practice.* Bentham Science Publishers Pte. Ltd.

Substance Abuse and Mental Health Services Administration (SAMHSA) (2014) Available from: http://store.samhsa.gov/shin/content//SMA14-4884/SMA14-4884.pdf

Substance Abuse and Mental Health Services Administration (2014) Available from: https://store.samhsa.gov/sites/default/files/d7/priv/sma14-4816.pdf

Thomas, MS, Crosby, S & Vanderhaar, J (2019) Trauma-informed practices in schools across two decades: An interdisciplinary review of research. *Rev Res Educ,* 43, 422-52.
[http://dx.doi.org/10.3102/0091732X18821123]

Tuckett, A, Winters-Chang, P, Bogossian, F & Wood, M (2015) 'Why nurses are leaving the profession … lack of support from managers': What nurses from an e☐cohort study said. *Int J Nurs Pract,* 21, 359-66.
[http://dx.doi.org/10.1111/ijn.12245] [PMID: 24571860]

Turner, S & Harder, N (2018) Psychological safe environment: A concept analysis. *Clin Simul Nurs,* 18, 47-55.
[http://dx.doi.org/10.1016/j.ecns.2018.02.004]

Varma, MM, Kelling, AS & Goswami, S (2016) Enhancing healthcare quality by promoting work-life balance among nursing staff. *J Hosp Adm,* 5, 58-62.
[http://dx.doi.org/10.5430/jha.v5n6p58]

Walker, LO & Avant, KC (2011) *Strategies for theory construction in nursing.* Springer.

Wedgeworth, M (2016) Anxiety and education: An examination of anxiety across a nursing program. *J Nurs*

Educ Pract, 6, 23-6.
[http://dx.doi.org/10.5430/jnep.v6n10p23]

Wheeler, K & Phillips, K E (2019) The development of trauma and resilience competencies for nursing education. *Journal of the American Psychiatric Association,* 1-12.
[http://dx.doi.org/10.1177/1078390319878779]

Wolf, ZR (2019) Wounded healers, second victims, caring environments. In: Wolf, Z.R., (Ed.), *Int J Hum Caring,* 23, 272-4.
[http://dx.doi.org/10.20467/1091-5710.23.4.272]

GLOSSARY

Accomplishment in well-being theory is the ability to use our strengths and gifts to achieve something that gives us deep satisfaction.

Acute stress disorder occurs when emotional reactions to a stressor linger over time and results in persistent post-traumatic disturbing symptoms that interfere with a person's everyday life.

Adverse childhood experiences (ACEs) refer to traumatic experiences that children are exposed to. Types of ACEs include abuse, neglect, household violence, caregiver mental illness or drug use, parental abandonment, parental death, and parental divorce or separation.

Advocacy can be on behalf of a cause or for an individual. At the personal level, it involves being the voice for a client/patient to address their needs, especially if they feel disempowered or too afraid to act on their own.

Appreciation involves recognizing or admiring someone's good qualities or noble actions.

Being cared for is described as living through suffering within a secure and trusting environment and being helped to live a fulfilling life more harmoniously.

Being present requires that we be fully absorbed in the other person and our desire for their well-being.

Bias consists of prejudice, stereotypes, and discriminatory behaviours.

Boundary violations happen when the actions between two people go against well-accepted social expectations.

Burnout is depicted by physical and mental exhaustion due to longstanding exposure to emotionally demanding and stressful working conditions.

Caring in nursing can be described as actions and motivation directed toward a person, for their protection, their overall welfare, and their enhancement of well-being in the physical, emotional, psychological, and spiritual realm.

Caring pedagogy uses caring components in nursing education to create a community of learning that is student-focused, inclusive, engaging, and prioritizes transpersonal caring relationships.

Caring practice consists of the nurse prioritizing the on being cared for, by seeking to understand what they need.

Caritas processes in nursing consist of ways to demonstrate sensitivity toward oneself and others by fostering spiritual practices that support loving, caring relationships.

Civility consists of polite, respectful, and courteous behaviours that are exhibited in all forms of communication.

Clear expectations in trauma-informed care consist of being honest and upfront about what the person can reasonably expect concerning all aspects of assessment and treatment.

Client-centered trauma-informed care puts the person who we are caring for, and their goals and hopes, at the centre of all that occurs.

Cognitive behavioral therapy (CBT) teaches a person to recognize negative beliefs, to challenge those ideas with the truth, and to think of themselves in a more positive way.

Coherence refers to making sense of one's life and the direction being taken.

Collaboration involves an unwritten contract between the caregiver and client that ensures the person's preferences are seriously considered in their plan of care.

Colonization refers to the way in which foreign nations invaded other nations, forced their values and ways of living on their people, accompanied by exploitation of resources, and other forms of harm.

Compassion is the ability to identify with the suffering of another person.

Compassion fatigue develops quite acutely when a caregiver becomes too emotionally involved with the suffering experienced by people in their care, results in caregiver emotional exhaustion, and interferes with their ability to act in empathetic ways to avoid further psychological trauma.

Compassion satisfaction refers to the positive feelings and gratification experienced by a caregiver from doing a good job of caring for others.

Confidentiality concerns protecting and safeguarding the privacy of a client/patient's history, care, and treatment.

Confirmation consists of acknowledging and inspiring the best in us and in everyone else.

Constructive feedback is a form of criticism with the goal of a positive outcome. It consists of an unbiased critique of performance and correcting any errors.

Creative visualization is a process where you use your mind's eye to imagine a scenario, with your eyes closed, with the general goal of assisting you to better manage your emotions or problems.

Critical incident debriefing is conducted by a trained professional after a traumatic event has occurred that is outside of normal human experience. It is used to help those who have been affected to sort through their feelings and other emotional stress.

Cultural awareness consists of the desire to want to understand the beliefs and values of people from differing cultures.

Cultural competence is a tool that assists health professionals in attaining the necessary skills to practice inclusivity when caring for diverse populations.

Cultural humility aims to offset power difficulties that occur through intentional actions of empowerment, excellence in care, and an atmosphere of inclusivity and mutual respect.

Cultural safety addresses power imbalances that exist in health care and aims to foster an environment that is free of all forms of discrimination.

Cultural sensitivity incorporates a person's cultural beliefs into practice.

Dementia as a general term is used to describe a person's impaired capacity to function in everyday life due to memory loss, impaired language skills, and being incapable of thinking clearly enough to problem solve.

Dialogue involves a dynamic exchange of opinions and ideas.

Dignity in practice consists of the recognition that everyone possesses intrinsic worth and value and should be treated with respect.

Education is described as "learning for its own sake," which means you participate because you want to, and not because you are required to.

Elder abuse consists of one or more acts or a lack of appropriate and helpful action, that causes harm or distress to an older adult, that may occur within any relationship where there is an expectation of trust.

Embracing diversity involves a willingness to accept ways of living and believing that may differ from your own.

Emotional appraisal is an emotional regulatory process that consists of restructuring of the meaning associated with a situation, to view its outcome more optimistically.

Emotional intelligence refers to the ability to be aware of our feelings and those experienced by other people.

Emotional strain refers to emotional exhaustion and related responses due to prolonged exposure to stressful situations that result in an inability to cope.

Emotional suppression is an emotional regulatory process that consists of avoidance of all displays of negative emotions.

Empathy is the ability to identify with all the experiences of another person and to understand what they have gone through.

Empathy-based stress is due to trauma exposure. It is accompanied by an affective reaction that causes a strain in empathetic capacity, where the caregiver is no longer able to identify with the experiences of another person.

Empowerment assists the individual in realizing that they have the skills, confidence, ability, and fortitude to make their own choices in life and to follow through with those choices.

Engagement in well-being theory is the ability to be fully engrossed in the activities of one's life.

Ethics of care is a special feature of nursing ethics that values relationships, context, meaning making, the interconnectedness of all of life, and the self-worth of every person. It does not tolerate discrimination and expects nurses to do what they can to end human suffering.

Existential reevaluation is an explanatory model of posttraumatic growth following adversity that consists of inner work, pursuing meaning, and being awakened to the precious aspect of life.

Flourishing is a term that describes how Positive Psychology can enhance a person's life by increasing happiness, improving relationships, increasing purpose, and assisting them in pursuing their dreams.

Flow is a term in Positive Psychology where you are so fully absorbed in an activity that you love that nothing else matters, and time stands still.

Gender identity refers to a person's individual description of their own personal experience of gender, and their gender identity may be the same or different than that assigned at birth.

Generativity is about investing in the well-being and future of members of the profession.

Gratitude is an action of being thankful and appreciative of people, situations, or things in your life.

Guilt consists of feeling bad after making a mistake, but it co-exists with a belief that because behavior is not a permanent part of one's personality, it can be altered or changed.

Heterosexuality refers to the feelings of a person toward others of the opposite sex and is only one of several designations associated with sexual orientation.

High-fidelity patient simulation (HFPS) in nursing utilizes human resembling manikins to create life-like simulations for learning.

Historical trauma affects the history of a specific group of people who have been oppressed and often contributes to systemic racism.

Hope consists of the belief that something better is possible and attainable in the future.

Human connection consists of the bonds that people develop with others that they value and esteem.

Humility consists of human character traits that are void of arrogance, which entails refusing to act with an attitude of superiority.

Implicit bias involves prejudicial attitudes and beliefs directed at a specific group of people.

Incivility is the direct opposite of civility and consists of disrespecting others through rudeness, condescending attitudes, and a refusal to consider views that differ from your own.

Indigenous is a word used to refer to people who consider themselves to be related to, or historically connected to, "First Peoples" whose civilizations predate a time before invasion or colonization by others.

Inherent bias is the assumption that the cause of something may or may not be based on actual fact but is presumed to be true.

Intimate partner violence (IPV) consists of violent sexual or physical acts inflicted by a person who has a relationship with the survivor, either currently or in the past.

Joy in work is comprised of positive components in the work environment that contribute to a content, highly productive, and vigorous workforce.

Kindness on purpose consists of actions that are thoughtful, caring, genuine, offer warmth and are respectful, and benevolent.

Knowledge competence is the ability to apply what one knows to the situations at hand. For nurses, it is about ensuring that our actions are evidence-based and align with best practices.

LGBTQ2S is an acronym that represents different sexual orientations or gender identities and stands for lesbian, gay, bisexual, transgender, queer, and two-spirited.

Logotherapy is a type of psychotherapy that focuses on the meaning of human life and man's search for meaning as a way to help people to heal from situations that were traumatic.

Meaning in well-being theory involves being of service to a cause or belonging to something that gives you purpose.

Meaning-making is the way in which a person makes sense of what has happened in their life, while also discovering and pursuing something that gives them purpose.

Meditation consists of exercises in the form of either uttering a mantra or using breathing to become calm, to shut out the outside world, and to sustain a heightened level of awareness.

Method in research refers to the actual way in which data is collected includes the sequencing, techniques, and strategies that were utilized.

Methodology in research refers to the approach used in the study to acquire, categorize, and analyze data.

Microaggressions consist of casual innuendos that may be intentional or unintentional, that are belittling, insulting, uncaring, or inconsiderate.

Mindfulness is a form of awareness that is increasingly being used to decrease personal suffering and cultivate personal growth.

Mindful self-compassion combines mindfulness and being fully present with self-compassion in the form of caring and loving thoughts directed at oneself.

Mutuality consists of clear lines of communication between the caregiver and the person seeking treatment.

Myth consists of a false assumption or belief that cannot necessarily be substantiated by fact.

Narratives are a form of phenomenology that consists of personal stories of actual life experiences as told by the people living through them.

Negative emotions are feelings that cause you to feel distressed or uncomfortable and may decrease life satisfaction. Fear, anger, disgust, and sadness are some common examples.

Neuroplasticity refers to the brain's intrinsic ability to change by developing new neural connections that are experience-based.

Ontology explores the nature of what is and focuses on gaining a better understanding of human beings and their journey.

Other-focused listening is more than ordinary listening. It requires us to be fully present, and to listen deeply and compassionately to what the other person is sharing.

Palliative care is an approach that aims to improve the quality of life of patients of all ages and their family members, while they are dealing with problems associated with a life-threatening illness.

Participatory leadership is cooperative in approach, transparent, and builds consensus.

Pedagogy refers to the process of teaching and includes specific designs, methods, and strategies that facilitate the acquisition of knowledge.

Peer support consists of the help and encouragement received from others who have lived through similar experiences.

People of color are used to describe groups of people who identify as 'non-white,' and the designation includes but is not limited to, Blacks, Latinos, Mexicans, Jamaicans, Chinese, Indigenous people, Asians, Southwest Asians, and Arabs.

Perception of reality is a specific stage of coping during post-traumatic growth that consists of self-deception by adopting unrealistic optimism and hope about what happened.

PERMA are the five original elements of Positive Psychology well-being theory that are comprised of positive emotion, engagement, relationships, meaning, and accomplishment.

PERMA+4 is a framework for work-related well-being in Positive Psychology that consists of these four additional elements, physical health, economic security, mindset, and environment.

Person-centered care that is trauma-focused provides services to people with acute and chronic health issues. Not unlike client-centered care it is built on the premise of putting the person at the center of all that occurs. It also involves a collaborative relationship between healthcare professional and recipient, and provides compassionate service.

Person-centered communication is a form of engagement that honors the person and their family's point of view, values their input, and seeks their active involvement in decisions related to their care.

Phenomenology is a theoretical perspective that emphasizes the very substance of human experiences as lived by humans.

Philosophy and Science of Caring as an adjunct to a material and physical ontological world, makes relational ontology its basis. It also reveres human connectedness to a source known as a universal essence.

Physical safety consists of an absence of harm or injury in one's environment.

Positive emotions in well-being theory contribute to life satisfaction and happiness and consist of the capacity to feel happy, and experience joy, love, and gratitude.

Positive Psychology involves the empirical study of what is good about humans and their capacity for strength, growth, and endurance.

Positive psychotherapy is a therapeutic approach derived from Positive Psychology that creates balance in therapy by focusing on a person's strengths and weaknesses, and by utilizing their strengths as the means to well-being.

Post-migration trauma consists of the hardships experienced by refugees and immigrants due to barriers to access to essential services.

Post-traumatic growth consists of positive change that happens in a person's life because of their personal struggle to carry on after experiencing trauma.

Post-traumatic stress disorder (PTSD) occurs due to exposure to a traumatic event or a series of stressful situations. Some of the symptoms associated with PTSD include reliving the incident in dreams or flashbacks, experiencing fearful thoughts, anger, irritability, and an inability to cope.

Potential psychologically traumatic events (PPTEs) consist of any distressing experience that includes, but is not limited to death, severe injury, or violence.

Professional boundary in nursing is a limit that is set on how far a relationship can go, and when it is unacceptable to continue.

Promising keeping in trauma-informed care consists of ensuring that we deliver the service we have suggested in a timely manner and that we follow through with commitments that we make.

Psychological personal protective equipment (PPE) consists of individual and system-wide measures that support and safeguard the mental health of employees.

Psychological preparedness is an explanatory model of posttraumatic growth following adversity that consists of becoming better able to deal with traumatic events when they happen in the future.

Psychological safety in trauma-informed care is the ability to feel safe from being harmed emotionally.

Psychological safety in the educational setting sets out to create a positive atmosphere for learning to occur without fear of retaliation, by demonstrating that it is okay to take personal risks, speak up when concerns arise, and freely ask questions and share ideas.

Psychological trauma refers to a disturbing event that is unexpected and beyond what would normally be anticipated, and results in a large array of physical, emotional, and psychological responses.

Purposeconsists of a person's reason for getting up in the morning and knowing where they are headed. It entails having clear goals and pursuing and achieving them.

Qualitative research in the Social Sciences focuses on gathering information about people through experiential means.

Racial microaggressions are commonplace everyday occurrences, that are intentional or unintentional, and consist of offensive verbal or behavioral actions that communicate derogatory racial slights or insults toward people of color.

Racial trauma is race-based trauma that is experienced personally or witnessed.

Recovery-orientated care that is person-centered values healing relationships as an essential component of addressing the needs of people with chronic conditions.

Reflective journalling is about freely writing about your values, beliefs, and attitudes to discover hidden aspects of your personality and to sort through your experiences.

Relationships in well-being theory that are healthy and loving, contribute to our happiness.

Religion involves the worship of a being or greater power outside of human material existence. It may consist of following sacred texts, books, and rules, offering formal prayers, or engaging in worship.

Rescuing is a form of helping in a professional capacity that is not beneficial for the recipient. It consists of doing things for a person, rather than helping them become more self-sufficient or empowered.

Residential schools were boarding schools created by the Canadian Government and operated by people of the Christian faith, to forcibly remove native children from their families, with the goal of destroying the "Indian," in the child.

Resilience is the ability to carry on and bounce back to original functioning after experiencing a trauma. It consists of constructive attributes of endurance, strength, and the will and motivation to move forward, despite what has occurred.

Resisting re-traumatization in trauma-informed care involves doing our best to avoid exposing people to situations that remind them of a particular adversity or event.

Respect for self-worth views each human being as deserving of honour and dignity, no matter what their circumstances.

Role modelling requires being a good example for others to follow.

Safety plan is designed to assist someone who is suicidal to identify their warning signs, ways to keep themselves safe, anchors for living, and people to call when they are in crisis.

Secondary trauma occurs because of close contact with people who are traumatized or due to direct exposure to adverse events.

Secondary traumatic stress (STS) is a condition that develops due to ongoing exposure to people who have directly experienced adversity. It manifests after viewing, hearing about, or being involved in traumatic stressors. Direct personal exposure to trauma is not necessary for STS to develop.

Self-awareness involves the process of purposefully examining the motives behind our actions.

Self-compassion entails purposefully viewing yourself with the same degree of empathetic concern that you would offer someone else in a similar situation.

Self-confidence consists of the self-assurance in your inherent abilities to acquire personal and professional ambitions and goals.

Self-reflection is the process of taking deliberate action to truthfully want to know why you think and act the way that you do.

Servant leadership is an altruistic stewardship and caring style of leadership that invests in followers' professional and personal development and well-being.

Sex refers to a person's biological designation based on the genitalia that they were born with.

Sexual orientation refers to the way that a person feels toward other people physically, sexually, romantically, or emotionally.

Shame is usually experienced as an intrinsically flawed character attribute that a person believes to be unchangeable.

Signature strengths in Positive Psychology consist of character strengths that are closely aligned with who we are, and what is vitally important to us.

Significance is the belief that somehow one's life is worthwhile, means something, and has something to look forward to.

Social intelligence is a part of emotional intelligence and consists of the capacity to feel and act in a socially acceptable manner.

Social safety refers to the emotional environment of the health care setting, where the expectation is that the person seeking help will be protected from harm or injury.

Somatization refers to emotional responses that surface as physical symptoms in the body.

Spirituality emphasizes the energy that exists within the person and their connection with a universal source of power that is a part of all of life.

Stranger rape consists of sexual assault that happens where the perpetrator of the assault and the victim do not know one another.

Strength-based trauma-informed strategies assist people to understand that they have gained new strengths and skills from surviving adversity that make them better equipped to deal with life's troubles when they arise.

Strengths due to suffering is an explanatory model of post-traumatic growth following adversity and occurs in the form of self-reassessment and questioning one's belief system.

Stress-hardy refers to a personal characteristic that enables a person to respond to demanding situations in an adaptive manner.

Structural trauma consists of violence toward specific populations by design (e.g., race, ethnicity, gender, sexual identity and orientation, and persons with disabilities).

Student-focused learning concentrates on the experience of learning that is cooperative, creative, and sensitive to the learner's needs.

Sturdy mindset involves a commitment to being fully engaged with life. It is about having a reason to get up in the morning and looking forward to the challenges of the day.

Subjective well-being is a personal and individualized measure of a person's feelings and moods, including sorrow or joy.

Survivor-centered approach to intimate partner violence works co-operatively with survivors, is client-centered, and prioritizes their choices, needs, strengths, and their ability to cope.

Systemic racism is harmful and consists of actions, practices and policies that perpetrate unjust prejudicial attitudes that target specific racial, ethnic, or other special populations.

Therapeutic relationship in nursing consists of the capacity of the nurse to know and understand their client/patient in such a way, as to be able to connect with them in a human and meaningful manner.

Theory in research is used to generalize and offer explanations of the relationships between the phenomena under study.

Transcultural caring in nursing is more than just being sensitive to cultural differences and involves intentionally seeking to understand and respect how a person's behaviors, wants and needs are influenced by culture.

Transference occurs when a person projects strong feelings that they may have had for someone else in their life, usually in childhood, toward the healthcare professional who is treating them.

Transgenerational trauma, which is also referred to as **intergenerational trauma,** consists of a transposition of prejudicial attitudes and behaviors from one generation to another.

Transparency in trauma-informed care consists of an openness to providing information about the care that is provided and ensuring that there are no hidden agendas.

Trauma refers to an event or series of circumstances that are harmful, threatening, or a danger to one's life, and have lasting adverse effects on the person's ability to function on a mental, physical, or spiritual level.

Trauma-informed involves the ability to recognize the ways that various forms of adversity have negatively impacted the lives of people.

Trauma-informed care endeavours to help people who have experienced trauma and targets change at the organizational and clinical level with the aim of improving client/patient outcomes. It focuses on prevention, intervention, and treatments that are evidence-based, and adaptable to the needs of those who have experienced past or present adversity.

Trauma-informed educational approaches value respectful interpersonal relationships, supportive learning environments, emotional intelligence, effective communication, empathy, caring, and compassion.

Trauma-responsiveness is concerned with every aspect of the delivery of services once a person has interfaced with a health care setting, with the key goal of avoiding unintentional harm.

Trauma-sensitivity in clinical practice consists of being aware and responsive to a person's history of adversity or interpersonal violence.

Traumatic stress response usually consists of a specific but normal neuropsychological reaction to an abnormal event. It may include a sequela of emotional responses that usually subside with time.

Trauma trigger refers to a perceptual stimulus involving the senses that causes a link to a previous traumatic experience.

Unconditional positive regard consists of the action of caring for someone without any conditions. The person does not need to be perfect to deserve care.

Validation consists of being able to communicate that you fully accept and want to understand, another person's experience.

Vicarious traumatization consists of a distressing emotional response after directly witnessing trauma or hearing the stories of people who have had adverse experiences.

Victim blaming holds a person responsible for their set of circumstances without considering other contributing factors like life circumstances or social injustices.

Violent traumas include all forms of abuse, are personal, and occur due to circumstances that affect a person directly.

Well-being theory in Positive Psychology consists of elements that are measurable and are comprised of what people are willing to choose as contributing to life satisfaction.

Will to meaning in life as a primary motivator, that is unique, valued, and specific to the individual, and can only be fulfilled by them. It is also what assists a person to endure and overcome pain and suffering.

Work-life balance consists of attaining a balance between work commitments and personal lifestyle.

SUBJECT INDEX

A

Abuse 9, 10, 13, 16, 17, 19, 32, 36, 39, 60, 72, 77, 157, 163, 165, 167
  domestic 9
  elder 10, 16, 17
  emotional 19
  financial 17
  sexual 9, 10, 13, 77, 157
  terrible 165
Abuser 100, 121
  drug 100
Abusive relationship 59, 93
Accidents, motor vehicle 160
Acts, aggressive 182
Acute distress disorder 23
Acute stress 1, 2, 4, 23, 39
  disorder 1, 4, 23, 39
  response 2
Adverse childhood experiences (ACEs) 2, 8, 9, 10, 11, 24, 36, 39, 65, 100, 227
Aesthetics 159, 203
Aggression, emotional 34
Ailing relatives 200
Alliance, therapeutic 96
Alzheimer's association 98
Anger 7, 23, 28, 54, 72, 102, 150, 181, 185, 200, 201, 212
  transform 150
Angry outbursts 183, 214
Anxiety 7, 10, 23, 24, 26, 28, 29, 36, 37, 100, 101, 104, 117, 181, 190, 200, 201, 234
  developing 104
  disorders 10
  display 190
Approach(s) 2, 32, 40, 50, 58, 82, 87, 88, 118, 123, 136, 251
  disease-obsessed 136
  resilience-focused 87, 88, 123
  strength-based 50, 58, 82, 118
  trauma-informed nursing education 251
  trauma-sensitive 2, 32, 40

Athletes, professional 104
Attributes of resilience 103

B

Behaviors 10, 22, 103, 105, 114, 195, 198, 199, 200, 201, 202, 208, 210, 211, 215, 230
  automatic 114
  courteous 199
  dangerous 10
  self-destructive 22
Biological homeostasis, normal 7
Boundary violation 87, 112, 114, 115, 124
Brain 23, 130, 133, 134
  function 23, 130, 133
  neuroplasticity 134
  plasticity 134

C

Caregiver(s) 10, 29, 30, 34, 55, 61, 63, 68, 71, 75, 112, 113, 180, 186, 190, 191, 223, 240
  adult 68
  primary 10
  professional 113
  role 190
  teaching 34
Caring 30, 177, 178, 190, 191, 192, 195, 196, 197, 198, 215, 229, 244
  activities 197
  behaviour 229
  trauma-informed 190
  communication skills 229
  fashion 196
  learning environment 177, 178, 191, 195, 198, 215
  nurses 244
  pedagogy & trauma-informed educational practices 192
  skills 198

www.ingramcontent.com/pod-product-compliance
Lightning Source LLC
Chambersburg PA
CBHW050815220326
41598CB00006B/212